# Methods
# in Pulmonary
# Research

Edited by  S. Uhlig
A. E. Taylor

Springer Basel AG

Editors:

Dr. Stefan Uhlig
Department of Pulmonary Pharmacology
Forschungszentrum Borstel
Parkallee 22
D-23845 Borstel
Germany

Professor Aubrey E. Taylor
Department of Physiology
College of Medicine
University of Southern Alabama
Mobile, AL 36688
USA

Library of Congress Cataloging-in-Publication Data
  Methods in pulmonary research/edited by S. Uhlig, A. E. Taylor.
      p. cm.
  Includes bibliographical references and index.
  ISBN 978-3-0348-9803-4        ISBN 978-3-0348-8855-4 (eBook)
  DOI 10.1007/978-3-0348-8855-4
  1. Respiratory organs--Research--Methodology. 2. Respiratory organs--Cytology--Research--
  Methodology. I. Uhlig, S. (Stefan), 1957– . II. Taylor, Aubrey E.
  QP121.M573 1998                      98-14358
  612.2'07'24--dc21                    CIP


Deutsche Bibliothek Cataloging-in-Publication Data
  Methods in pulmonary research/edited by S. Uhlig, A. E. Taylor.
  Springer Basel AG, 1998
  ISBN 978-3-0348-9803-4

Cover illustration: Taken from «Physiologie der Atmung», with the friendly permission of © 1980 Boehringer Ingelheim Pharma KG.
Cover design: gröflin. Graphic Design, Basel

ISBN 978-3-0348-9803-4


9 8 7 6 5 4 3 2 1

# Contents

# Airways

# Vessels

# Edema

## 9   Neurogenic inflammation in the airways: Measurement of microvascular leakage  . . . . . . . . . . . . . . . . . . . 231

*M.G. Belvisi and D.F. Rogers*

# Airway liquid

# Cell culture

# Histology

# Further methods

# List of corresponding authors

**Dr. Sam Bayat**
TIM C-PRETA, UMR CNRS 5525,
Dept. de Physiologie, Faculté de Médecine de Grenoble
F-38700 La Tronche, France

Tel. 0033 476 6371-38, Fax 0033 476 6371-86, E-mail: Sam.Bayat@imag.fr

**Dr. Maria Belvisi**
Rhône-Poulenc Rorer Research & Development
Dept. of Pharmacology, Dagenham Research Centre
Rainham Road South, Dagenham, Essex, RM10 7XS, UK

Tel. 0044 181 919-2075, Fax 0044 181 919-2497, E-mail: m.belvisi@ic.ac.uk

**Dr. Michel R. Corboz**
Dept. of Physiology, MSB 3024, Univ. of South Alabama, College of Medicine
Mobile, AL 36688-0002, USA

Tel. 001 334 460-7826, Fax 001 334 460-6464
E-mail: mcorboz@jaguar1.usouthal.edu

**Dr. Christopher Dawson**
Dept. of Physiology, Medical College of Wisconsin, Research Service 151
5000 West National Avenue, Milwaukee, WI 53295-1000, USA

Tel. 001 414 384-2000 ext. 1440, Fax 001 414 384-0115
E-mail: dawson@vms.csd.mu.edu

**Dr. Robert E. Drake**
Dept. of Anesthesiology, The University of Texas,

Health Science Center at Houston
6431 Fannin, TX 77030, USA

Tel. 001 713 792-5566, Fax 001 713 794-4157


**Prof. David Eidelman**
Meakins Christie Laboratories, McGill University
Montreal, Canada H2X 2P2

Tel. 001 514 398-3864, Fax: 001 514 398-7483
E-mail: david@meakins.lan.mcgill.ca


**Dr. Manfrid Eltze**
BYK Gulden Lomberg Chemische Fabrik
Byk-Gulden-Str. 2 - FP2, Postfach 10 03 10, D-78403 Konstanz, Deutschland

Tel. 0049-7531-84-2617, Fax 0049-7531-84-2474


**Dr. Heinz Fehrenbach**
Institut für Pathologie, Universitäts-Klinikum Gustav Carus
Fetscherstr. 34, D-01307 Dresden, Germany

Tel. 0049 351 458-5277, Fax 0049 351 458-4328


**Prof. Roy G. Goldie, Ph.D.**
Dept. of Pharmacology, University of Western Australia
Nedlands, WA, 6907

Tel. 0061 9 346-2812, Fax: 0061 9 346-3469
E-mail: rgoldie@receptor.pharm.uwa.edu.au


**Dr. Gerd Hoymann, Prof. Dr. Uwe Heinrich**
Frauenhofer-Institut für Aerosolforschung
Nicholai-Fuchs Str. 1, D-30625 Hannover, Germany

Tel. 0049 511 5350-404, Fax: 0049 511 5350-155
E-mail: hoymann@ita.fhg.de

**Dr. Wolfgang Koch**
Frauenhofer-Institut für Aerosolforschung
Nicholai-Fuchs Str. 1, D-30625 Hannover, Germany

Tel. 0049 511 5350-117, Fax: 0049 511 5350-155


**Dr. Jamson Lwebuga-Mukasa**
Lung Biology Research Program, Pulmonary and Critical Care Division
Dept. of Internal Medicine, SUNY at Buffalo School of Medicine
Buffalo General Hospital
100 High Street, Buffalo, New York 14203, USA

Tel: 001 716 859-3682, Fax: 001 716 859-3620
E-mail: jlwebuga@ubvm.cc.buffalo.edu


**Dr. Rene P. Michel**
Dept. of Pathology, McGill University, Lyman Duff Medical Sciences Bldg.
3775 University St., Montreal, PQ, Canada H3A 2B4

Tel. 001 514 398-7194, Fax 001 514 398-7446
E-mail: michel@pathology.lan.mcgill.ca


**Dr. Else Müller-Schweinitzer**
Dept. of Internal Medicine, Clinical Pharmacology, University of Basel
Petersgraben 4, CH-4031 Basel, Switzerland

E-mail: muellere@ubaclu.ch


**Dr. Daniela Negrini**
Instituto di Fisiologica Umana 1, Univesrita di Milano
Via Magiagalli 32, I-20133 Milano, Italy

Tel. 0039 2 7063-8768, Fax 0039 2 7063-0032


**Dr. Bengt Robertson**
Div. for Experimental Perinatal Pathology, Karolinska Hospital
S-171 76 Stockholm, Sweden

Tel. 0046 8 729-6160/6161, Fax 0046 8 729-6165

**Dr. Rod Scott**

Dept. of Biomedical Sciences, Marischal College, Aberdeen University
Aberdeen AB9 1AS, Scotland, UK

Tel. 0044 1224 2730-51, Fax 0044 1224 2730-19, E-mail:
rod.scott@abdn.ac.uk

**Dr. Troy Stevens**

Dept. of Pharmacology
MSB 3130, University of South Alabama, College of Medicine
Mobile, AL 36688-0002, USA

Tel. 001 334 460-6497, Fax 001 334 460-6798
E-mail: tstevens@jaguar1.usouthal.edu

**Dr. Stefan Uhlig**

Division of Pulmonary Pharmacology, Research Center Borstel
Parkallee 22, D-23845 Borstel, Germany

Tel. 0049 4537 188-478, Fax 0049 4537 188-778
E-mail: Suhlig@fz-borstel.de

**Dr. Peter von Wichert**

Klinikum der Philippis-Universität Marburg
Baldingerstrasse
D-35043 Marburg, Germany

Tel. 0049 6421 28-6451, Fax 0049 6421 28-8987

# Preface

Pulmonary diseases have increased in incidence over the last 40 years and it is obvious that basic and clinical pulmonary research must be intensified in order to understand the underlying mechanisms that cause each particular disease. This book affords renowned experts the opportunity to present a broad range of methods now used in pulmonary research. The techniques span the range from evaluating cell mechanisms in endothelial and epithelial cell cultures to those studying the inflammatory responses of *in situ* lungs. The theoretical background of each technique is presented in some depth whenever possible. The major emphasis of this book lies in the practical application of the methods and it constitutes a valuable guide for investigators not familiar with basic pulmonary measurements that can be incorporated into experiments within their laboratories.

The first part of the book describes techniques used to study lung mechanics and airway smooth muscle. The first four chapters describe *in situ* lung preparations, isolated perfused lungs, lung explants and classical tracheal preparations. The techniques described in these chapters using perfused lungs and lung explants can easily be extrapolated to study pulmonary vessels. Chapters 5 to 7 provide important new methods for studying the pulmonary vasculature in great detail, such as intravital microscopy, pulmonary vascular occlusion techniques and bronchial circulation studies. Since edema formation is a broad and important field in pulmonary research, the edema section begins with a review on the methodology in this field. Chapters 9 to 11 describe in detail how microvascular leakage can be assessed, how intravital microscopy can be applied to interstitial studies and what techniques are now available to study the lymphatic system. The next three chapters then present methods to evaluate airway secretion and their contents *in vitro*, using bronchoalveolar lavage and surfactant activities. The lung consists of more than 40 different cell types, some of which are isolated into cultures and monolayers in many laboratories. With regard to harvesting and culturing techniques, only type II alveolar epithelial cells and endothelial cells are considered in chapters 15 and 16. Basic histological techniques are presented in chapters 17 and 18. Chapter 19 explains how to generate aerosols and how to introduce them into the respiratory tract. Finally, chapter 20 explains how lung tissue can be preserved over long periods of time to maintain its structure and even function.

Obviously, many other techniques, such as those used in biochemistry or molecular biology, are now extensively used in lung studies, and are described in detail in many other excellent books. In this work we have presented only those techniques useful to evaluating the lung function at the organ level in order to stimulate continued pulmonary research in organs and relate these measures to data collected at the cellular level.

Stefan Uhlig          Aubrey E. Taylor          October 1997
Borstel, Germany      Mobile, AL, USA

# Airways

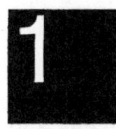

# Measurement of lung function in rodents in vivo

*H.G Hoymann and*
*U. Heinrich*

Examination of pulmonary function is a nondestructive procedure of assessing the functional consequences of alterations of lung structure or (temporary) changes in the tonus of airway smooth muscle cells, providing information on the presence, the type, and the extent of alteration. The principles governing ventilation, air flow, lung volume, and gas exchange are common among most if not all mammals [3]. There is a considerable quantity of literature describing the methodology, physiological principles and typical values of lung function tests in man and experimental animals. Reviews of the methods used for rodents have been presented by Mauderly and Likens [10, 12], Costa and Tepper [3], and Murphy [13]. The tests used at present are the result or unique adaptations of clinical lung function tests to small animals.

In this chapter we will present methods of noninvasive pulmonary function measurement in rodents in our laboratories, and we will present typical examples of their use. Our main working fields are the preclinical evaluation of drugs using nonallergic and allergic asthma models, lung function tests to assess and to monitor lung alterations in inhalation studies (e.g. in legally prescribed toxicity tests), and the investigation of pulmonary diseases (e.g. fibrosis, asthma, or organ rejection after lung transplantation). These studies can be performed according to the guidelines of Good Laboratory Practice (GLP). Conscious guinea pigs are used in preclinical efficacy studies, primarily in asthma studies. The experimental design of this model is relatively simple so that four animals can be examined at the same time. The disadvantages are that movement artifacts sometimes disturb the measurements and that only a few spontaneous respiration parameters can be measured. Therefore, in toxicological and some of the pharmacological questions not enough end points and sensitivity are available. In *anaesthetised* rats, the whole range of lung function tests available in the clinic can be performed. This animal model is thus used in preclinical studies as an asthma model, in safety pharmacology and toxicity studies when more end points and a higher resolution of measurement are needed (extended lung function).

The methodology of noninvasive pulmonary function measurement in the anaesthetised rat [6, 8, 9] is based mainly on methods reported by Likens and Mauderly [11]. Anaesthesia permits measurement of lung compliance and resistance and yields the ability to perform involuntary breathing manoeuvres to achieve an extended functional characterisation (e.g. by forced expiratory flow-volume curve or quasistatic manoeuvre). The lung function tests can be performed before and after treatment and/or challenge of the animal (e.g. as an asthma model), all on the same occasion or in different phases of a study (used in long-term studies). To test for non-specific bronchospasmolytic potency of drugs or as a hyperreactivity test, an acetylcholine challenge can be performed, which is a useful bronchial provocation test for small rodents. As a model for allergic asthma, the animal can be sensitised (by ovalbumin) and challenged by the respective antigen.

## Spontaneous respiration

Plethysmography is the most common approach to function testing in small animals [12]. Respiratory flow rates (F) are calculated from pressure differences measured across a pneumotachometer. A pneumotachometer consists of a resistance element fixed in a gas flow path, creating a pressure difference between the upstream and downstream sides of the resistance. The measured pressure difference is proportional to flow rate in a given frequency range as long as the flow is laminar (*see* also Section on *Material and equipment*). Respiratory volume changes (e.g. tidal volume, $V_T$) are determined by electronic integration of the flow rates. In addition, respiratory frequency (f) is obtained from the flow signal.

Transpulmonary pressure ($P_{TP}$), the driving force of respiration, is the pressure difference between the pleural surface and the mouth. The intrapleural pressure can be measured indirectly as oesophageal pressure. Measurement of changes in $P_{TP}$ is necessary for calculating dynamic lung compliance ($C_{dyn}$) and lung resistance ($R_L$), for example, based on the method of Amdur and Mead [1].

Lung resistance includes tissue forces, but in healthy animals almost entirely reflects airway resistance, representing particularly the large airways [12]. $C_{dyn}$

reflects the elasticity of lung tissue but also contains the force needed to overcome airflow resistance and therefore is also decreased in bronchoconstriction, especially in the small airways.

For measurement of the functional residual capacity (FRG), which represents the lung volume at the end of tidal exhalation, the barometric method is applied [4]. This is the most rapid technique and is most frequently used for anaesthetised rodents in plethysmographic measurements. Boyle's law ($P_1 V_1 = P_2 V_2$ under isothermal conditions) is applied to recorded changes of volume and pressure in the lungs caused by the breathing efforts of the animal against the occluded airway.

## Pulmonary manoeuvres

Several involuntary pulmonary manoeuvres, also called extended lung function tests, can be performed in anaesthetised animals. Initially, to produce a brief apnoea triggered by the Hering-Breuer reflex, the animal is hyperventilated several times. During the resulting apnoea, an involuntary inspiration and expiration can be performed comparable to the respective voluntary manoeuvres carried out by patients in lung function examinations. Forced expiratory flow-volume manoeuvre, quasistatic pressure-volume manoeuvre, nitrogen washout test and CO diffusion test are methods based on such breathing manoeuvres.

A forced expiratory flow-volume (FEFV) manoeuvre can be performed to detect early signs of bronchial obstruction or bronchoconstriction/-dilation, distinguishing between small peripheral and large central airways. A slow inspiration to total capacity is followed by a fast expiration to residual volume. A $P_{TP}$ of $+25$ to $+30$ cm $H_2O$ is most commonly used to define the total lung capacity, based on the fact that the pressure-volume curve is flattened at this pressure [12]. In the quasistatic pressure-volume manoeuvre, the same inspiratory procedure is followed by a slow expiration in which volume and pressure changes are recorded. Total lung capacity (TLC) is calculated by adding the functional residual capacity (FRC) to the inspiratory volume change. The subvolumes of TLC are derived by subtraction (*see* Section on *Methods*). Maximum quasistatic lung compliance ($C_{qs}$) is calculated as the steepest slope of the pressure-volume curve.

In rats as well as in humans, the $N_2$ washout curve has been used to characterise lung disease and the uniformity of distribution of ventilation [6, 11, 12].

Starting from residual volume, the lung is inflated with pure oxygen as the tracer gas to replace – or wash out – the original gas in the lung (*see* Section on *Methods*). During expiration, the $N_2$ concentration and lung volume are measured. Phase I of the resulting $N_2$ washout represents the dead space gas, phase II a mixture of dead space and alveolar gas, and phase III primarily represents the alveolar gas. The slope of phase III indicates inequalities in regional ventilation caused by increased numbers of lung units with increased time of filling and emptying (which can be caused by narrowing of bronchioles). The onset of phase IV is called "closing volume"; in rats this occurs rarely and is then thought to represent the point of emptying of poorly filled ventilating units [11, 12].

The diffusing capacity of the lung for CO (DLCO) – sometimes called CO transfer factor – is a very sensitive and common approach to evaluate alterations in gas exchange. In a single-breath manoeuvre, the animal is inflated by a gas volume containing CO and additionally Ne as an inert gas relatively insoluble in blood (to calculate the initial CO concentration in the lung decreased by dilution with the FRC). The DLCO is measured as the volume of CO which is absorbed by the lung in $ml_{STPD}$ per mmHg of actual air pressure per minute (*see* Section on *Methods*). In contrast to $O_2$, the high affinity of CO for hemoglobin eliminates the problem of dependence of the transfer on the capillary perfusion. Since an increased lung volume elevates the area for diffusion, the specific CO diffusing capacity (DLCO/VA) is calculated by dividing the DLCO by the actual lung volume.

## Material and equipment

Different devices for measuring lung function in rodents with different levels of sophistication are available. The following companies supply complete systems for tests in rodents: Buxco Electronics Inc., Sharon, CT, USA, and Hugo Sachs Elektronik, March-Hugstetten, Germany.

In our lung function laboratories both the conscious and the anaesthetised animal models are established: Firstly, for lung function tests on *conscious* guinea pigs a system with four double-chamber plethysmographs (Buxco El. Inc.) is used to measure spontaneous breathing parameters in four animals at the same time. The thoracic and nasal chambers are each equipped with a pneumotachometer (*see* below) and a differential pressure transducer. The primary pressure signals are enhanced by amplifiers and processed by hard- and software. In addition, an aerosol generation system is used for provocation tests or inhalation treatment (*see* Chapter 19). Secondly, for the extended lung function tests as performed on patients, a complex set of measurement devices is needed additionally. In our labs these tests are usually performed on *anaesthetised* rats. A plethysmograph for the measurement of the spontaneous respiratory activities as well as involuntary pulmonary manoeuvres is used. For the latter, a pressure system is applied. If the animal is anaesthetised by inhalation, a special anaesthetic system (evaporator with tube system and air and vacuum sources) is connected. For provocation tests or inhalation treatment an aerosol generation system is used and for nitrogen washout test and CO diffusion test further instrumentation (nitrogen analyser, gas chromatograph) is used. Surface activity of BAL or surfactant samples can be measured with a Pulsating Bubble Surfactometer (PBS, Electronetics Corp., New York City, NY, USA).

## Lung function laboratory

Taking our set-up for lung function of the rat as an example, we will describe the different parts of equipment in detail (Fig. 1.1). For the measurements on rats we use a 2.6-l whole-body plethysmograph ($L \times W \times H$: $28 \times 13 \times 7$ cm, perspex; Fraunhofer ITA), which is used as a flow-type plethysmograph with volume displacement and for the measurement of the functional residual capacity (FRC) as a constant volume-type plethysmograph (*see* Section on *Methods*). For very large rats (male Wistar rats older than 5 months) we use a 4.2 l whole-body plethysmograph ($34 \times 17 \times 7$ cm; Fraunhofer ITA). A pneumotachometer (a round orifice, inner diameter 18 mm, containing seven to eight layers of wire cloth with 400-mesh per inch) is inserted in the rear wall of the chamber. The breathing port – a Luer fitting – is inserted in the front wall of the chamber. On the side wall, a differential pressure transducer (MP45, Validyne, Northridge, CA, USA) is connected with the inside of the chamber. The pneumotachometer-transducer system results in linearity ($\pm 2\%$) of the

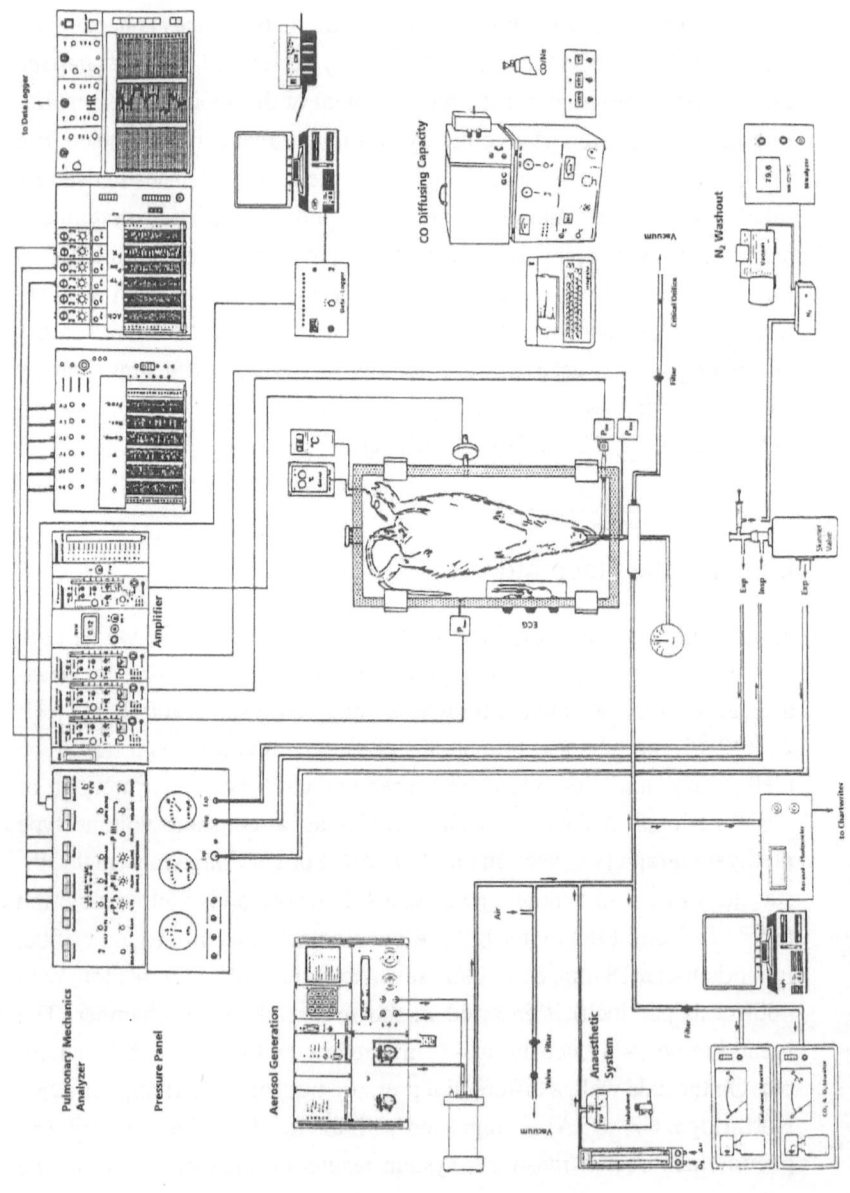

*Figure 1.1. Setup of equipment used for extended lung function tests in anaesthetised rats*

volume signal in a frequency range from below 20 to over 300 breaths per minute which is not exceeded by the animals in any of the experimental designs ($-9\%$ at $420\,\mathrm{min}^{-1} = 7\,\mathrm{Hz}$).

The plethysmograph is kept warm by means of a heating pad below the bottom plate with a thermostat to protect the anaesthetised animal from loss of body heat. The temperature of the bottom of the plethysmograph is controlled by means of a digital thermometer. Rectal temperature is measured by means of a Ni-Cr-Ni sensor connected to another digital thermometer (needed especially for CO diffusion test). For recording of the heart rate, a triple ECG-electrode is used connected to a ECG/Rate coupler (type 576, in a three-channel recorder Graphtec-Watanabe Linear corder mark VII WR 3101, Hugo Sachs Elektronik, March-Hugstetten, Germany).

For measurements of oesophageal pressure a water-filled PVC tube (13 cm, outer diameter 1.6 mm, inner diameter 1.0 mm, open-tipped with two small side holes near the tip to reduce the likelihood of plugging) is connected to a pressure transducer (P23Db, Gould Statham Instr. Inc., Hato Ray, Puerto Rico) via a Luer fitting inserted in the side wall of the chamber. For measurements of airway pressure an air-filled pressure transducer (W101/RFT, Meßgerätewerk Zwönitz, Germany) is connected to a side branch directly outside the breathing port. On a side wall of the plethysmograph, a fourth pressure transducer (W101/RFT) is connected to the inside for measuring chamber pressure when performing FRC measurements (*see* Section on *Methods*).

The tracheal cannula for intubation of rats is made from a 14-gauge intravenous catheter (Cathlon IV 14 g, Nr. 4428, Jelco, Raritan, NJ, USA; inner diameter 1.78 mm, outer diameter 2.1 mm, length reduced to 52 mm). The outer edge of the tube is smoothed carefully by very fine emery paper to prevent lesions of the trachea. The needle of the Jelco-catheter is cut to fit and the tip is made round by a drop of glue, needed for inserting the cannula into the trachea. For large rats (e.g. male/female Wistar rats over 4/12 months) we use a catheter with OD 2.4 mm (ID 1.78 mm, length 57.2 mm).

The four pressure transducers are connected to an amplifier system (Plugsys type 603, Hugo-Sachs Elektronik): oesophageal, airway and chamber (FRC) pressure transducers to three direct current bridge amplifier modules (DBA 660), the differential pressure transducer for air flow to a carrier frequency bridge amplifier module (CFBA 677). A module of the amplifier system subtracts the oesophageal pressure from the airway pressure to obtain transpulmonary pressure changes ($P_{TP}$) and reduces the amplification when forced manoeuvres are performed. The amplified transducer signals are analysed by a Pulmonary Mechanics Analyzer (model 6, Buxco Electronics Inc., Sharon, CT, USA), which calculates lung function parameters such as compliance and resistance and controls the pulmonary manoeuvres. The analogue values are monitored continuously as tracings on a chart recorder (Watanabe Linear corder mark VII, WR 3101, six channels, Hugo Sachs Elektronik). An analogue-digital convertor (Data Logger DL-12, Buxco El. Inc.) digitises and averages the signals from the analyser in adjustable time intervals (e.g. 6 or 12 s) and transfers the data to a personal computer. By means of special lung function evaluation programs (Branch Technology, Dexter, MI, USA, and Fraunhofer ITA) a primary printout is produced online, the data are stored, summarised, statistically analysed, and transfer files are produced for generating tables and graphics for reports.

For the involuntary manoeuvres, a pressure panel (Buxco El. Inc.) is used which controls sources of compressed air, oxygen, and vacuum. Three 10 l reservoirs connected to the pressure panel serve as the pressure sources for inflation with air or pure oxygen and for deflation. They are controlled at pressures of +40 and −50 cm $H_2O$, respectively. Inspiratory and expiratory flow rates of the manoeuvres are limited by needle valves. A solenoid valve (V52DA3012, Skinner, New Britain, CT, USA) with a Luer fitting is used for opening the respective pressure source to the airway, triggered by the pulmonary mechanics analyser.

For inhalation anaesthesia and oxygen supplementation of the animal, two anaesthetic systems are installed: A halothane evaporator (Vapor 19.3, Drägerwerk AG, Lübeck, Germany) is connected to a compressed air supply and to a cylinder with compressed pure oxygen, providing the animal with a gas mixture of halothane in 30–50 % oxygen via a tube system (ID = 1 cm). The end of the tube is connected to a perspex cylinder in which the breathing port of the plethysmograph protrudes, and the animal can breathe air freely and spontaneously out of this cylinder. The pressure in this cylinder should be very close to ambient pressure (*see* below and Section on *Troubleshooting*). At the outlet of the cylinder the gas mixture is sucked off to protect the laboratory personnel. Another compressed air supply is connected to a second halothane evaporator producing anaesthetic gas for a small perspex box (about 2 l) to initiate anaesthesia before intubation of the animal. Flowmeters are used to adjust and control the flows and concentrations of $O_2$ and anaesthetic gas in these systems, resulting in a constant end flow at the breathing port (normally 2.5 l/min). To adjust a constant flow in this air supply – which is especially important in inhalation treatment – a critical orifice is connected to a vacuum source downstream of the animal port. Since this system has advantages in performing inhalation treatment (*see* below), we use this as the standard assembly.

In a side branch as near as possible to the animal breathing port, monitors for halothane and oxygen concentration are supplied with a probe flow of the anaesthetic gas via a glass fibre filter to protect against aerosols (Normac AA 102, Normocap CD-102/$O_2$, Datex Instr. Corp., Helsinki, Finland / Hoyer Medizintechnik, Bremen, Germany). The output signal for the anaesthetic gas concentration is recorded together with the spontaneous breathing values by means of the lung function software.

In addition, for provocation tests or inhalation treatment, an aerosol generation system is installed. Ultrasonic or jet driven nebulisers are commercially available for this purpose. We use a jet-driven aerosol generation system (Bronchy type III, Fraunhofer ITA; available at Buxco El. Inc.) developed primarily for challenge tests in our labs, which can work with very small fluid quantities and can be controlled by computer. Aerosols are generated by means of a nozzle into a buffer chamber (800 ml) and are mixed with oxygen or anaesthetic gas mixture downstream of this chamber. Before and after treatment the Bronchy III delivers clean air to the system. In this assembly a side branch connected to vacuum (via filter and an open side branch) collects the overflow of the aerosol system upstream of the point of mixing of the two streams and compensates small pressure changes. In addition, the pressure in the breathing port of the animal measured continuously by means of a pressure gauge is held very close to ambient pressure (*see* Section on *Troubleshooting*). This aerosol delivery system has the advantage of good control of the flows and their mixing relation and therefore produces stable exposure conditions. Silica gel can be added if necessary to ensure dry and well defined particle diameters and therefore reproducible exposure conditions and lung deposition. To evaluate aerosol concentration, a scattering light aerosol photometer (SAD, Fraunhofer ITA) is connected with a side branch as near as possible to the animal breathing port using a sample flow of 0.25 l/min. The signals of aerosol concentration and of the minute volume of the animal are recorded by a second computer and the dose inhaled by the animal is calculated and displayed using a dose control program.

For the nitrogen washout test and CO diffusion test, further instrumentation is used: a nitrogen analyser (Model 505 Nitralyzer, Med-Science Electronics Inc., St. Louis, MO, USA, with ionisation chamber, needle valve and vacuum pump) and a gas chromatograph.

# Methods

For many investigations 12-week-old female Wistar rats weighing about 220–240 g are used (e.g. as a nonallergic asthma model). For studies with allergy models we use 6 to 9-week-old Brown Norway rats or Dunkin Hartley guinea pigs (age at sensitisation). In toxicological studies the rat is the species of choice. In inhalation studies mostly Wistar or Fischer F344 rats are examined, usually at several time points (after some weeks up to 2 years). To obtain base values before treatment, the pulmonary function of the same animal should be tested after administration/exposure of the vehicle or after clean air exposure. The following descriptions apply to lung function measurement in rats.

## Preparation and calibration

First, a warming up of at least 30 min is necessary for most of the electronic equipment. The oesophageal catheter and its transducer are filled with gas-free water and calibrated in the position in which they are to be used (*see* also Section on *Troubleshooting*). Gas bubbles in this system have to be removed since they dampen the pressure signal. It is important that the screens of the pneumotachometer are clean (ultrasonic bath). Prior to a series of measurements, a validation of the system consisting of the pulmonary analyser, data logger, computer, and chartwriter is performed using calibration signals produced by the analyser. For the spontaneous respiration parameters, defined readings on the computer (e.g. a signal 2 V for 2 ml as "2.00") and on the chartwriter (e.g. 2 ml as 2 cm amplitude) are adjusted by means of the data logger and the chartwriter gain controls, respectively. Correspondingly, the forced manoeuvres can be simulated by the analyser and the results can be controlled. This validation ensures that signals received by the analyser are correctly stored by the computer and recorded by the chartwriter (documentation according to Good Laboratory Practice).

Next, the instruments are calibrated (once before a study). The transducers for oesophagus and airway pressure are calibrated using a calibrated pressure source (usually a Gauer column). The differential pressure transducer and the chamber pressure transducer are calibrated directly in volume units. Volumes of 1, 2, and 10 ml are injected into the breathing port of the plethysmograph (volume displacement mode) with a frequency of about 70 cycles per min using glass cylinder syringes. The amplification for the tidal volume signal (differential pressure transducer) is adjusted so that the correct value is recorded on the chartwriter (e.g. 2 ml injections as a 2 cm amplitude). The frequency response of the pneumotachometer-transducer system can easily be checked by oscillating 2 ml for example by means of the calibrating syringe with increasing frequencies into and out of the plethysmograph. After closing the pneumotachometer (pressure mode plethysmography), the chamber transducer used for FRC measurement is calibrated by performing slow injections into the breathing port by means of a 1 ml syringe.

The calibrations of the $O_2$-monitor and the nitralyser are done with room air. The anaesthetic gas monitor is calibrated using a calibration gas provided by the supplier of this device, and the gas chromatograph is calibrated daily by means of the CO/Ne-test gas (Messer Griesheim, Germany), according to the certified concentration values.

## Pulmonary function testing

The animals are anaesthetised initially with 4% halothane in a 2 l chamber with a flow of 2.5–3 l/min. Alternatively, e.g. in allergen challenge tests, we use pentobarbital sodium anaesthesia (40–60 mg/kg i.p.) which is also widely used in rodent lung function testing. When the anaesthesia is deep enough (i.e. when breathing frequency is visibly reduced), the animal is intubated orally with the tracheal cannula under visible control of the vocal cords using a small surgery lamp. The intubated animal is placed supinely in the whole-body plethysmograph and the tracheal tube is connected to the breathing port of the plethysmograph. The halothane concentration is adjusted individually between 1.5 and 3% (in 30% $O_2$, gas flow 2.5 l/min) to obtain similar respiratory frequencies for all animals (about 70 breaths/min). In bronchial challenge tests we use a gas mixture with 40 or 50% $O_2$ to prevent apnoea which can otherwise occur caused by a strong bronchoconstrictive response (and which is especially undesirable when a forced manoeuvre should follow). The sensor of the digital thermometer is inserted rectally to measure body temperature which is needed for CO diffusion tests. The ECG electrodes are fixed and heart rate (HR) is evaluated by the ECG/Rate Coupler from the recorded ECG signal.

The water-filled oesophageal catheter is now inserted into the oesophagus to a position in midthorax at which a maximum pressure signal is yielded (*see* also Section on *Troubleshooting*). The catheter can be inserted carefully until reaching the maximum signal or can be inserted almost to the depth of the stomach and then be withdrawn to the optimum position. Prior to the measurements, the trachea of the animal is aspirated to remove possibly existing mucus using a syringe with a very thin stiff catheter (OD = 1 mm, Teflon) which projects 2 mm over the tip of the tracheal cannula connected to the breathing port. After this, the animal is ventilated three times slowly by means of a syringe with a volume exceeding its tidal volume (2 to 2.5 ml for rats) to establish a uniform lung volume history (middle position of breathing), thus ensuring a representative volume at the end of expiration (FRC). Pulmonary function measurements are started when a steady state of the breathing pattern is reached – after about 3–4 min – and baseline drift in the volume signal between the breaths is eliminated.

First, the parameters of *spontaneous respiration* are recorded, usually for a period of 1–2 min. An example of a typical chart recorded from a rat is given in Figure 1.2. Respiratory flow (F), tidal volume ($V_T$), transpulmonary pressure ($P_{TP}$), dynamic compliance ($C_{dyn}$), lung resistance ($R_L$), breathing frequency (f), minute volume (MV), heart rate (HR), halothane concentration, and aerosol concentration during inhalation treatment are recorded simultaneously. The analogue signals are recorded on the chartwriter, displayed, digitised and averaged by the data logger, and stored in the computer by means of lung function evaluation

**a)**      **b)**

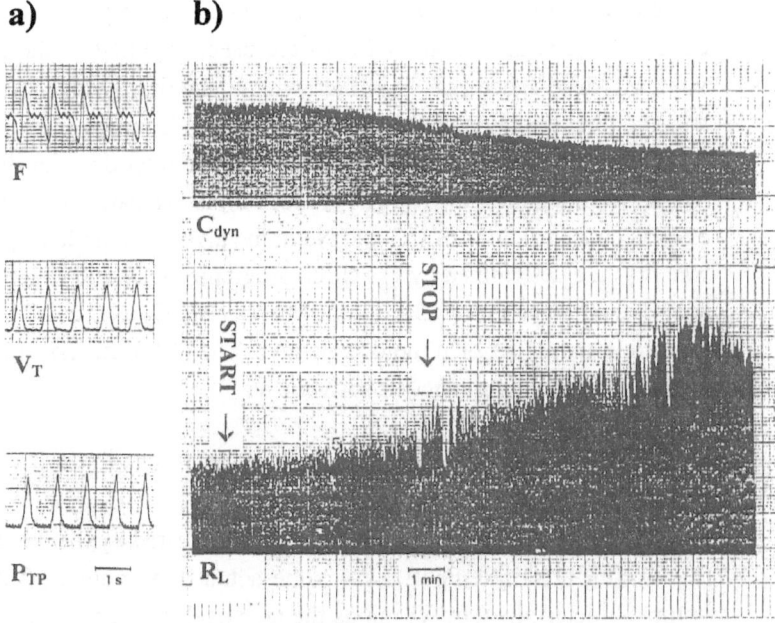

**Figure 1.2. Tracings of measurements of spontaneous breathing parameters**
*a) Respiratory flow, tidal volume, and transpulmonary pressure at rest; b) dynamic compliance and lung resistance during/after antigen challenge (ovalbumin aerosol, see arrows) performed on a 10-week-old ovalbumin-sensitised Brown Norway rat; (abbreviations see text).*

software (*see* below). These parameters can also be measured in challenge tests (*see* below).

The *CO diffusion test*, used typically in inhalation toxicity studies, is mostly performed as the first manoeuvre after recording spontaneous breathing since it takes some time to obtain results by means of gas chromatography. Prior to the manoeuvre, the animal is hyperventilated by means of a respiratory bag (ambubag) for infants with about 10–12 inflations to a $P_{TP}$ of 20 cm $H_2O$ to induce a temporary apnoea for about 12 to 15 s. When using inhalation anaesthesia, the ambubag is filled with the anaesthetic gas mixture. During apnoea, the inspiratory volume ($V_I$) required to increase the $P_{TP}$ to 20 cm $H_2O$ is determined using a gas-tight syringe filled with room air. In a second apnoea, an equal volume of test gas containing 0.4% CO ($F_ICO$) and 0.5% Ne ($F_INe$) in air is injected into the lungs from the larger of two gas-tight syringes (10 and 5 ml) connected by a three-way cock. In older rats the inspiratory volume can exceed 10 ml and then larger syringes are used. One-half of the injected volume ("dead-space gas") is withdrawn into the first syringe after about 4 s, and then the remainder ("alveolar sample") is removed into the second syringe. The "breath holding time" (t), the total time for diffusion for the second half of the test gas (about 7 s), is evaluated from $P_{TP}$ traces. Gas concentrations of CO and Ne in the alveolar sample ($F_ACO$, $F_ANE$; dry) are determined by gas chromatography. $CO_2$ and water vapour are separated on a Porapack column whereas Ne, $O_2$, $N_2$, and CO are separated in that order on a molecular sieve. The CO diffusing capacity is evaluated by the lung function software as

$$DLCO_{STPD} = [VA_{STPD}/t(P_{atm} - P_{H_2O})] \ln[F_0CO/F_ACO].$$

The CO concentration in the lung at t = 0 is indicated by the Ne dilution ($F_0CO = F_ICO \times F_ANe/F_INE$). VA is the actual lung volume ("alveolar volume") determined by $V_I$ minus the technical dead space volume $V_D$ divided by the Ne dilution $F_ANE/F_INE$ and corrected for BTPS. The specific DLCO (DLCO/VA) and DLCO/body weight are also calculated. After this as well as after each involuntary manoeuvre, the animal is ventilated three times by 2 ml syringe. After an inspiration to TLC it takes about 3 to 6 min to reach a new steady state in spontaneous breathing.

A *forced expiratory flow-volume (FEFV) manoeuvre* can be performed subsequently. Prior to the manoeuvre, the airway of the animal is aspirated (*see* above), and then the animal is hyperventilated again (5–8 inflations to a $P_{TP}$ of 20 cm $H_2O$) to induce a temporary apnoea for about 8 to 12 s. Then the Skinner valve is connected to the breathing port, and the manoeuvre is started immediately. Controlled by the pulmonary analyser, the valve is opened to the first air reservoir (+40 cm $H_2O$) and the lungs are inflated up to a $P_{TP}$ of +30 cm $H_2O$ (–20 to +25 cm $H_2O$ for measurements of bronchoconstriction) using an inspiratory flow of 8–10 ml/s. At the selected cutoff pressure the inflation is stopped and the animal is subsequently deflated rapidly by means of the second air reservoir at a pressure of –50 cm $H_2O$ without intentionally limiting expiratory flow.

Flow-volume plot (Fig. 1.3) and volume-time plot ("spirogram") are printed out and are analysed electronically to determine the typical parameters. From the volume-time curve, the following "spirometric" parameters are evaluated: inspiratory capacity (IC), forced vital capacity (FVC), expiratory reserve volume (ERV), forced expiratory volume in 0.05, 0.1, 0.2, and 0.4 s ($FEV_{0.05...0.4}$) in ml or %FVC. From the flow-volume curve, the parameters peak expiratory flow (PEF) and forced expiratory flow at 75, 50, 25, and 10% of the FVC remaining to be expired ($FEF_{75}$ to $FEF_{10}$) are derived; the maximum mid-expiratory flow (MMEF) is calculated as the expiratory flow between 75 and 25% of FVC.

To determine the *FRC*, the plethysmograph is used in pressure mode: the pneumotachometer is sealed with a stopper. The breathing port is blocked after the end of a tidal expiration (breathing frequency below 70 breaths/min). Five to six inspiratory efforts of the animal are recorded and then the port is opened. If the breathing frequency is too high, the dose of inhalation anaesthetic must be increased or the measurement has to be performed during temporary apnoea. The changes of volume ($\Delta V$) and pressure ($\Delta P$) in the lungs caused by the inspiratory efforts of the animal against the blocked breathing port are recorded. The airway opening pressure is measured in the side branch of the breathing port and the volume changes are derived from pressure changes in the plethysmograph caused by the small expansions of the thorax. At the end of a normal ex-

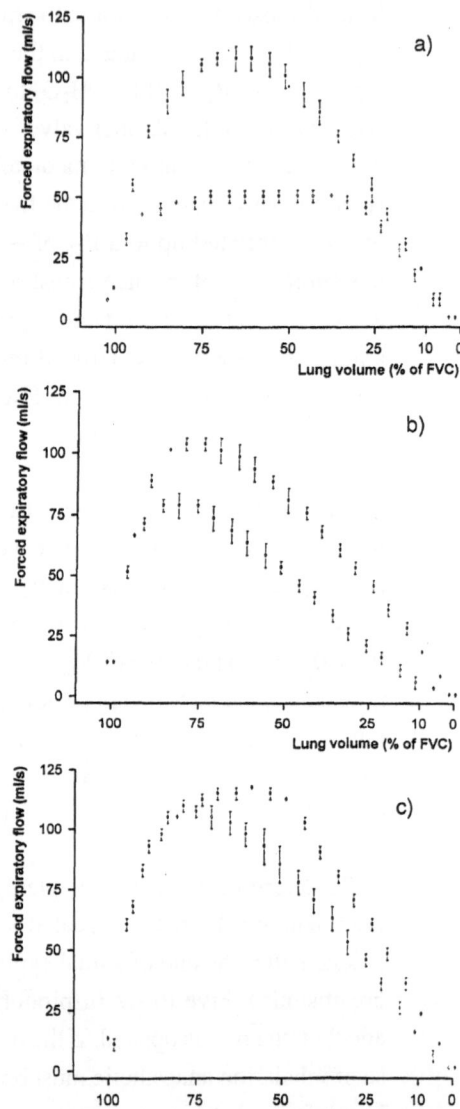

**Figure 1.3. Flow-volume curve of Wistar rats with different localisation of obstruction**

*a) Central airway stenosis (o) experimentally produced by narrowing of the lumen of the tracheal cannula, b) combined large and small airway bronchoconstriction (o) by inhalation exposure to acetylcholine aerosol (challenge test), and c) peripheral airway obstruction (o) after 12 months of isocyanate exposure (see text) compared to baseline measurement (a/b: •) or control group (c: •).*

piration the actual lung volume is the FRC and the actual pressure is the atmospheric pressure ($P_{atm}$) minus the water vapour pressure (47 mmHg at 100% saturation and 37 °C body temperature). $V_D$ is the dead space which is included in the measured volume.

$$FRC = \Delta V / \Delta P \times (P_{atm} - 47 \text{ mmHg}) - V_D$$

In another temporary apnoea to perform a *quasistatic pressure-volume manoeuvre*, the lungs are inflated (8–10 ml/s) up to a $P_{TP}$ of $+30$ cm $H_2O$ ($+20$ to $+25$ cm $H_2O$, *see* FEFV) and then deflated slowly, limiting the expiratory flow to 4 ml/s by means of a needle valve in the pressure panel. The pressure-volume plot and the derived parameters are printed out. Total lung capacity (TLC) and its different subvolumes – inspiratory capacity (IC), vital capacity (VC), expiratory reserve volume (ERV) and residual volume (RV) – are calculated by measuring the volume changes caused by this quasistatic manoeuvre and by adding the FRC (measured previously). Maximum quasistatic lung compliance ($C_{qs}$) is calculated as the steepest slope of the pressure-volume curve. Dividing by FRC yields the specific compliance ($C_{qs}$/FRC). The chord compliance ($C_{chord}$) is calculated as mean of compliance between 0 and 10 cm $H_2O$ of $P_{TP}$, encompassing the tidal breathing range.

In a further apnoea, the *single-breath nitrogen washout (SBNW)* test is performed. Prior to the manoeuvre, the nitrogen analyser is calibrated by room air nitrogen. Then a slow deflation from FRC to residual volume (4 ml/s) is followed by an inflation with 100% $O_2$ to a $P_{TP}$ of $+30$ cm $H_2O$ ($+20$ to $+25$ cm $H_2O$, *see* FEFV) using a flow of 8–10 ml/s and subsequently followed by a slow deflation (4 ml/s) back to residual volume. During the expiration the $N_2$ concentration and the volume of the expired air are recorded. $N_2$ concentration is measured by the nitrogen analyser collecting a small part of the expired volume with 3 ml/min (adjusted by means of a needle valve at the Luer fitting of the Skinner valve). The air probe is drawn by means of a vacuum pump. The vacuum is positioned very close to the breathing port (just downstream of the needle valve) so that the probe reaches the analyser very quickly. This is important to get the characteristic $N_2$ signal simultaneously to the volume signal. The resulting % $N_2$-volume curve (Fig. 1.4) and parameters calculated from that are stored in the computer (e.g. the slope of phase III of the $N_2$ washout curve).

Lung function measurements can be performed under *bronchial challenge* (in pharmacological efficacy examinations or hyperreactivity tests). To do so, the animal is exposed to a bronchoconstrictive aerosol

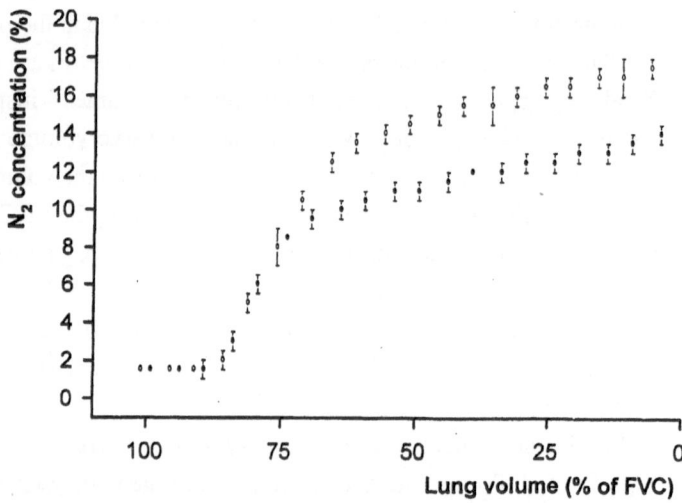

**Figure 1.4. Nitrogen washout curve of 20-month-old Wistar rats exposed to isocyanate (o) or clean air (•) for 17 months (see text)**

(e.g. from 1 to 10% aqueous solutions of acetylcholine chloride [ACh] or ovalbumin after sensitisation) using the aerosol generation system (*see* Section on *Material and equipment*). Before measurements, the aerosol photometer which monitors the concentration is calibrated gravimetrically, and the particle diameter (MMAD) is evaluated by means of a cascade impactor (Marple impactor). To reach the large as well as the small airways (bronchioles), in intubated rats we use particles of about 1.5–2 μm MMAD (in conscious nose-breathing guinea pigs a MMAD of about 1 μm is necessary, *see* Chapter 19).

Prior to challenge, the base values of spontaneous respiration are recorded. Then, the exposure is started while lung function recording is continued (Fig. 1.2b). The inhaled dose is controlled and displayed by the dose control program receiving signals of aerosol concentration and

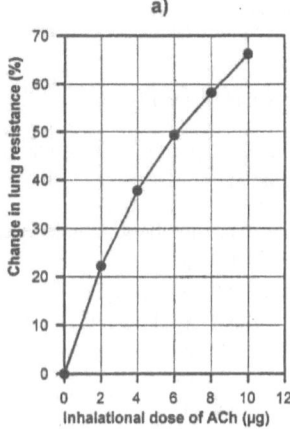
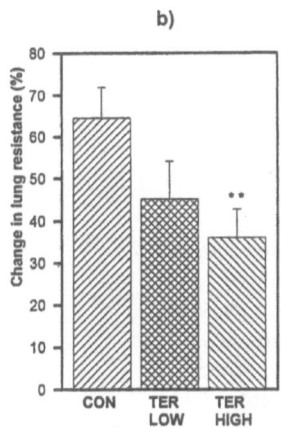

**Figure 1.5. Acetylcholine (ACh) challenge, single inhalation**
*a) Dose-effect relation of ACh on 13-week-old Wistar rats; b) effect of aerosolised low terbutaline and high terbutaline (0.27 and 0.54 mg/ml) versus vehicle (28-week-old Wistar rats; ** p<0.05).*

the minute volume of the animal. The breathing parameters at the end of exposure or at a selected inhaled aerosol volume – and therefore inhaled dose – or at $R_L$ maximum are evaluated and delta and delta % values related to base values are calculated. Typical parameters are the increase of resistance and the decrease of dynamic compliance as % of base value. There is a clear dose-effect relation between measured delta % value and the inhaled ACh concentration (Fig. 1.5a). A forced flow-volume manoeuvre can be added immediately. Since the bronchoconstriction decreases quickly after the end of ACh exposure, we use a prealarm of the dose control program to stop recording of spontaneous parameters at a predefined dose and to prepare for the manoeuvre whilst continuing the aerosol exposure (for about 25 s). In sensitised animals, IgE titer, eosinophilia and other immunologic parameters are measured additionally after challenge.

*Table 1.1. Lung function measurements in rats*

| Conditions, parameters | Values, facts | |
|---|---|---|
| Species | Rat | |
| Strains | Wistar, Brown Norway, Fischer | |
| Anaesthesia | Halothane 2–3%, pentobarbital sodium 40–60 mg/kg i.p. | |
| Typical values obtained for | 12-week- / | 12-month-old female Wistar rats |
| Tidal volume | 1.4 | 1.5 ml |
| Dynamic compliance | 0.21 | 0.24 ml/cm $H_2O$ |
| Lung resistance | 0.27 | 0.21 cm $H_2O$/ml/s |
| Total lung capacity | 12.5 | 15.5 ml |
| Vital capacity | 10.8 | 12.8 ml |
| Functional residual capacity | 2.8 | 3.8 ml |
| Quasistatic compliance | 1.0 | 1.3 ml/cm $H_2O$ |
| Expiratory peak flow (PEF) | 100 | 120 ml/s |
| Forced expiratory flow at 25% FVC | 45 | 55 ml/s |
| Phase 3 of nitrogen washout curve | 0.75 | 0.55% $N_2$/ml |
| CO diffusing capacity | 0.17 | 0.22 ml/mmHg/min |
| Pressure cutoff for inspiration manoeuvre | +30 cm $H_2O$ (+20 or +25 cm $H_2O$, *see* text) | |
| Pressure for expiration manoeuvre | −50 cm $H_2O$ | |
| Typical duration of preparation | 40–60 min once at the daily start and 10–20 min for anaesthesia/intubation/instrumentation (each rat) | |
| Typical duration of animal experiment | 30–60 min (different measurement sessions) | |
| Animals/day | 5–10 | |
| Papers that exemplify usage of these techniques | [8, 6, 9, 11, 12, 13] | |

Provocation tests such as ACh challenge can be performed as a single challenge, challenge before and after, for example, drug treatment, or with stepwise increasing the dose of bronchoconstrictive agent. In the latter protocol, usually steps with doubling of concentrations and doses are applied until the animal reaches a predefined resistance value (usually +150% baseline). The exposure time of any single step has to be short (about 30–60 s) and prior to the next step the animal is ventilated three times by 2 or 2.5 ml room air to reduce resistance and ensure a representative base level.

## Examples for applications

Pharmacological efficacy studies were performed in rats and guinea pigs using mostly inhalation exposure to acetylcholine or ovalbumin after sensitisation. The bronchospasmolytic effects of various test compounds such as phosphodiesterase inhibitors [8], $\beta_2$-sympathomimetics [7], or bronchodilating natriuretic peptides [5] have been examined in comparison with a control group and/or a control session before treatment. Resistance, dynamic compliance, and the parameters of forced expiratory manoeuvre were used to evaluate effects of the test compounds. Figure 1.5b shows an example of inhibition of acetylcholine-induced bronchospasm by terbutaline in Wistar rats [7]. In another study on Wistar rats [8], the selective PDE III/IV inhibitor zardaverine has shown a more than 30-fold bronchoprotective potency compared to theophylline. Lung resistance, dynamic compliance, and the parameters of the flow-volume curve (PEF, MMEF, $FEF_{25}$, $FEF_{50}$) measured before and after acetylcholine challenge before and after oral treatment were the most powerful parameters in this study.

The forced expiratory manoeuvre is used in studies detecting airflow obstruction with high sensitivity and with the advantage of distinguishing between effects on large (central) and small (peripheral) airways. Figure 1.3 shows the impact of a central (1.3a), combined (1.3b) or peripheral (1.3c) airway obstruction on the flow-volume curve of rats. A central stenosis (artifical narrowing of the lumen of the tracheal cannula in a position between larynx and top of trachea) reduced FEF between 95 and 30% of FVC (1.3a). Characteristically, $FEF_{75}$ and PEF were decreased markedly (each by 54%), and for comparison, $R_L$ was increased strongly (by 122%). FEF at $\leq$25% FVC as well as $C_{dyn}$ were not affected. In contrast, an obstruction of the small peripheral airways after isocyanate exposure (1.3c and *see* below) decreased $FEF_{25}$ and $FEF_{10}$ but not $FEF_{75}$ (as well as $R_L$ and $C_{dyn}$). As an example of "combined obstruction" (1.3b), after bronchial challenge with acetylcholine aerosol, PEF, $FEF_{75}$, $FEF_{25}$ and $FEF_{10}$ (as well as

$C_{dyn}$) were decreased ($R_L$ was increased). The MMAD of the aerosol was $1.9 \pm 1.2 \, \mu m$, which accounts for a deposition in large as well as in small airways. $FEF_{50}$ is affected in central as well as in peripheral obstruction (1.3a-b). Therefore, as in humans, $FEF_{75}$ and PEF are characteristic for central obstruction, $FEF_{25}$ for obstruction in the small airways.

In a long-term inhalation study to investigate the chronic toxicity of monomeric 4,4'-methylenediphenyl diisocyanate (MDI) in female Wistar rats, we performed lung function tests after 6, 12 and 17 months [9]. These examinations were carried out on the same groups of animals. The lung function measurements revealed a dose-dependent impairment of lung function indicating an ob-

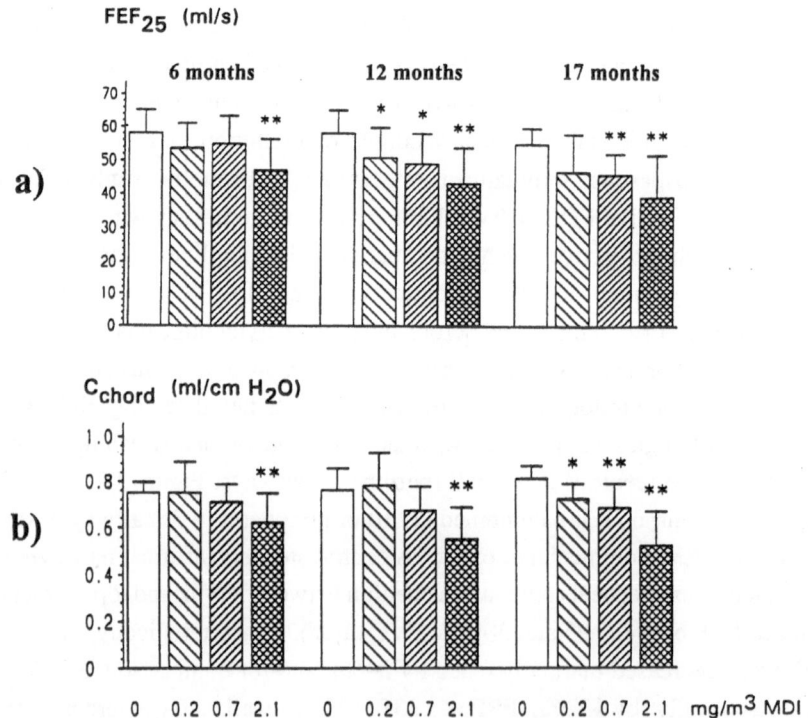

Figure 1.6. Decreased forced expiratory flow at 25% FVC (a) and decreased quasistatic chord compliance (b) in Wistar rats after 6, 12, and 17 months of isocyanate exposure (* p < 0.05, ** p < 0.01 compared to control group).

structive-restrictive malfunction with diffusion disorder, beginning earlier than 6 months of exposure and increasing at 12 months, but not much more at 17 months. This correlates very well to the dose-dependent interstitial and peri-bronchiolar fibrosis found in the histopathological examinations after 12 and up to 24 months of exposure. The forced flow-volume manoeuvres yielded significantly reduced values for $FEF_{50}$, $FEF_{25}$, $FEF_{10}$, and MMEF but not for $FEF_{75}$ (Fig. 1.3c and 1.6a). These findings increased with the dose and exposure time, indicating a significant increase in flow resistance in the small peripheral airways. The unchanged $FEF_{75}$ and resistance values at the same time show that there were no such alterations in the large airways. Both results correlated very well with the histopathological findings in the airways: narrowing fibrotic wall thickening exclusively in the very small peripheral bronchioles.

When recording the pressure-volume curve, both increasing MDI concentrations and time of exposure significantly reduced vital and total lung capacity, quasistatic chord compliance (Fig. 1.6b) and specific compliance. These results indicate a reduced distensibility and elevated elastic recoil of the lung tissue. The histological correlate of these restrictive alterations of the lung is the already mentioned fibrosis. The nitrogen washout test showed an increased inhomogeneity of the alveolar ventilation in the medium and high dose groups after 17 months of exposure (Fig. 1.4). After 12 and 17 months, the absolute and the specific CO diffusion capacities were decreased at the high concentration. These results indicate a reduced diffusion through the alveolar-capillary membrane, probably enhanced by a decreased area available for diffusion as a result of the elevated elastic recoil of lung tissue and the inhomogeneity of ventilation with poor gas mixing and obstruction of the small airways. These findings too correlate very well with the ascertained peribronchiolar and interstitial fibrosis, probably causing ventilatory inhomogeneity by narrowing of small airways and resulting in thickening of the alveolar-capillary membrane.

# Discussion

Functional responses of man and laboratory animals to different types of lung injury are similar and therefore pulmonary function tests in laboratory animals can be used to estimate the impact of responses to inhaled materials in man [12]. The known effects of many drugs as well as airborne pollutants on the respiratory system and worldwide regulatory requirements support the need for including pulmonary function evaluations in pharmacological, safety-pharmacological, and toxicological studies. When including lung function measurements in studies in which histological examinations are performed, direct correlations between function and morphology can add greater dimension to the relevance of the experimental pulmonary data to man [2].

Anaesthesia permits measurement of dynamic lung compliance and lung resistance and yields the ability to perform involuntary breathing manoeuvres to achieve an extended functional characterisation. Inhalation anaesthesia facilitates a fine adjustment of the respiratory frequency of the spontaneously breathing animal and produces very stable and reproducible values of the measured parameters. Anaesthesia alters breathing, but the breathing pattern of animals under consistent anaesthetic conditions can still have interpretive value [12]. Unanaesthetised animals are used to study patterns of uptake and distribution of inhaled toxicants. However, pulmonary function measurement in anaesthetised rodents is well established in most of the pharmacological and toxicological questions, and enables extended lung function with more than only one end point.

Changes in the mechanical properties and gas exchange function of the lung are classified as obstructive or restrictive disorders, bronchoconstricting/-dilating/-protective drug effects, or diffusion disorders. These can be evaluated in anaesthetised laboratory rodents by performing flow-volume and pressure-volume manoeuvres, nitrogen washout tests and CO diffusion tests. Measurements of the spontaneous breathing parameters are not as sensitive and indicative as the tests mentioned but are used when continuous monitoring of changes in lung function is necessary. Lung resistance and dynamic compliance in particular are indicative for obstructive and restrictive disorders as well as for bronchoconstricting or -dilating drug effects. In most cases, a combination of spontaneous breathing parameters and extended measurements will be the best approach.

Parameters measured during forced exhalation (expiratory flow-volume curve) are aimed at detecting airflow obstruction with greater sensitivity and descriptive value than measurements during tidal breathing and were first incorporated in lung function tests of rats in pharmacological and toxicological studies in 1977 [12]. A higher sensitivity compared to spontaneous breathing parameters is attributed to the fact that changes are measured at maximum attainable flow rates and volumes whereas $R_L$ or $C_{dyn}$ are measured at 10–20% of maximum [13]. In addition, this method provides functional endpoints comparable to measurements in humans. As in human subjects, flow-limiting behaviour is demonstrated in forced flow-volume curves at different negative driving pressures: At middle and low lung volumes flow is "effort-independent" and there is some evidence that, as in humans, diminished flows in this part of the curves are indicative of peripheral airway obstruction [12]: peak flow and $FEF_{75}$ represent large airway function, $FEF_{25}$ represent small airway function (*see* also Section on *Examples for applications*, Fig. 1.3 and 1.6a). In bronchial challenge tests, an inspiration to TLC partly reduces the bronchoconstrictive effect by temporarily dilating the airways. Therefore we terminate the inspiration at $P_{TP}$ of 25 or 20cm $H_2O$ resulting in smaller absolute flow values but a better ratio of pre- to post-challenge (% decrease of flow). However, according to Mauderly [12] and from our experience also, the forced expiratory test also has good sensitivity when starting the exhalation below TLC (below $P_{TP}$ of 30cm $H_2O$) and is still useful in situations in which inflation to maximal lung volume is undesirable (for example emphysema or bronchoconstriction).

The barometric method for measuring the FRC most probably includes the total FRC especially in the presence of poor gas mixing. This means that the gas volume in alveoli which are partially or completely separated from gas exchange by obstruction of the feeding airways are included in the FRC value obtained by this method. The open-circuit $N_2$ washout method and the gas dilution method (*see* above, CO diffusion test) underestimate the FRC in the presence of poor gas mixing and therefore the barometric measurement procedure is the method of choice, especially in animals with airflow limitation and air trapping. For comparison, these methods can be combined with the barometric method to assess the volume of poorly ventilated regions.

In fact, increased FRC values were found in obstructive lesions of the lung (measured e.g. after isocyanate exposure in rats, *see* Section on *Examples for applications*). A decrease in FRC was measured in restrictive lung disorders (e.g. after long-term exposure with $SiO_2$ or toner particles in rats [6]).

Restrictive lesions or diseases of the lung increase the elastic recoil of the lung tissue which is the main reason for the decrease in total lung capacity and vital capacity usually measured by the quasistatic pressure-volume manoeuvre. Both the dynamic and the quasistatic lung compliance depend on the composition of the lung tissue and the surface tension of the surfactant. A number of lung diseases or long-term exposure to air pollutants can increase the elastic recoil by changing the composition of the surfactant and by accumulation of fluid, cells and collagen (fibrotic lesions) in the lung tissue. Since the quasistatic compliance is almost unaffected by the pulmonary frictional resistance, it reflects the elasticity of the lung better than the dynamic compliance. However, the compliance of the lung also depends on the volume at which the tidal breathing cycle or the breathing manoeuvre starts: the FRC. If the FRC is decreased – as measured in restrictive lung disorders (*see* above) – the compliance is decreased due to reduced starting volume. In these cases, the specific quasistatic compliance ($C_{qs}$/FRC) can indicate that part of reduced compliance which is due to an increased elastic recoil.

A reduction in DLCO may indicate the loss of alveolar surface area, thickening of the alveolar-capillary membrane by accumulation of fluid, cellular infiltration and collagen or increased coating of the alveolar surface by various materials and cells. But it has to be kept in mind that the DLCO is a non-specific but sensitive parameter: Inequalities in regional ventilation may result in a reduced DLCO caused by regions of poor gas mixing and trapped air. To assess the part of the decrease in DLCO which is really due to changes in the alveolar-capillary membrane and alveolar surface lining, the SBNW can be performed additionally to determine the inhomogeneity of ventilation.

The specific DLCO is aimed at indicating the diffusion changes independent of changes in alveolar area. This area cannot be determined directly and so dividing the DLCO by the actual lung volume is an accepted estimate for the volume-independent DLCO. However, this obviously overestimates the area effect a little, since volume changes of the lungs exceed the related area changes.

Provocation tests can be performed as a single test comparing treatment groups to a control group or as a "double challenge test", performing a challenge before and an identical challenge after, for example, drug treatment. The latter method yields the advantages of intraindividual comparison and exclusion of "low responders" and "hyperresponders". To reduce variation in bronchoconstrictive effect due to biological variability, the provocative dose can also be adjusted approximately to the reaction of the animal in the first challenge and this dose is repeated in the second challenge. Another type of challenge test is a protocol with stepwise increasing (doubling) the dose of bronchoconstrictive agent until the animal has reached a predefined rise in resistance. This is a well-established test, especially when the bronchoconstrictive response is not predictable or as a test on non-specific hyperreactivity (e.g. after allergen challenge). Since the exposure time of the single step and the provoked bronchospasm has to be short to ensure fast recovery, a flow-volume manoeuvre can hardly be performed reproducibly during a very brief reaction (*see* Section on *Methods*).

---

## Troubleshooting

The frequency response of the volume signal depends strongly on the transducer-pneumotachometer system chosen. Alinearity of the volume signal within the frequency range of the breathing of the animals can be corrected, for example, by reducing the number of screens in the pneumotachometer. This also reduces the measured pressure difference over the pneumotachometer and the sensitivity, and therefore a new calibration is necessary.

Except in very large rats, the oesophageal catheter should not exceed 1.6 mm OD. Especially in very young rats, a 2 mm catheter would press against the non-intubated part of the trachea and increase tracheal resistance to flow. We measured an increased lung resistance and decreased flow-volume curve (PEF) when using a 2 mm catheter in 10-week-old Wistar rats.

However, a critical point is the insertion of the water-filled oesophageal catheter. Sometimes the pressure signal is small, which mostly results from dampening by gas bubbles or material such as mucus or food particles in the tip of the catheter. The catheter should be removed, flushed with water, and inserted again as described. Another possibility is to inject about 0.1–0.3 ml water to flush the catheter in the oesophagus but from our experience this is successful only in few cases. Alternatively, an air-filled catheter can be used which reduces the problem mentioned above but also certainly decreases the frequency response of the pressure signal.

The pressure in the breathing port should be very close to the ambient pressure. A significant pressure difference ($> \pm 0.3$ cm $H_2O$) resulting, for example, from a markedly higher flow than used here (*see* Section on *Methods*) has to be avoided since that would change the level of breathing (FRC) of the animal.

Leaks in the plethysmograph, the transducers, the device for the manoeuvres or the connecting tubes can reduce the flow or pressure signals and disturb the forced manoeuvres. Particularly in the forced manoeuvres, a leak is undesirable since they are more sensitive for that than the spontaneous breathing. During a forced manoeuvre, a leak inside the plethysmograph will have impact on the flow signal since it reduces the pressure difference over the pneumotachometer by bypassing. A leak in the tracheal cannula (not connected tightly to the breathing port or to the trachea) will be detected by slowing down the inspiratory phase or prevention of reaching the final inspiratory $P_{TP}$ (e.g. 30 cm $H_2O$) and by the fact that the volume measured at the end of expiration is above the FRC level. A leak outside the plethysmograph, e.g. in the valve or the tubes for forced manoeuvres, will also be detected by slowing down the inspiratory phase or preventing the final inspiratory $P_{TP}$ being reached but has no direct impact on the flow signal. Depending on the symptoms observed, the leak can be localised and removed. Leaks are, however, very rare and problems can be avoided by checking the system before performing studies (e.g. by generating pressure in the system and checking the tightness by measuring the pressure drop after closing the system or by using leakage spray). In the forced manoeuvres, the tracings of volume and pressure give information about the correct course.

## References

1 Amdur MO and Mead J (1958) *Am. J. Physiol.* **192**: 364

2 Costa DL (1985) *Fund. Appl. Toxicol.* **5**: 423

3 Costa DL and Tepper JS (1988) Approaches to lung function assessment in small mammals. In: *Toxicology of the Lung*, Gardner DE, Crapo JD and Massaro EJ (eds), p. 147, Raven Press New York

4 DuBois AB, Botelho SY, Bedell GN, Marshall R and Comroe JH, Jr. (1956) *J. Clin. Invest.* **35**: 322

5 Flüge T, Hoymann HG, Hohlfeld J, Heinrich U, Fabel H and Wagner TOF (1994) *Eur. J. Pharmacol.* **271**: 395

6 Heinrich U, Muhle H, Hoymann HG and Mermelstein R (1989) *Exp. Pathol.* **37**: 248

7 Hohlfeld J, Hoymann HG, Molthan J, Fabel H and Heinrich U (1997) *Eur. Respir. J.* **10**: 2198

8 Hoymann HG, Heinrich U, Beume R and Kilian U (1994) *Exp. Lung Res.* **20**: 235

9 Hoymann HG, Creutzenberg O, Ernst H and Heinrich U (1998) In: *Relationships Between Respiratory Disease and Exposure to Air Pollution.* Brain JD, Driscoll KE, Dungworth DL, Grafström RC, Harris CC and Mohr U (eds), ILSI Press Washington D.C., (in press)

10 Likens SA and Mauderly JL (1979) Respiratory measurements in small laboratory mammals: A literature review. *Inhalation Toxicology Research Institute* (Rep. LF-68; available from Nat. Tech. Inform. Serv., Springfield, VA, USA)

11 Likens SA and Mauderly JL (1982) *J. Appl. Physiol.: Respirat. Environ. Exercise Physiol.* **52(1)**: 141

12 Mauderly JL (1989) Effect of inhaled toxicants on pulmonary function. In: *Concepts in Inhalation Toxicology.* McClellan RO and Henderson RF (eds), p. 347, Hemisphere Publishing Corp., New York

13 Murphy DJ (1994) *Drug Dev. Res.* **32**: 237

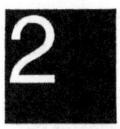

# The isolated perfused lung

*S. Uhlig*

The lung has developed dedicated structures and cell types to accomplish its particular functions. An elaborate exchange of both information and matter takes place between the lung and other organs of the body, which in total is a system of utmost complexity. In order to be able to study this perplexing system at least some of the complexity has to be eliminated. In this sense the isolated perfused lung represents a system much less complicated than the whole animal while preserving most of the integrity of the organ. As an experimental approach the isolated perfused lung (IPL) stands in between experiments *in vivo* with whole animals and *in vitro* with cultured cells. As such it combines assets and shortcomings of both. The present chapter will describe a set-up for the isolated perfused rat lung that allows to study four important aspects of lung physiology: respiratory mechanics, vessel mechanics, gas exchange and edema formation. Here, we will focus on the perfused rat lung, however, most of the equipment can also be used for isolated lungs from rabbits [1] or guinea pigs [2]. In a number of aspects the present text supplements our previous papers on the method of the rat IPL [3, 4]. A good compilation of earlier papers on perfused lungs is given in the introduction of the paper by Kröll et al. [2]. Previous reviews on the method of the isolated lung can be found in [5–9]. In addition, more specialized systems such as single lung perfusion [10] or perfusion through the bronchial artery [11] have also been described.

## Advantages and disadvantages of perfused lungs

Unlike experiments with cell cultures or homogenates, physiological parameters can be determined. It is a distinct advantage of the perfused lung that studies are performed in an intact organ, with physiological cell-to-cell contacts and native intracellular matrix. Examples are known of experiments with homogenates or with lung strips not predicting the results in perfused lungs or intact animals. For instance, platelet activating factor which is a potent constrictor of airway smooth muscle *in vivo* and in the perfused lung [12, 13] fails to contract the isolated trachea [14]. Another example is the endotoxin-induced release of thromboxane which occurs in pulmonary tissue *in vivo* [15] and in the perfused lung [16], but neither in lung slices [15] nor in isolated lung cells [17]. Thus, it is clear that many important properties are preserved in perfused lungs.

While *in vivo* experiments may provide good evidence that a certain substance affects the lung, only the testing of this substance in perfusion experiments allows the definitive assessment of its impact on the lung. The concentrations of the added substances can be very well controlled and multiple samples from the perfusate may be obtained easily and frequently. Unlike experiments in intact animals, perfusion experiments allow the investigator to retain control over several experimental parameters such as perfusion pressure or composition of the perfusate. In addition, measurement of lung mechanics in rodents is only possible after procedures not less laborious than the preparation of perfused lungs (*see* Chapter 1). Perfused lungs allow continuous monitoring of many aspects of lung physiology (airway resistance, pulmonary vascular resistance, edema formation, gas exchange) at the same time, which is, as yet, not possible *in vivo* in small laboratory animals. In addition, the isolated perfused lung preparation also offers the opportunity of investigating administration of multiple agents by different routes and in different physical forms.

The principal limitation imposed by the isolated perfused lung preparation is the short duration of study, since lung mechanics deteriorate with time. This progressive decline of lung mechanics can be significantly retarded if regular hyperinflations are carried out [4], but even then such lung preparations cannot be maintained for more than 8 h. Another limitation is the fact that the IPL is deprived of nervous regulation and lymph drainage, the effects of which are largely unknown.

## Theoretical background

### Vascular resistance

Lungs are perfused with either buffer or blood through the pulmonary artery by constant flow or constant pressure. The relationship between vascular pressure ($P_V$) and flow (Q) is given by

$$P_V = R_V \cdot Q \qquad \text{(Eq. 1)}$$

where $R_V$ represents vascular resistance. If constant flow perfusion (Q=constant) is used, to obtain $R_V$ vascular pressure ($P_V$) must be recorded. In case of constant pressure perfusion ($P_V$=constant), perfusate flow rate (Q) must be measured. Under these two conditions, vasoconstriction is detected as increased vascular pressure or decreased perfusate flow rate, respectively. The advantages of the two ways of perfusing lungs will be discussed below. $P_v$ can be measured with pressure transducers, Q with an electromagnetic flow probe or with Doppler methods.

### Respiratory mechanics

The lung can be envisaged as a small tube (airways) to which a balloon (alveolar space) is connected. In order to fill this balloon with air, two forces must be overcome, namely resistive forces to move air through the small tube (airway resistance; $R_L$) and elastic forces to inflate the balloon (compliance, $C_L$). This relationship is depicted in the following equation

$$P = \frac{1}{C_L} V + R_L \frac{dV}{dt} \qquad \text{(Eq. 2)}$$

where P is the pressure that forces the volume V at the velocity dV/dt into the lung. Generally, it is assumed that resistance is a parameter related to the airways, whereas compliance is related to the parenchyma [18]. Measurement of $C_L$ and $R_L$ is possible if P, V and dV/dt are known. P can be measured by pressure transducers and airflow velocity (dV/dt) by a pneumotachometer (*see* Chapter 1). Volume can be obtained by integrating dV/dt, the maximum volume representing the tidal volume. Compliance can by calculated at points where dV/dt equals zero by $C_L = \dfrac{\Delta V}{\Delta P}$, resistance by looking up the airflow (dV/dt) at isovolumetric points during inspiration and expiration (e.g. at 70 % tidal volume) according to $R_L = \dfrac{\Delta P}{\Delta dV / dt}$ [19]. Alternatively, $C_L$ and $R_L$ can be calculated from one complete breath by obtaining the coefficients of Eq. (2) by multiparametric regression.

## Material and equipment

Most of our equipment was from Hugo Sachs Electronics (HSE, March Hugstetten, Germany). However, not all experimenters may need all the options described here. The equipment required can be divided into that needed for ventilation, perfusion, weight measurement and assessment of blood gases. The complete set-up is shown in Figure 2.1. Please note that all data are transmitted to a computer via an A/D converter (for example Metrabyte DASH16). Depending on the system, calculation of lung mechanics may take some time. In most experiments we record one complete data set every 10 s. In addition, most of the parameters are also recorded on two Graphtec linear recorders WR3310 (HSE).

*Figure 2.1. The set-up for the isolated perfused rat lung*
B: Weight transducer; F: fleisch pneumotachogramm tube; L: liquid level sensor; P: pressure transducer for thorax chamber; Q: electromagentic flow probe; $V_Q$: valve to adjust perfusate flow; $P_{art.}$: pressure transducer for arterial pressure; $P_{ven.}$: pressure transducer for venous pressure; T: temperature probe; 1: electrode venous pH; 2: electrode venous $O_2$; 3: electrode venous $CO_2$; 4: electrode arterial pH. Modified with permission from [4].

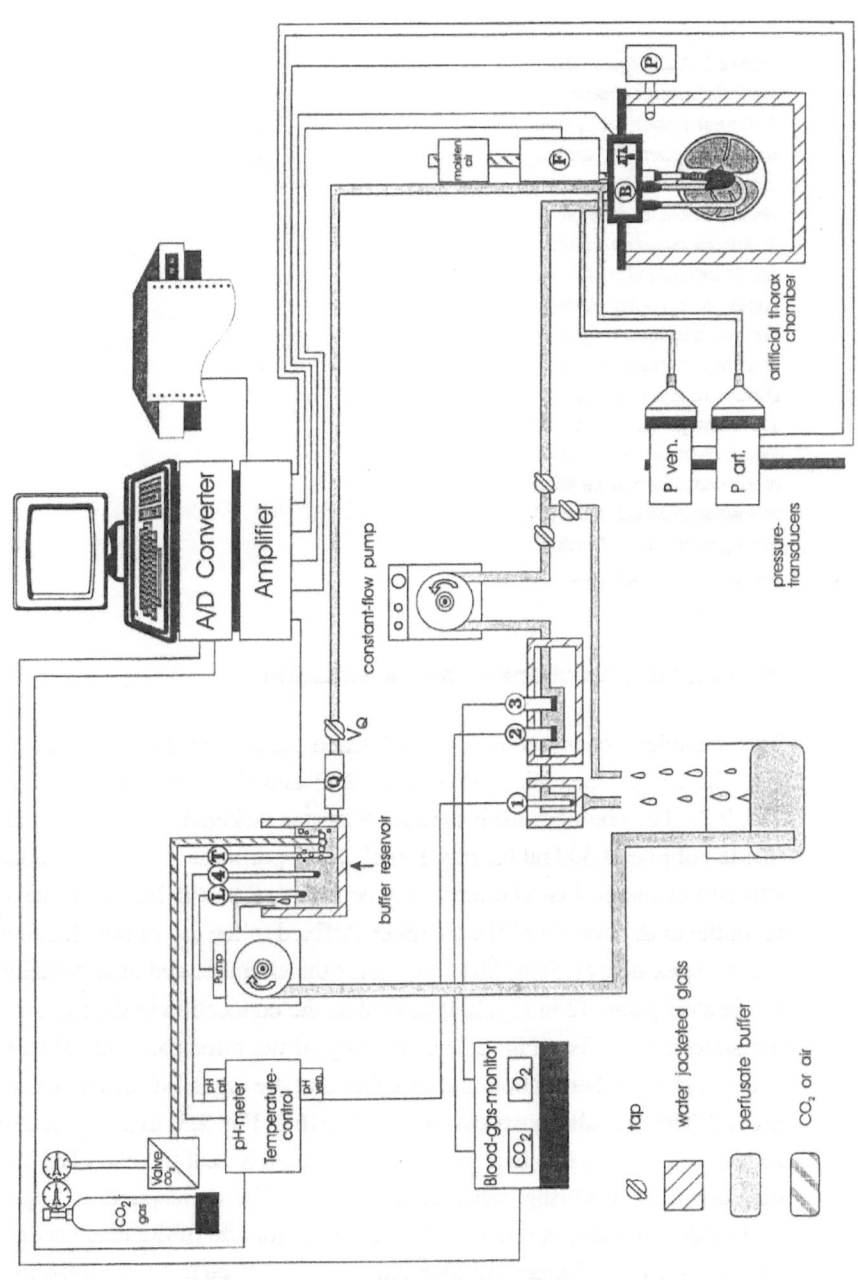

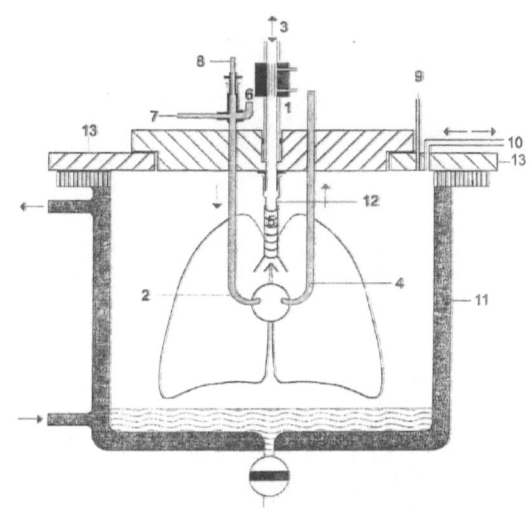

**Figure 2.2. Design of the artificial thorax chamber**
1: Organ holder with pneumo-tachometer; 2: arterial cannula; 3: air flow; 4: venous cannula; 5: trachea; 6: to arterial pressure transducer; 7: arterial inflow; 8: Luer conus for syringes (remove bubbles and inject drugs); 9: to chamber pressure transducer; 10: to venturi gauge; 11: water-jacketed artificial thorax chamber. The bottom of the chamber may be filled with water to provide a humid atmosphere. 12: Tracheal cannula. 13: Plexiglas disc.

## Artificial thorax chamber and ventilation

The complete chamber consists of three parts: the chamber (11 in Fig. 2.2), a perspex disc (13 in Fig. 2.2) and the organ holder (1 in Fig. 2.2). The chamber itself is made of water-jacketed glass and has an inside volume of 300 ml for rats. For cleaning purposes, but also because sometimes the perfusion circuit may be a bit leaky, it is helpful to have an outlet at the bottom of the chamber. Affixed to the top of the chamber is a perspex disc (1.5 cm thick) that seals the chamber and also contains the venturi gauge (2 in Fig. 2.3) as well as the connection to the pressure transducer. This disc (Fig. 2.3) is the only of the three parts that always stays in place, whereas both the chamber and the organ holder can be removed. The disc also hosts two metal clips (6 in Fig. 2.3) that are used to fix the chamber to the disc; in order to completely seal the chamber, the disc contains an O-ring, whereas the glass on the corresponding upper part of the chamber is roughed. A hole in the middle of the disc accommodates the organ holder. Another pair of clips is used to fix the holder to

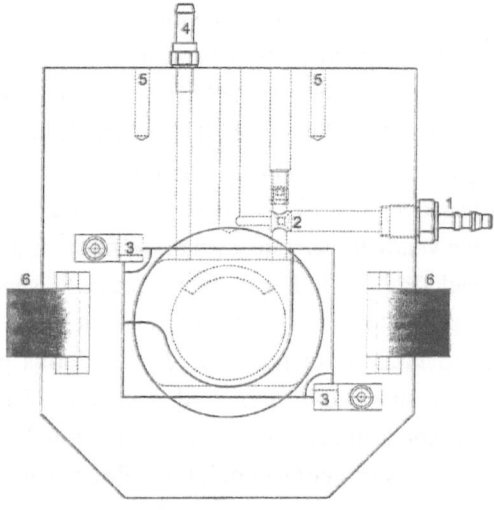

**Figure 2.3. The perspex disk that seals the thorax chamber and holds the organ holder**

*1: To respirator; 2: venturi gauge; 3: clip to fix organ holder; 4: to pressure transducer for chamber pressure; 5: hole for screws to mount the disk to the stand; 6: metal clip to fasten thorax chamber.*

the disc (3 in Fig. 2.3). The organ holder (1 in Fig. 2.2) has an outlet that fits onto the luer lock of the tracheal cannula (1 in Fig. 2.4) by which the lungs are suspended. The tracheal cannulas are made of stainless steel and have an inner diameter of 2.2–3.3 mm, depending on the size of the lungs.

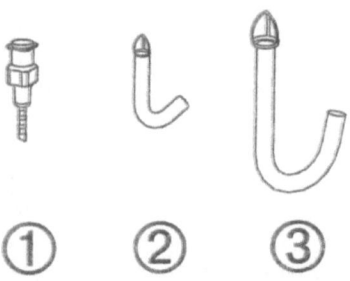

**Figure 2.4. The tracheal (1), arterial (2) and venous (3) cannula**

*The cannulas are made of stainless steel. The tripod on top of the arterial and venous cannula prevents occlusion of the cannula by tissue.*

During surgery the organ holder is removed from the chamber to the OP-table; the tracheal and also the arterial and the venous cannulas (by silicon tubing) are connected to the disc. After surgery the organ holder with the lung hanging on it is transferred to the chamber. Fig. 2.2 shows a schematic representation of the whole chamber with the organ holder already in place. The holder has three openings, for airflow, arterial inflow and venous outflow. In addition, the holder may include the weight transducer (HSE LS30) which has been described in detail elsewhere [3].

The design of the whole chamber allows ventilation to be performed by either positive or negative pressure. For positive pressure ventilation (PPV), the line from the ventilator is connected to the tracheal line via a special ventilation head (Fig. 2.5). For negative pressure ventilation (NPV) the ventilator is connected to the venturi gauge in the perspex disc. The venturi gauge is operated by compressed air, transforms positive pressure into negative pressure and is connected to the artificial thorax chamber. The shorter the connection between venturi gauge and chamber the quicker the chamber pressure (Pc) can build up; please note that the absolute values for compliance or resistance depend – among other things – also on the speed by which the pressure builds up. A simple valve (not

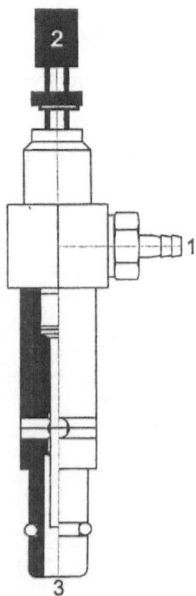

**Figure 2.5. The ventilation head**
1: To respirator; 2: control of respiration; 3: outflow of air.

shown in Fig. 2.1) allows to switch between positive and negative pressure ventilation. The ventilator should i) be able to generate pressures of at least ($\pm$)25 cm $H_2O$ end inspiratory pressure, ii) have the possibility to set end expiratory and end-inspiratory pressure, iii) allow for a frequency of at least 100 breaths/min and iv) support the regular execution of sighs (deep breaths). We use the HSE VCM module which has been designed to meet all these demands, but at least for positive pressure ventilation other ventilators such as from Harvard Apparatus may also be used.

For measurement of lung mechanics it is necessary to relate pressure to airflow and lung volume (*see* above). Airflow: Since lung volume can always be derived by integration, it is sufficient to measure airflow. Airflow velocity is assessed with a pneumotachometer (*see* also Chapter 1) connected to a differential pressure transducer (Validyne DP45-14). Mostly, a Fleisch type pneumotachometer tube, for rats type 0000, is used. The Fleisch pneumotachometer is made of solid metal and requires continuous heating to avoid condensation of water. However, it is also possible to use pneumotachometers made of perspex (HSE PTM type 378/1.2), which are cheaper, since due to the lack of water condensation no heating is required. Pressure: the pressure represents the force that is applied to the lung and is measured with a Validyne DP45-24 pressure transducer. During NPV this is the negative pressure inside the thoracic chamber, during PPV tracheal pressure can be used. While during NPV Eq. (2) may be used to calculate pulmonary resistance, this is somewhat problematic during PPV as tracheal pressure may not always represent alveolar pressure [20]. However, changes in positive inspiratory pressure can be used as a good indicator of bronchoconstriction during PPV [21, 22]. Both pressure transducers (for airflow and pressure) are connected to a carrier frequency bridge amplifier (CFBA, HSE).

## Perfusion

As a perfusion medium we use filtered Krebs-Henseleit buffer (37 °C) (in mM; NaCl 118, KCl 4.7, $KH_2PO_4$ 1.2, $MgSO_4$ 1.2, $CaCl_2$ 2.5, $NaHCO_3$ 13 mM) that also contains 2% albumin (fraction V standard grade from Serva, Heidelberg, Germany), 0.1% glucose and 0.3% HEPES. The osmolality of this buffer as determined by freezing point depression is 310 mOsm. The endotoxin content of the buffer is <5 ng/ml (determined with Coattest, Kabivitrum GmBH, Munich, FRG). This concentration of endotoxin may be sufficient to stimulate release of tumor necrosis factor from rat lungs, which however is not a problem for most applications. If, however, cytokine responses are of interest, the use of low-endotoxin grade albumin is recommended.

A stainless steel cannula (2 in Fig. 2.4) is used to cannulate the pulmonary artery. The venous return is collected in the left atrium by another cannula (3 in Fig. 2.4) that prevents occlusion of the opening by the tender atrium tissue. These cannulas are connected via silicon tubing (diameter 2.8 mm ID) to the perfusion system. In case of perfusion with constant pressure, the height of the buffer reservoir above the lung determines the arterial pressure. The relative height of the opening of the venous effluate determines the venous pressure. Referenced to the lung hilum, we normally use an arterial pressure of 12 cm $H_2O$ and a venous pressure of 4 cm $H_2O$, thus the driving pressure is 8 cm $H_2O$. This results in a perfusate flow rate of about 25 ml/(min·g lung tissue) and 15 ml/(min·g lung tissue) during NPV and PPV, respectively. Perfusate flow velocity is measured with a Narcomatic RT 500 flow probe connected to a Narcomatic flowmeter. Perfusate pressure is measured at sideports of the perfusion system with pressure transducers. It is important that the side port connecting tubings are thin (ID 1 mm, OD 2 mm) and of very stiff material (PE tubing). It is difficult to find pressure transducers that are ideally suited to measure the low venous pressure. We use pressure transducers available from HSE to measure both arterial ($P_a$) and venous pressure ($P_V$). The venous effluate is collected in a beaker and by means of a roller pump pumped up into the buffer reservoir. During constant pressure perfusion hydrostatic pressure has to be maintained constant, so this pump must be controlled by a level sensor that senses the perfusate level in the upper reservoir. Finally, the pH of the buffer must be controlled. Most researchers use carbonate-buffered salt-solutions. With this buffer system the lung exhales $CO_2$ and the effluate pH is more alkaline then the inflowing pH. Therefore, the exhaled $CO_2$ must be replenished. This can be done either on demand (a pH-meter controls a valve that is connected to a $CO_2$-supply as shown in Fig. 2.1) or by continuously gassing the buffer with 5% $CO_2$, or carbogen gas, i.e. 5%/95% $CO_2/O_2$, in an oxygenator. One such device that might be used is a glass oxgenator (available from HSE) that also minimizes foaming that may present a problem if protein-containing solutions are to be gassed. Another alternative, i.e. ventilating the lungs with carbogen, is not recommend since increased alveolar concentrations of both oxygen [23–25] and carbon dioxide [26–30] may have unwanted side-effects in the lungs.

## Weight measurement

Edema formation represents an important problem in pulmonary research. Monitoring the lung weight is a sensitive (1 µl = 1 mg) method to follow edema formation. During positive pressure ventilation weight is usually measured by suspending the lung from a weight transducer. In case of negative pressure ventilation weight measurement has not been possible until recently. We have developed a weight transducer that works also under conditions of negative pressure ventilation. The details of this device (HSE LS30) have been published [3] and shall not be re-iterated here.

Usually it is of interest to know whether the edema originates from hydrostatic or permeability changes. In case of hydrostatic edema capillary pressure is the driving force. In perfused lungs, capillary pressure can quite conveniently be determined by the so-called double occlusion technique (see Chapter 7). A useful indicator for changes in vascular permeability is the filtration coefficient, which can be measured by gravimetric and other methods (see Chapter 8).

## Gas exchange

The ultimate goal of the lung is to organize and accomplish the gas exchange. In principle, oxygen and carbogen dioxide can be monitored both in the inspired and expired air, as well as in the perfusate. In our model, we can continuously monitor $pO_2$ and $pCO_2$ in the venous effluate. Since measurement of $pO_2$ and $pCO_2$ is flow dependent, we use a peristaltic pump (ISM827, HSE) to divert a small but constant fraction of the whole perfusate flow (4 ml/min) to a thermostated measurement block that houses the gas electrodes.

In addition, since we use a carbonate buffer the pH of the buffer before and after passage through the lung can be used as an index of $CO_2$ exhalation. In line with this, Kröll et al. [2] using a similar set-up as described here have demonstrated in perfused guinea pig lungs that the $pCO_2$ in the venous perfusate is lower than the arterial one. Further insight into the homogeneity of gas exchange can be obtained by measuring the ventilation/perfusing mismatch or carbon monoxide diffusion washout (*see* Chapter 1).

# Methods

## Surgery and setting up the lung

The whole surgery procedure takes no longer than 15 min. The OP-table should allow to perform the surgery at about the same height as the lung will finally hang; this reduces the risk of hydrostatic edema and also helps to keep tubings as short as possible. Rats are anaesthetised with i.p. pentobarbital sodium (60 mg/kg). After wetting the fur with 70% ethanol, the trachea is exposed and cut between the fourth and fifth cartilaginous ring. The tracheal cannula is inserted and secured by a ligature. The tracheal cannula is then connected to the organ holder which is held in position by a small clamp which is mounted on the OP-table. Already at this time, positive pressure ventilation with 80 breaths/min room air and a tidal volume of approximately 1.5 ml is started. Please note, that since the lung is already fixed to the organ holder, there is no need to disconnect breathing during the whole experiment. After laparotomy the diaphragm is removed and heparin sodium (2000 IU/kg) injected into the right ventricle. After waiting for about 30 s to allow for distribution of the heparin, the animals are exsanguinated by a cut in the vena cava inferior. Now the chest is completely opened by cutting along the sternum and hooks are fixed on both sides of the rib bows to hold open the thoracic cavity. The thymus is removed and one loose ligature is placed around the pulmonary artery and the aorta. To avoid air embolism before inserting the cannula it is important to open the valve that controls perfusate flow ($V_Q$ in Fig. 2.1) just enough to maintain a little dripping of buffer from the arterial cannula. An incision is made in the right ventricle and the arterial cannula (Fig. 2.3b) is inserted through the semilunar valve into the pulmonary artery. Then, the ligature is drawn tight to simultaneously fix the cannula in the pulmonary artery and close the aorta. Now, since the aorta is clamped off, arterial pressure begins to rise slowly. To avoid excessive hydrostatic pressure, the apex of the heart should quickly be removed. Then, the left atrium is cannulated by advancing the venous cannula (Fig. 2.3c) through the mitral valve. A ligature around the heart keeps this cannula in place. The venous outflow is now connected to the assigned opening in the organ holder. Please note that successful connection requires that all the tubings have been primed with buffer. In addition, the tubing supposed to receive the venous effluate must have been closed by a valve (or clamp), which is opened only after the venous line has been connected. At this stage, the lungs are perfused at a flow rate of 5 ml/min in a non-recirculating manner. Once perfusion is established the heart and lungs are removed *en bloc*. To do so, gently lift the organ holder (with the trachea connected) and then trim and tease the fascia that connect the trachea, esophagus and lungs to the dorsal area of the thoracic cavity. Having finished this, the lungs should be above the animal, but still attached to the dorsal aorta. Cut the dorsal aorta close to the heart and remove any ligaments that may have remained, but be careful not to touch the lungs with the scissors. Since the lung is already connected to the organ holder via the trachea, one can now lift the holder and transfer the lung from the OP-table to the perspex disc. The organ holder is secured by two clips and finally the thoracic chamber is affixed to the lower part of the disc by the metals clips.

When the chamber is sealed negative pressure ventilation is initiated and the ventilation head is removed and replaced by the pneumotachometer for the measurement of respiratory flow. In order to obtain zone 3 conditions [31], the lungs are perfused by a constant hydrostatic pressure of 12 cm $H_2O$ and a venous pressure of 4 cm $H_2O$ resulting in an average flow of 25 ml/g lung. Our respiratory settings during NPV are 80 breaths/min, 50% of the duty cycle inspiratory, oscillating chamber pressure between −2 cm $H_2O$ and −6 cm $H_2O$, in order to achieve an initial tidal volume of about 2 ml. To improve the functioning of the lung, regular sighs should be exerted; we perform such a hyperinflation (−16 cm $H_2O$) every 5 min. Humidifying the inspired air also has a modest positive effect on lung mechanics. Once the perfusate is clear of cells and debris, which usually requires perfusion of about 200 ml of buffer, it is recirculated. The final total volume of circulating buffer in our model is 100 ml.

*Table 2.1. Checklist for perfused rat lung*

| Species | Rat (200–300 g) |
|---|---|
| Buffer/medium | Krebs-Ringer |
| Temperature | 38 °C |
| Values preset at | |
| Endexpiratory pressure | −2 cm $H_2O$ |
| Endinspiratory pressure | −6 cm $H_2O$ |
| Arterial pressure | 12 cm $H_2O$ |
| Venous pressue | 4 cm $H_2O$ |
| Typical values obtained | |
| Tidal volume | 2 ml |
| Perfusate flow rate | 25 ml/min |
| Pulmonary compliance | 0.5 ml·cm $H_2O^{-1}$ |
| Pulmonary resistance | 0.2 cm $H_2O \cdot min \cdot ml^{-1}$ |
| $pO_2$ | 130 mm Hg |
| $PCO_2$ | 30 mm Hg |
| Criteria for quality of preparation | No edema formation; breathing mechanics are stable |
| Time to set up experiment | 20 min |
| Typical duration of preparation | 3 h |
| Papers that exemplify usage of this technique | [2, 12, 16, 21, 22, 32, 70] |
| Cost per unit | $ 60 000 |
| Experiments/day/unit | 1–2 |

## Criteria for viability

Criteria for success of perfused lung preparations have not generally been agreed upon. First of all, the lung should look homogeneously white, unless blood is perfused. Second, no overt signs of edema should be visible. Biochemical criteria, such as release of cytosolic enzymes, e.g. lactate dehydrogenase, appear not to be sensitive enough. Thus, we recommend to rely on physiological parameters. Their values should not only be within a certain range (*see* Tab. 2.1), but also remain stable. Interestingly, vascular resistance remains frequently stable, even in the presence of edema formation or bronchoconstriction. Therefore, this parameter appears not to be suited for quality control. In contrast, lung mechanics and weight gain appear to be sensitive and large irregularities or marked changes in these parameters usually indicate bad preparations. In untreated lungs, we observe a linear decay in lung function over time, here expressed in percent changes per hour: tidal volume 4–8 % (decrease $\Downarrow$), compliance 6–8 % ($\Downarrow$), resistance 1–2 % ($\Uparrow$), and lung weight 2–10 % ($\Uparrow$). Though the factors that limit perfusion time are unknown, the fact that compliance is reduced while resistance remains almost stable suggests that edema formation or surfactant production may be limiting factors. In this respect it is of interest that after 150 min of perfusion no edema (except around the big vessels) was observed, while surfactant stores in type II pneumocytes were depleted [32].

## Cleaning the apparatus

For cleaning the apparatus, before and after each experiment, we thoroughly rinse the parts of the apparatus where the buffer flows with at least 2 l of deionised water. Over night, the apparatus is filled with 1 % mucasol. However, we never leave vascular pressure transducers in mucasol, as their membranes may dissolve. Others have recommended 0.1–1.0 N NaOH [7].

## An example application

Figure 2.6 shows changes in a number of parameters that were monitored after injection of a bolus of 5 nmol platelet activating factor (PAF) into the perfusate. PAF is a useful substance to probe a perfused lung system since it affects many different lung functions. PAF increases pulmonary resistance and vascular resistance, indicating both broncho- and vaso-constriction. The bronchoconstriction, of course, also shows as a decrease in tidal volume, which in turn explains the decrease in venous $pO_2$ and the increase in venous $pCO_2$. It can also be seen that the difference of the pH before and after passage through the lung shows nearly identical changes as the venous $pCO_2$. This demonstrates that in fact the pH-difference can be used instead of $pCO_2$ measurements. It can further be seen that PAF elicits an increase in lung weight. By measuring capillary pressure and the vascular filtration coefficient we demonstrated that this edema formation is caused by increased vascular permeability and not by a hydrostatic mechanism [12]. Having established these responses, this model can then be used to study the mechanism of the PAF-induced alterations of lung function. Such studies demonstrated that the PAF-induced vaso- and bronchoconstriction are mediated by thromboxane and leukotrienes [12], whereas the mechanism of the PAF-induced edema formation remains unknown [12, 33].

Figure 2.6 contains also the time-course of weight changes after PAF infusion. The graph shows two curves for the weight measurement. The lower one is the curve that has actually been measured. However, the vasoconstriction evoked by PAF causes the vascular volume to decrease which in turn lowers lung weight. Therefore, as a result of the vasoconstriction lung weight decreases. Since, however, we are interested in weight gain due to edema, at the beginning of each experiment we always record the relation between vascular filling and lung weight and use this relationship to compute a corrected weight that takes into account the effective vasoconstriction [3]. At least in the case of PAF this procedure seems possible, since PAF does not alter vascular compliance [33].

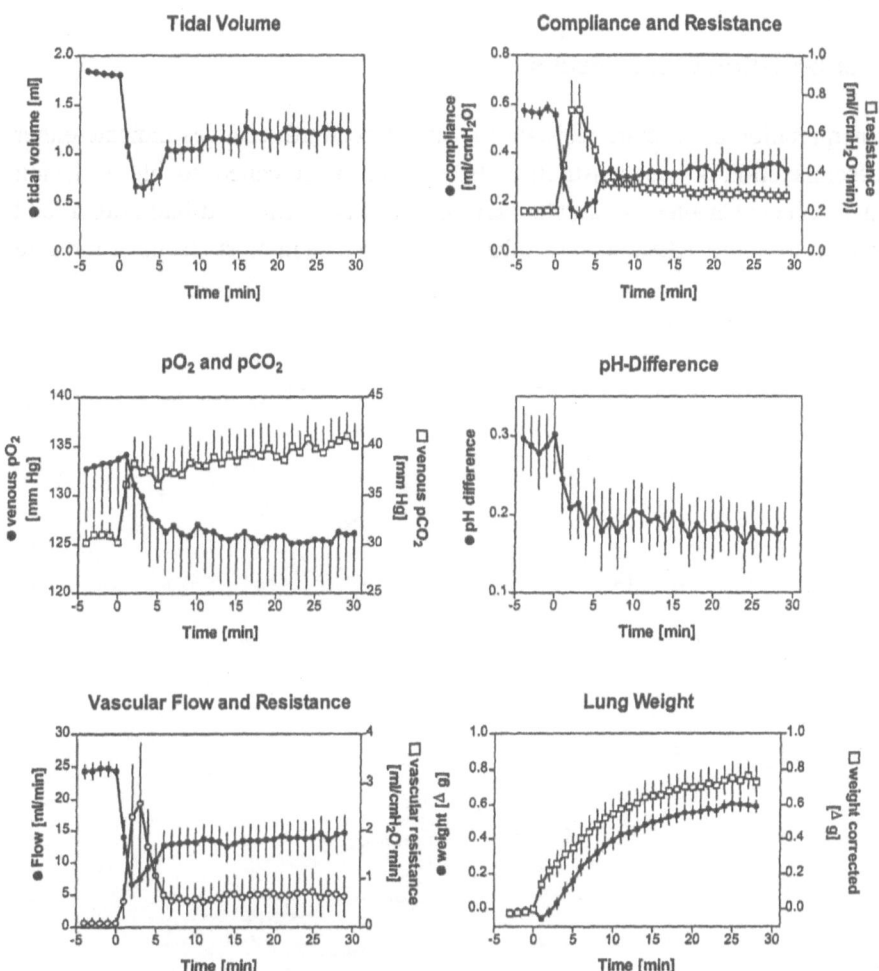

**Figure 2.6. Responses of the isolated perfused rat lung exposed to a bolus injection of 5 nmol PAF into the pulmonary artery**

PAF was injected at the time point indicated a 0. Shown is the mean±SEM of five independent experiments. The parameters shown are explained in the text. The legends to the plots are shown at the ordinate axis.

# Discussion

## Interpretation of the results

Interpretation of vascular resistance is straightforward; changes indicate either vasorelaxation or vasoconstriction. By help of the so-called double occlusion method (*see* Chapter 7) vascular resistance can be partitioned into arterial and venous pressure. Alterations in pulmonary resistance in most instances indicate

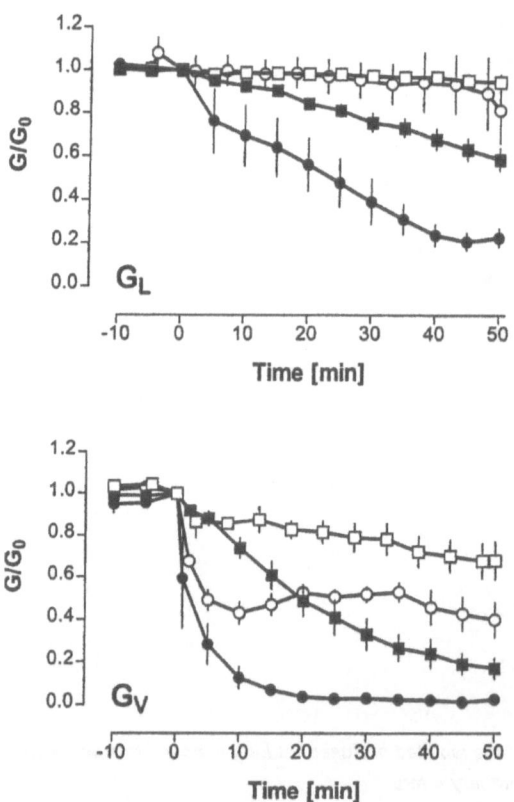

**Figure 2.7. Circulating versus non-circulating perfusion: The effect of endothelin-1 (ET-1)**
*Responses of the perfused rat lung to ET-1. 1 nmol (□, ■) or 3 nmol (○, ●) ET-1 was injected into the pulmonary artery. Shown are pulmonary ($G_L$) and vascular ($G_V$) conductance in experiments where buffer was either recirculated (■, ●) or not (□, ○). Data are mean ± SEM from at least three different experiments. $G/G_0$, conductance normalised to the time of ET-injection, i.e. time point 0.*

bronchodilation or bronchoconstriction. However, one should always keep in mind that pulmonary resistance includes both airway and tissue resistance. When evaluating data for vascular or pulmonary resistance it may be profitable to look at the inverse of resistance, i.e. conductance (Fig. 2.7). In case of vascular or airway constriction resistance can become infinitesimally large, while conductance approaches zero. The advantage of using conductance is twofold: it represents the physiological situation of reduced flow rates and it results in lower statistical variance of the data. Pulmonary compliance reflects the elasticity of the lower airways and is affected by, for example edema or fibrosis. However, this is perfectly true only for static compliance. The compliance measured by application of Eq. (2) yields dynamic compliance, which is a mixed parameter, since it is also influenced by resistance [18]. Thus, changes in dynamic compliance are only of interest if resistance remains stable. Such a situation can be obtained if edema is induced by perfusion with detergents such as linoelaidic acid [3, 34]. The formation of edema can best be followed by measurement of weight gain. This method is quite sensitive since 1 μl of water corresponds to 1 mg of weight. Alternatively, the wet/dry ratio of lungs [35], which can only be determined at the end of the experiment, has frequently been used to assess edema. Usually it is of interest to differentiate between hydrostatic and permeability types of edema. Frequently, this question is addressed by measuring the change in capillary pressure and the vascular filtration coefficient [36, 37]. A more complete analysis would also include measurement of the protein reflection coefficient (*see* Chapter 8). Vascular permeability can also be addressed by looking at the pulmonary distribution of high molecular weight substances such as albumin, which may be labeled or not.

## Constant flow (CFP) *versus* constant pressure perfusion (CPP)

Although constant flow perfusion may mimic the *in vivo* situation more closely, the choice depends on the purpose of the study. In studies related to the metabolism and kinetics of added or released compounds CFP is preferable because the interpretation of concentrations detected in the perfusate is not confounded by changes in flow velocity. Bjernaes and Hauge compared CFP *versus* CPP during hypoxic vasoconstriction [38]. They observed that changes in vascular resistance were much more pronounced during CPP than during CFP, suggesting that the former condition is more sensitive. This advantage, however, was offset by the fact that in some lungs perfusate flow completely stopped and that if normoxia was reinstated the change in vascular resistance was not completely reversible. Therefore, despite its lower sensitivity these authors recommended CFP for studies of vascular reactivity owing to its better reproducibility.

The major disadvantage of CFP is the formation of hydrostatic edema that inevitably occurs if vascular resistance increases and flow is maintained. Since edema itself may increase vascular resistance [39, 40], airway resistance [41] and pulmonary elastance [42], it is suggested to perform cumulative dose-response curves only if lung weight is recorded, too. The occurrence of hydrostatic edema makes the CFP less suitable for studies of permeability edema that recently have received much interest. Many substances that alter vascular permeability, such as reactive oxygen species, PAF, complement factors, histamine or thrombin, also increase vascular resistance. Therefore, some investigators interested in permeability edema have used vasodilators such as papaverine to prevent the vasoconstriction. However, since papaverine itself may alter vascular permeability [43], such experiments may be difficult to interpret. Therefore, in experiments with CFP it may not be easy to distinguish between hydrostatic and permeability edema. For this reason, in our studies with PAF we always have employed CPP [12, 33]. Moreover, the ever pending edema formation during CFP causes investigators to choose lower flow rates during CFP than CPP. This may be relevant since lower flow rates may reduce vascular responsiveness [44], protein synthesis and the metabolism of compounds such as serotonin [45]. In addition, when lungs are perfused at flow rates much lower than that which normally occur, estimation of *in vivo* drug clearance is difficult.

A short comment regarding the use of pulsatile perfusion which has been used only rarely is in order: Pulsatility does not cause edema, because the pressure pulses build up predominantly in the pulmonary artery [46]. It was further shown that oxygenation of the perfusate is similar under constant flow or pulsatile conditions, in normal lungs, while in edematous lungs pulsatile perfusion may perform slightly better [47].

## Negative or positive pressure ventilation

Both positive and negative pressure ventilation have been used. It was reported that NPV produces less edema formation [48] and higher cardiac output [49] than PPV. Another concern is that during inspiration in the case of PPV the vessels are compressed while they are expanded during negative pressure ventilation. Therefore, in order to mimic more closely the *in vivo* situation, negative pressure ventilation has been considered preferable [2, 4, 50]. On the other hand, *in vivo* left atrial pressure falls with pleural pressure as during PPV, but not during NPV. In most perfused lung set-ups ventilated by negative pressure the venous effluate will exit in the ambient atmosphere, thereby generating an artificially high transmural pressure (pressure difference between the intra- and extravascular space). To circumvent this problem, it has been recommended to place the venous exit inside the artificial thorax chamber [51, 52]. Alternatively, an equilibration chamber may be used that connects the oscillating chamber pressure to the venous outflow pressure.

In addition, it is assumed that NPV allows the regular induction of hyperinflations of the lung to be carried out more safely. Such maneuvers, which are habitual *in vivo*, are very valuable since it has been known for many years that lung compliance falls with time unless regular hyperinflations are performed [53, 54]. Hyperinflations (sighs) reopen atelectatic lung areas, enhance release of surfactant [55, 56] and may help to resolve small edema [57]. Another advantage of physiological ventilation is that lung mechanics are more easily studied. Until recently, however, there was one major drawback of NPV, i.e. the inability to measure lung weight (as an index of edema) in the presence of alternating negative chamber pressures. To overcome this limitation, we have recently developed a weight transducer that can be used during negative pressure ventilation [3].

## Choice of perfusate

Most experimenters have used artificial perfusate media based on Krebs-Ringer solution. From a number of studies [58–60] it is quite clear that salt buffers must be supplied with plasma expanders of at least 1%, better 2% or even 4% [58] in order to prevent edema formation. Most frequently, albumin has been used. Alternatively, some investigators have used ficoll or dextran. Though this question has not systematically been investigated, there are some hints to suggest that dextran may be toxic for rats [7]. For stabilization of pH we have included HEPES as a buffering agent in all our experiments, Recently, however, a study demonstrated that HEPES at 12 mM alters endothelial permeability [61] and hence it may advisable not to use it.

Of course, the most natural perfusion medium would be whole (heparinized) blood, though supply usually is a problem with smaller animals. Since blood is a very complex system it confounds interpretation of experiments. Further variables are introduced by the unknown state of the donor's blood (circulating mediators, etc.). Therefore, in cases where similar responses can be obtained in the absence of blood, the use of artificial media is suggested. Sometimes, however, blood appears to be indispensable [62, 63] and in other cases responses may be different when blood is used [64–67]. Some investigators have reported pulmonary hypertension during perfusion with blood, an effect which appears to be mediated by thromboxane [60, 68].

Comparing the responses in blood-free perfused lungs to those *in vivo* or in blood-perfused lungs can help to answer which responses of the lung depend on blood-derived leukocytes or not. If this question is important, the presence of marginated leukocytes should be checked. Unfortunately, different groups have made different observations: in our model, we have found virtually no leukocytes, neither marginated nor in the perfusate [32], which is in contrast to others [69]. The reasons for this difference is not quite clear, but may relate to our using higher perfusion rates, i.e. 25 ml/min *vs*. 10 ml/min, the application of NPV compared to PPV or the amount of buffer that is used to wash the lungs before recirculation is started.

## Recirculating *versus* non-recirculating perfusion

Experiments in perfused lungs can be performed with the perfusate being either recirculated or not. Recirculating perfusion has been criticized, because under *in vivo* conditions mediators released from the lung may be cleared in the systemic circulation and therefore not act on the lung again. This criticism, however, may not be relevant for short-lived mediators such as thromboxane. Another advantage of non-recirculating perfusion is that the concentration of compounds in the venous effluate reflects production of the lung at the time the sample is drawn.

On the other hand, this may also be a disadvantage, if concentrations are below the detection limit. In such cases recirculation may be advantageous since here the perfusate concentration represents the integral and not the rate of production. In addition, during recirculating perfusion an equilibrium between the perfusate and the tissue is established, which parallels the *in vivo* situation. Over all, however, the most weighty argument against non-recirculating perfusion is that of cost. Non-recirculating perfusion at flow rates of about 25 ml/min requires 1500 ml of buffer in 1 h; owing to the cost of albumin this is too expensive for routine experiments.

We have compared the effects of circulating *versus* non-circulating perfusion in three different models, i.e. perfusion with PAF, endothelin-1 (ET-1) and endotoxin. In these models, bolus injection of the compound elicits bronchoconstriction and vasoconstriction (not in the case of endotoxin), although with a different time-course. The PAF-induced pressor responses occur almost instantaneously after injection of PAF. These responses, which are largely mediated by cyclooxygenase-1 and thromboxane [12, 16], are nearly the same during recirculating and non-recirculating perfusion (data not shown). Recirculating perfusion with endothelin causes a long lasting vaso- and bronchoconstriction (Fig. 2.7) that is only partly mediated by thromboxane [70, 71]. Figure 2.7 shows that if non-recirculating perfusion is employed vasoconstriction is much weaker and bronchoconstriction hardly occurs at all. Similar observations were made with endotoxin, where bolus injection in a non-recirculating system showed no effect on the lung (not shown). This seems reasonable since endotoxin-induced bronchoconstriction commences only after at least 30 min of perfusion [32] and depends on induction of cyclooxygenase-2 and subsequent thromboxane formation [16]. Thus it appears that responses which develop over time require continuous exposure to the stimulating agent. This may reflect the *in vivo* situation where concentrations of compounds such as PAF, ET-1 or endotoxin are usually increased for longer periods of time.

## Additional experimental options

The isolated perfused lung system described here can be extended in a number of ways. Capillary pressure can be assessed by the so-called double occlusion technique (*see* Chapter 7). The capillary filtration coefficient and the vascular compliance can also be routinely measured [37]. We have made additional use of the perfused lungs in order to prepare isolated pneumocytes [72] or precision cut lung slices [73] (*see* Chapter 3).

## Troubleshooting

The isolated perfused lung preparation is usually very stable and reproducible once the experimenter is familiar with it. If more than three subsequent preparations fail, there may be a technical problem and the following points should be considered. 1) Buffer quality. Check osmolality, pH and bacteria growth as well as endotoxin content and pH. A good general check for the perfusate is osmolality: if the buffer composition is wrong, it will show here. In line with observations made in the 1970s [5], we also find that for unknown reasons some albumin preparations cause edema formation and/or a sudden decline in lung mechanics, sometimes only after 1 h of perfusion. Therefore it is a good idea to keep a charge of a working albumin on stock. 2) Avoid overinflations of lungs during surgery. 3) Thorough cleaning of the apparatus is very important. 4) Ventilation. Are all tubes tight? Avoid twisting of tubings. Is the ventilator still working properly? 5) It is imperative to avoid air bubbles in the perfusate, because perfused lungs are prone to air embolism. Even small air bubbles can spoil an otherwise good preparation. 6) Animals. Has the batch/litter of animals changed? Are the animals infected?

## Final comments

Compared to experiments with isolated organ preparations, cell culture or many *in vivo* studies, experiments with perfused lungs are much more time consuming, since only one or two preparations can be done per day. In addition, an expensive apparatus and a skilled experimenter are required. However, when fully equipped the isolated perfused lung system provides a wealth of information such as tidal volume, pulmonary compliance, pulmonary resistance, vascular resistance, vascular compliance, weight gain, filtration coefficient and blood gases from each single experiment. This gives an integrated view on the totality of lung function that repays all the effort involved in setting up the experiment.

# References

1 Seeger W, Walmrath D, Grimminger F, Rosseau S, Schütte H, Ermert L and Kiss L (1994) *Meth. Enzymol.* **233**: 549

2 Kröll F, Karlsson JA, Nilsson E, Persson CGA and Ryrfeldt Å (1986) *Acta Physiol. Scand.* **128**: 1

3 Uhlig S and Heiny O (1995) *J. Pharm. Tox. Meth.* **33**: 147

4 Uhlig S and Wollin L (1994) *J. Pharm. Tox. Meth.* **31**: 85

5 Longmore, WJ (1982) The Isolated Perfused Lung as a Model for Studies of Lung Metabolism. In: *Lung Development: Biological and Clinical Perspectives, Vol 1,* McClellan RO and Henderson RF (eds), p. 101, Academic Press New York

6 Mehendale HM, Angevine LS and Ohmiya Y (1981) *Toxicology* **21**: 1

7 Roth RA, McClellan LJ and Carpenter RO (1989) Potential Role of Phagocytic Cells as Mediators of Chemically Induced Lung Injury: Use of Isolated Lung Preparations in Evaluating Pneumotoxicity. In: *Concepts in Inhalation Toxicology, Vol E: 1,* p. 445, Library of Congress Washington D.C.

8 Smith BR and Bendf JR (1981) *Meth. in Enzymol.* **77**: 105

9 Rhoades RA (1984) *Environ. Health Perspect.* **56**: 43

10 Weksler B, Schneider A, Ng B and Burt M (1993) *J. Appl. Physiol.* **74**: 2736

11 Munoz NM, Chang SW, Murphy TM, Stimler-Gerard NP, Blake J, Mack M, Irvin C, Voelkel NF and Leff AR (1989) *J. Appl. Physiol.* **66**: 202

12 Uhlig S, Wollin L and Wendel A (1994) *J. Appl. Physiol.* **77**: 262

13 Desquand S, Touvay C, Randon J, Lagente V, Vilain B, Maridonneau-Parini I, Etienne A, Lefort J, Braquet P and Vargaftig BB (1986) *Eur. J. Pharmacol.* **127**: 83

14 Vargaftig BB, Lefort J, Chignard M and Benviste J (1980) *Eur. J. Pharmacol.* **65**: 185

15 Feuerstein N and Ramwell PW (1981) *Br. J. Pharmacol.* **73**: 511

16 Uhlig S, Nüsing R, von Bethmann A, Featherstone RL, Klein T, Brasch F, Müller K-M, Ullrich V and Wendel A (1996) *Mol. Med.* **2**: 373

17 Uhlig S and Wendel A (1995) Lipid Mediators in Perfused Lung. In: *Interdisziplinäre Aspekte der Pneumologie,* von Wichert P and Siegenthaler W (eds), p. 66, Georg Thieme Verlag Stuttgart

18 Drazen JM (1984) *Environ. Health Perspect.* **56**: 3

19 Amdur MO and Mead J (1958) *Am. J. Physiol.* **102**: 364

20 Valta P, Corbeil C, Chasse M, Braidy J and Milic-Emili J (1996) *Am. J. Respir. Crit. Care Med.* **153**: 1825

21 Hamasaki Y, Mojarad M, Saga T, Tai HH and Said SI (1984) *Am. Rev. Respir. Dis.* **129**: 742

22 Lal H, Woodward B and Williams KI (1995) *Br. J. Pharmacol.* **115**: 653

23 Fisher AB, Dodia C, Tan ZT, Ayene I and Eckenhoff RG (1991) *J. Clin. Invest.* **88**: 674

24 Winter PM and Smith G (1972) *Anesthesiology* **37**: 210

25  Zocco J, Wilk J, Crute SL and Greenfield LJ (78) *Surgery* **85**: 400

26  Cander A (1989) *Am. J. Physiol.* **257**: L354

27  Longmore WJ, Niethe C, Sprinkle DJ and Godinez RI (1973) *J. Lipid Res.* **14**: 145

28  Baudouin SV and Evans TW (1993) *Crit. Care Med.* **21**: 740

29  Gibbs JM, Tait AR and Sykes MK (1976) *Brit. J. Anaesth.* **48**: 629

30  Hyman AL and Kadowitz PJ (1975) *Am. J. Physiol.* **228**: 397

31  West JB, Dollery CT and Naimark A (1964) *J. Appl. Physiol.* **19**: 713

32  Uhlig S, Brasch F, Wollin L, Fehrenbach H, Richter J and Wendel A (1995) *Am. J. Pathol.* **146**: 1235

33  Uhlig S, Featherstone RL, Wilhelms O-H and Wendel A (1996) *Naunyn-Schmiedeberg's Arch. Pharmacol.* **354**: 684

34  Uhlig S (1995) Analysis of Edema Formation in Isolated Perfused Rat Lungs Ventilated by Negative Pressure. In: *FFB 9: Pharmacological Evaluation of Cardioprotective Substances*, Biomesstechnik Verlag March Germany (ed.), p. 152

35  Collins JC, Newman JH, Wickersham NE, Vaughn WK, Snapper JR, Harris TR and Brigham KL (1985) *J. Appl. Physiol.* **59**: 592

36  Drake R, Gaar KA and Taylor AE (1978) *Am. J. Physiol.* **234**: H266

37  Uhlig S and von Bethmann AN (1997) *J. Pharm. Tox. Meth.* **37**: 119

38  Bjertnaes L and Hauge A (1980) *Acta Physiol. Scand.* **109**: 193

39  Hillyard R, Anderson J and Raj JU (1991) *Lung* **169**: 97

40  Ngeow YK and Mitzner W (1983) *J. Appl. Physiol.* **55**: 1154

41  Hogg JC, Agarawal JB, Gardner AJS, Palmer WH and Macklem PT (1972) *J. Appl. Physiol.* **32**: 20

42  Seeger W, Wolf HRD, Stähler G and Neuhof H (1983) *Respiration* **44**: 273

43  Swanson JA and Kern DF (1993) *J. Appl.*

Physiol. **75**: 2326

44  Tucker A and Rodeghero PT (1981) *Respiration* **42**: 228

45  Watkins CA and Rannels DE (1987) *Anesthesiology* **67**: 916

46  Saito O, Lamm JE, Hildebrandt J and Albert RK (1995) *J. Appl. Physiol.* **78**: 914

47  Hauge A and Nicolaysen G (1980) *Acta Physiol. Scand.* **109**: 325

48  Dritsas KG, Brown D and Couves CM (1969) *Surgery* **65**: 611

49  Skaburskis M, Michel RP, Gatensby A and Zidulka A (1989) *J. Appl. Physiol.* **66**: 2223

50  Niemeier RW and Bingham E (1972) *Life Sci.* **11**: 807

51  Permutt, S. (1977) Mechanical Influences on Water Accumulation in the Lungs in Pulmonary Edema, Fishman, AP and Renkin, EM (eds), p. 175, American Physiological Society

52  Culver BH and Butler J (1980) *Annu. Rev. Physiol.* **42**: 187

53  Huang YC, Weinmann GG and Mitzner W (1989) *J. Appl. Physiol.* **65**: 2040

54  Mead J and Collier C (1959) *J. Appl. Physiol.* **14**: 669

55  Nicholas TE and Barr HA (1983) *Respir. Physiol.* **52**: 69

56  Nicholas TE, Power JHT and Barr HA (1982) *Respir. Physiol.* **49**: 315

57  Dreyfuss D, Soler P and Saumon G (1992) *J. Appl. Physiol.* **72**: 2081

58  Rippe B, Townsley MI and Taylor AE (1985) *J. Appl. Physiol.* **58**: 1521

59  Chang RSY, Wright K and Effros RM (1981) *J. Appl. Physiol.* **50**: 1065

60  Kraft SA, Fujishima S, McGuire GP, Thompson JS, Raffin TA and Pearl RG (1995) *J. Appl. Physiol.* **78**: 499

61  Douglas GC, Swanson JA and Kern DF (1993) *J. Appl. Physiol.* **75**: 1423

62  Adkins WK, Barnard JW, May S, Seibert AF, Haynes J and Taylor AE (1992) *J. Appl. Physiol.* **72**: 492

63  Raj JU and Anderson J (1991) *Circ. Res.* **68**:

1108

64 Selig WM, Noonan TC, Kern DF and Malik AB (1986) *J. Appl. Physiol.* **60**: 1972

65 Hakim TS and Malik AB (1988) *Respir. Physiol.* **72**: 109

66 Hinshaw LB, Kuida H, Gilbert RP and Visscher MB (1957) *Am. J. Physiol.* **191**: 293

67 Rodman DM, Stelzner TJ, Zamora MR, Bonvallet ST, Oka M, Sato K, Obrien RF and Mcmurtry IF (1992) *J. Cardiovasc. Pharmacol.* **20**: 658

68 Patterson GA, Rock P, Mitzner WA, Adkinson NF and Sylvester JT (1985) *J. Appl. Physiol.* **58**: 892

69 Seibert AF, Haynes J and Taylor A (1993) *Am. Rev. Respir. Dis.* **147**: 270

70 Uhlig S, Bethmann AN von, Featherstone RL and Wendel A (1995) *Am. J. Respir. Crit. Care Med.* **152**: 1449

71 Uhlig S and von Bethmann A (1995) *J. Cardiovasc. Pharmacol.* **26**: S111

72 Bundschuh DS, Uhlig S, Leist M, Sauer A and Wendel A (1995) *In Vitro Cell. Dev Biol. – Animal* **31**: 684

73 Martin C, Uhlig S and Ullrich V (1996) *Eur. Respir. J.* **9**: 2479

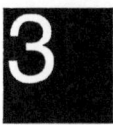

# Lung explants

E.A. Cowley and
D.H. Eidelman

Elastic recoil is a fundamental physiological characteristic of lung tissue. Unfortunately, this mechanical property has proved a major impediment to establishing culture systems for mature lung tissue. While fetal lung tissue is relatively easy to handle with standard culture techniques, mature lung slices are more difficult to manipulate because this intrinsic elasticity leads the tissue to roll up rather than lie flat on a culture dish. A number of approaches have been proposed to overcome this problem, but recently we [1–5] and others [6–14] have adapted the technique of slicing agarose-filled lungs. This concept was initially described by Hackney [12], and improved by Guerrero [13], and eliminates alveolar collapse within the tissue, while maintaining a high degree of anatomical and structural integrity. Variations on this technique have successfully been used in studies of the bronchi, pulmonary vessels and the lung parenchyma.

The concept behind these slices, or explants, depends upon the physical properties of agarose, specifically its temperature hysteresis. Agarose can be both a sol and a gel at body temperature. Therefore, lungs can be inflated with liquid agarose solution, which can then be cooled to form a gel. Agarose-filled explants will lie flat because the agarose within them resists the recoil of the alveolar walls, thus enabling them to be cultured using conventional techniques.

# Material and equipment

## Preparation of culture media

All procedures must be performed under sterile culture conditions. Explants are cultured in bicarbonate-buffered culture medium (BCM), pre-

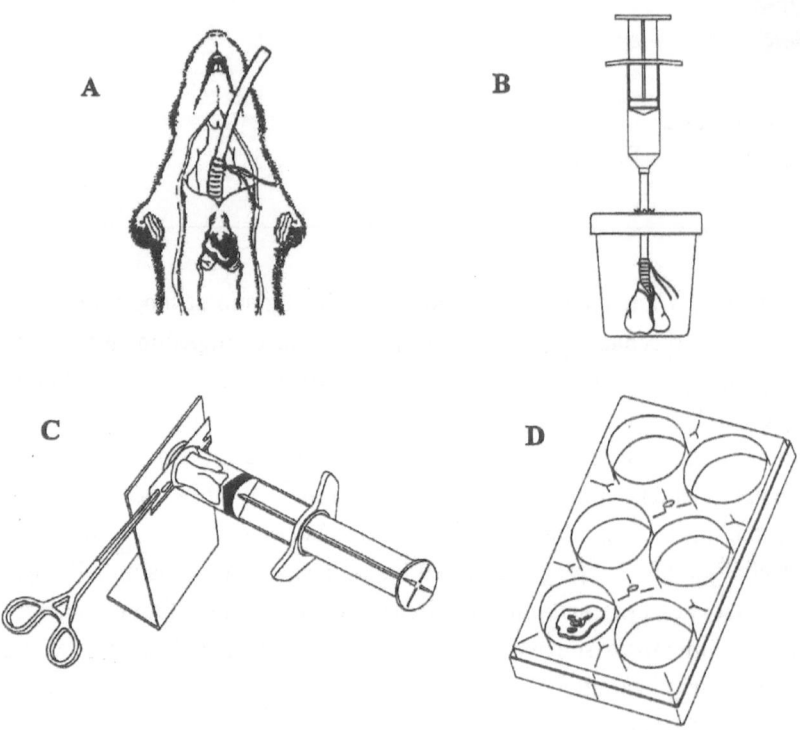

**Figure 3.1 Fundamentals of the explant technique**

*The animal is intubated (A) and the dissected lungs inflated with agarose within a sterile container (B). Lungs are then placed in a 35 ml syringe and surrounded with 4% agarose solution, resulting in an agarose-lung block, which can be clamped horizontally and cut by hand (C). Following their overnight culture, explants suitable for study are placed in a six-well plate (D) and examined under the microscope.*

pared from minimal essential medium (MEM) powder with Earle's salts and L-glutamine, further supplemented with 2.2 g/l sodium bicarbonate, 1x MEM amino acid solution, 1x vitamin solution, 0.1 µg/ml vitamin A, 50 µg/ml gentamicin, 10 ml/l 100 mM sodium pyruvate solution, 0.1 µg/ml bovine insulin and 0.1 µg/ml hydrocortisone. Additionally, a BCM with double the amounts of the above additives must also be prepared. Solutions should be filter sterilised (0.22 μm filter) and have a final pH of 7.3. Store at 4°C.

## Preparation of agarose

The agarose used to inflate the lungs is Type VII low gelling temperature (Sigma Chemicals). This is prepared in 100 ml BCM (without the supplements) at 4% wt/vol, sterilised by autoclaving and stored at 4°C. Both the culture solutions and the agarose must be used within 1 week of their preparation.

## Preparation of animals

Animals are administered a lethal dose of anaesthetic, placed supine in a laminar flow hood, and their necks, thorax and abdomens soaked with 70% ethanol (Fig. 3.1A). They are then intubated by tracheotomy with a length of sterile polyethylene tubing (for rats, PE-240; for mice, PE-90, Intramedic, Becton and Dickson, Parsippany, NJ) and exsanguinated by cutting the inferior vena cava. For routine studies, we have found it unnecessary to perfuse the lungs free of blood: however, if desired, blood can be removed by perfusion with $Ca^{2+}$ and $Mg^{2+}$ free Hank's buffer [14] via a catheter placed in the pulmonary artery. The anterior chest wall is removed and the heart and lungs excised *en masse*. For rats and guinea pigs, these organs are placed in a sterile container with a hole punctured in the lid through which the tracheal tube protrudes (Fig. 3.1B), while for mice the lungs are typically inflated *in vivo*, and the entire animal placed in a sterile Petri dish.

## Preparation of explants

On the day of the experiment, the 4% agarose solution in BCM is melted in a microwave, and allowed to cool to 37°C. An equal volume of this is then mixed with the BCM (prepared with the double supplements and pre-warmed to 37°C), resulting in a 2% agarose/BCM mixture. It is this mixture which is slowly instilled into the lungs with a syringe, until the desired lung inflation is achieved. The tracheal tube is then clamped and the inflated lungs placed at 4°C for 30 min, which allows the liquid agarose solution to gel. After cooling, the heart, trachea and all remaining tissue are dissected away, and the lung tissue (typically the left lung alone for guinea pigs and rats, or both lungs for mice) is placed upright in a sterile 35 ml syringe, from which the needle end has been cut away. A 4% agarose solution is then poured into this syringe to surround the lung tissue, prior to placing the syringe at 4°C for 30 min to gel the agarose. The result is a lung-agarose block, which can be clamped so that the syringe lies horizontally. By applying pressure to the base of the block,

*Table 3.1. Summary of explant preparation*

| Species: | Small mammals | |
|---|---|---|
| Buffer: | Bicarbonate-buffered medium: | |
| | Base: | MEM<br>Earle's salts + L-glutamine |
| | Additives: | Sodium bicarbonate<br>50X MEM amino acid solution<br>100X vitamin solution<br>Vitamin A<br>Gentamicin<br>Sodium pyruvate<br>Bovine insulin<br>Hydrocortisone |
| Temperature: | 37°C | |
| Time to prepare solutions: | 1–2 h | |
| Time to prepare explants: | 2–3 h | |
| Culture period: | 24 h | |
| Cost per experiment | $40–$100* | |

*This cost varies depending upon the amount of agarose used and whether the explants are supported on culture plate inserts*

the agarose will begin to protrude out of the top of the syringe, allowing the block to be cut into transverse sections (typically between 0.5–1.0 mm thickness). In our laboratory, slices are now cut by hand with a microtome blade (model 02118, Surgipath, Winnipeg, Manitoba) (Fig. 3.1C). Alternatively, it is possible to use a commercially available microtome to produce the explants (Krumdieck Tissue Slicer, Alabama Research and Development, Munford, AL), which typically produces explants of 0.2–0.3 mm thickness [14].

Any residual agarose must be carefully removed from the airway lumen. We find that by gently bending the explant to and fro, this agarose can easily be removed with fine forceps, at least from relatively large airways and vessels. The resulting explants are then placed in a 100 mm Petri dish containing 3mls BCM (Fig. 3.1D). Our original protocol called for explants to be supported during their culture on 30 mm culture plate inserts (PICM 030 50: Millipore, Bedford, MA) within six-well plates. However, we have found that because our culture period is so short, these inserts are not essential. Explants are then incubated overnight at 37°C in a 5% $CO_2$ / 95% air mixture (Tab. 3.1).

## Image acquisition

Explants suitable for further study are transferred to six-well plates containing 2 ml of BCM and placed on the stage of an inverted microscope. Imaging of airways or vessels can be achieved using a conventional video camera attached to the microscope and images stored on optical disc. For quantification, it is then necessary to connect the video camera to a digitising board attached to a personal computer. Many software packages, including some available on the Internet (for example, Image PC by Scion Corporation or Uthscsa Image Tool for the PC, NIH Image for Macintosh) can then be used to measure various parameters such as luminal area (Fig. 3.2).

For measurements of ciliary beat frequency, we have taken advantage of the interlaced nature of conventional television signals. Using the approach of Romet et al. [15], we count odd and even scans as sequential measurements of the same location, which increases the effective

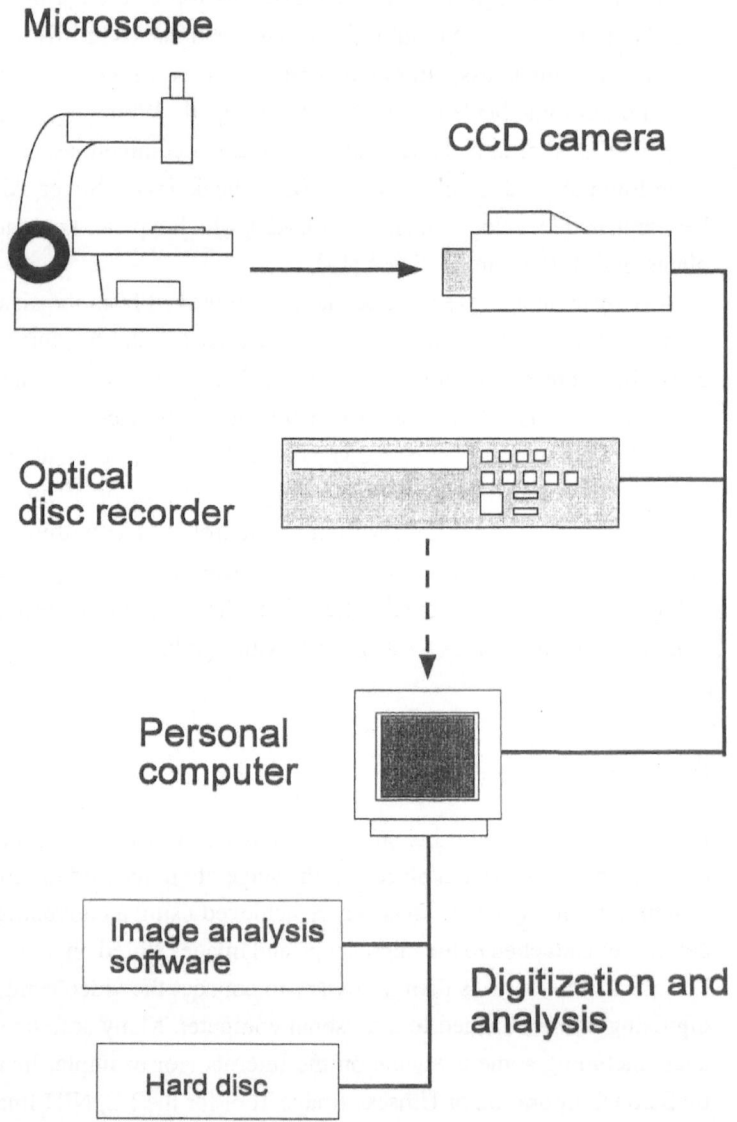

**Figure 3.2. Typical video microscopy set-up**

*Images are recorded from the microscope to an optical disc recorder via a conventional video camera. Stored images can then be transferred to a personal computer and analysed using suitable image analysis software.*

sampling rate from 30 Hz to 60 Hz [2]. This approach requires the development of custom software, and interested parties should contact the authors.

## Variations on this technique

A number of other authors have adapted this technique to study various aspects of pulmonary biology. Fisher and Placke [9–11] prepared explants inflated with 0.5 % agarose, cultured on a sterile gelatin support sponge saturated with media. Importantly, these explants are not submerged in liquid. This gas-liquid interface reportedly decreases the toxicity associated with the high $O_2$ concentration required for extended periods in culture. By supporting explants in this manner, explants could be cultured for up to 28 days.

This culture period was prolonged even further by Siminski et al. [7] by culturing on a gelatin support and gently turning the explants over every other day, so reducing the tendency of the lung cells to adhere to the support. In this way, explants can be cultured for up to 60 days, with normal parenchymal architecture being maintained. However, the integrity of the pulmonary vasculature and endothelial cells are not maintained beyond the seventh day in culture. Martin et al. [14] have developed another culture technique, in which the explants are placed in a dynamic roller culture system so that the explants are continuously turned. Using this approach, explants are viable for at least 70 h.

# Applications

## Effects of bronchoconstriction

Lung explants prepared in this way provide a convenient means to directly measure and thus quantify the response of individual airways during bronchoconstriction [1, 14]. Explants must contain an airway in cross-section (Fig. 3.4), with the entire epithelial-luminal junction in focus. Ideally the explant will con-

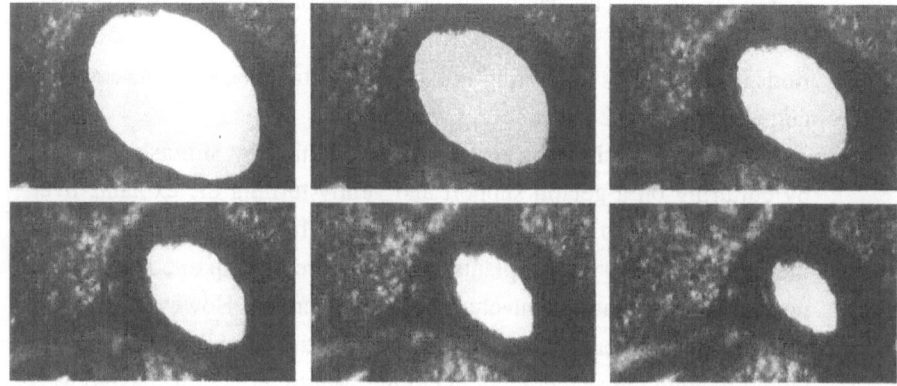

**Figure 3.3. Lung explant before and after addition of methacholine**

Bronchoconstriction induced by methacholine in a lung explant inflated to 75% TLC with 1% agarose solution. Frames show baseline luminal area followed by 2, 5, 10, 20 and 180 s exposure to $10^{-2}$ M methacholine.

tain a range of airway sizes, so any differential effects of bronchoconstrictors on airways of different diameters will be evident. By recording baseline images of all the airways to be studied prior to the addition of increasing concentrations of the agent, a dose-response curve can be produced.

Studies using this technique have determined that the maximal response to methacholine is dependent both upon the degree of lung inflation as well as the concentration of agarose used, suggesting that airway-parenchymal interdependence mechanisms are involved during bronchoconstriction. Inflation with a 1% agarose concentration at 75% of the predicted total lung capacity appears to produce optimal methacholine induced bronchoconstriction [1].

Recently, Galen et al. [16] have used the same imaging approach to study constriction in the trachealis. Although this technique obviates the requirement for agarose, it is not suitable for the study of peripheral airways.

## Measurements of mucociliary clearance

Ciliary motion can easily be detected in lung explants, even at low magnification. Clearance of particles and bacteria by the mucociliary elevator plays an important role in primary host defence, and lung explants provide a tool to investigate ciliary function in a variety of small and large calibre airways [2]. Both ciliary beat frequency (CBF) and particle transport may be examined in explants,

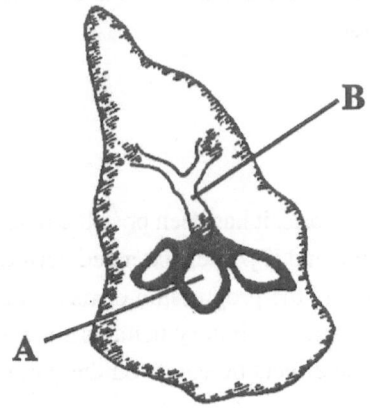

*Figure 3.4 Schematic illustration of a lung explant*
Airways may either be cut in cross-section (A) or tangentially (B). Cross-sections can be used for measurements of ciliary beat frequency, while those cut tangentially are useful for particle transport studies.

depending upon the orientation of the airway.

CBF is measured using explants which contain airways cut in cross-section (Fig. 3.4), clear of tissue debris and agarose. Digitisation is reduced to a narrow band containing the image of the beating cilia, and at each sampling location the power spectrum of variation in light intensity is calculated using fast Fourier transformations. The frequency with the highest value in the power spectrum is taken as the CBF.

The transport of particles by the mucociliary clearance mechanism can also be measured by adding a small amount (<5 µl) of a charcoal-BCM mixture to tangentially sliced airways. Images of the particle's path can then be recorded onto videocassette. This technique allows physiological and pharmacological investigations into the factors involved in these important defence mechanisms.

## Measurements of pulmonary vasculature

Since blood vessels are found in close proximity to airways, lung explants can also be used to investigate the pulmonary vasculature. It is possible, therefore, to identify pulmonary vessels based on their anatomical location and appearance. Dose response curves can therefore be constructed by studying the degree of vessel constriction or relaxation. Using explants prepared from human lung tissue, there appears to be significant differences between the responses of airways, veins and arteries to histamine and 5-HT [4]. Furthermore, studies in guinea pig explants demonstrated a difference in the rate of contraction induced by these agonists in a model of postobstructive pulmonary vasculopathy produced by arterial ligation *versus* control (non-ligated) vessels [5].

## Long term explant culture techniques

By supporting explants upon gelatin-sponge supports, it has been possible to extend the culture period to 28 days [9–11] and beyond [7]. Such extended periods of culture enable toxicological investigations, and the progression of tissue damage has been described for a number of classical respiratory irritants such as asbestos [10], silica [11] and oxygen [6, 8]. The effects of agents on the parenchyma can be investigated in such long term cultures, although the integrity of other pulmonary cell types is not maintained.

## Investigations of protein and gene expression

We have demonstrated that explants can be used for measurements of protein and mRNA expression, in which it is possible to directly correlate *in vitro* physiological measurements with markers of cellular activation. Explants may be fixed in 10% buffered formalin, paraffin-embedded and sectioned for routine histology or morphometry. Protein expression can be investigated by either snap freezing the tissue in liquid nitrogen, or fixation in 4% paraformaldehyde prior to immunocytochemistry, while fixation in 4% paraformaldehyde followed by 15% sucrose/PBS washes and freezing gives tissue suitable for *in situ* hybridisation [3].

## Troubleshooting

During the course of our studies, a number of problems have been encountered and are discussed briefly here. The concentration of agarose used to inflate the lungs is important, as this will have an effect upon contractility of the airways. Therefore, on each microwave melting of the agarose solution, it is important to completely dissolve all agarose and then mix by inversion several times. This will ensure that a uniform concentration is used in all experiments. Additionally, we have found that using a 1% agarose solution for inflation is the lowest concentration which can provide the support required to slice the lungs, while minimising the rigidity and loss of contractility seen with higher agarose concentrations. It is also important to ensure that the agarose solution used to inflate the lungs is at 37°C – this will eliminate clotting of the agarose and subsequent airway blockage resulting in damage to the lung structure.

The thickness of the explant is also important to the success of each experiment: explants which are too thick (over 1 mm) are generally more difficult to image successfully, while those that are too thin (less than 0.5 mm) often do not have examples of intact airways or vasculature. Obviously, if it is impossible to acquire a good image of the structure to be examined, then it will be impossible to accurately measure any of the parameters of interest. The use of an automated tissue slicer, such as that described by Martin et al. [14], may allow the production of thinner explant slices with a larger number of intact airways.

If freshly cut explants are examined under the microscope, the presence of air bubbles within the parenchyma makes good image acquisition difficult. This is overcome in our laboratory by culturing the explants overnight, which reduces the amount of air seen. Another potential approach to reduce this problem would be to degas the lungs prior to the beginning of the experiment.

## Discussion

Lung explants have been successfully used in our laboratory to study a variety of physiological parameters. Explants are relatively inexpensive to produce and a large number may easily be prepared from a single animal – typically around 10 explants per mouse; 25 per rat; and 35 per guinea pig. Thus this system makes it possible to study a number of different parameters. This preparation provides an important intermediary between *in vivo* measurements of pulmonary function, which are by definition indirect, and *in vitro* cell culture studies, in which cells are removed from their normal environment. The main advantage of explants is that pulmonary structures can be visualised within the framework of an intact, supported parenchyma. For example, using this system one can study bronchoconstriction at the level of the single bronchiole, eliminating contractile elements other than airway smooth muscle, which may be present in parenchymal strip preparations. Similarly, measurements of mucociliary function can be made in airways other than the trachea and proximal airways, typically used in other studies.

Explants can be prepared from any species, though in our laboratory we have restricted their preparation to human, dog, guinea pig, rat and mouse lung. In particular, they have proved useful in the study of rat and mouse lung, as the small size of these airways makes them more difficult to be studied with other techniques.

Investigation into the viability of these slices reveals that they illustrate a reasonable representation of the *in vivo* situation, provided certain parameters are adhered to. Long-term culture of explants in a gas-liquid interface system has demonstrated that inflation of the parenchyma with agarose prevents the atelectasis and necrosis typically seen in other culture techniques, presumably by increasing the surface area available for nutrient gas exchange. Such studies have reported normal anatomical appearance when explants are cultured in MEM or M199 for up to 4 weeks, with a normal cellular complement identifiable. However, the choice of culture medium is crucial for successful long-term culture. Placke and Fisher [9] provide a detailed discussion of the effects of eight commonly used culture media on tissue viability, several of which lead to severe tissue degeneration and ultimate autolysis. When MEM or M199 are used however, a normal histology is maintained along with protein and nucleic acid levels comparable to those seen prior to culture. The reason for this strict dependence of viability in culture on the type of medium used is not obvious.

One important disadvantage of lung explants is that inflation of the lungs with agarose and the subsequent slicing potentially produces a high degree of mechanical trauma in the tissue. While Placke and Fisher [9] have demonstrated normal histology in explants, a result we have replicated, the potential release of cellular factors in response to this trauma, and the effects these may have on lung physiology, remains to be addressed.

Another disadvantage relates to the obvious differences in the mechanical properties of agarose when compared to air. It is extremely important that after slicing, all traces of agarose are removed from the large airways. If not, this will act as a physical barrier to bronchoconstriction. However, it is extremely difficult to remove all traces of agarose from smaller diameter airways, and it is possible that residual agarose may alter the responses of smaller airways.

In conclusion, lung explants demonstrate a number of advantages over other *in vitro* systems, most importantly that the structural relationship between parenchyma and airways is maintained and can be easily visualised. It provides a unique opportunity to examine aspects of lung physiology which would otherwise be extremely difficult to undertake.

# Acknowledgements

The authors thank Dr Chong-Gang Wang for helpful discussion and Mr Travis Webber for the artwork. This work was supported by the Medical Research Council of Canada, the Canadian Cystic Fibrosis Foundation and the J.T. Costello Memorial Fund.

# References

1  Dandurand RJ, Wang CG, Phillips NC and Eidelman DH (1993) *J. Appl. Physiol.* **75**: 364

2  Kurosawa H, Wang CG, Dandurand RJ, King M and Eidelman DH (1995) *J. Appl. Physiol.* **79**: 4

3  Eidelman DH, Minshall E, Dandurand RJ, Schotman E, Song YL, Yasruel Z, Moquel R and Hamid Q (1996) *Am. J. Resp. Cell Molec. Biol.* **5**: 582

4  Shi W, Wang CG, Dandurand RJ, Eidelman DH and Michel RP (1995) *Am. J. Resp. Crit. Care Med.* **151**: A625

5  Michel RP, Shi W, Hu F and Eidelman DH (1995) *Am. J. Resp. Crit. Care Med.* **151**: A735

6  Shapiro PS, Casty FE, Stirewalt WS, Leslie KO, Absher MP and Evans JN (1994) *Am. J. Physiol.* **267** (*Lung Cell. Mol. Biol.* **11**): L720

7  Siminski JT, Kavanagh TJ, Chi E and Ragnu G (1992) *Am. J. Physiol.* **262** (*Lung Cell. Mol. Biol.* **6**): L105

8  Martin WJ, Gadek JE, Hunninghake GW and Crystal RG (1981) *J. Clin. Invest.* **68**: 1277

9  Placke ME and Fisher GL (1987) *Toxicol. Appl. Pharmacol.* **90**: 284

10  Placke ME and Fisher GL (1987) *Drug Chem. Toxicol.* **10**: 133

11  Fisher GL and Placke ME (1987) *Toxicology* **47**: 71

12  Hackney JD, Bils RF, Takahashi Y, Rounds DE and Collier CR (1967) *Am. Rev. Resp. Dis.* **95**: 871

13  Guerrero RR, Rounds DE and Booher J (1977) *In Vitro* **13**: 517

14  Martin C, Uhlig S and Ullrich V (1996) *Europ. Resp. J.* **9**: 2479

15  Romet S, Schoevaert D and Marano F (1991) *Biol. Cell.* **71**: 183

16  Galens S, Munoz NM, Rabe KF, Herrnreiter A, Mayer D, Morton B, McAllister K and Leff AR (1995) *Am. J. Physiol.* **268** (*Lung Cell. Mol. Biol.* **12**): L519

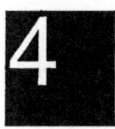

# Tracheal preparations

*M. Eltze*

The guinea pig is a commonly employed species for studying the effect of drugs on respiratory smooth muscle and airway dynamics and shows a surprisingly broad pharmacological similarity to airway function in man. In both species two main neuronal mechanisms, i.e. cholinergic nerves using acetylcholine, and excitatory noncholinergic, nonadrenergic (e-NANC) nerves using tachykinins as neurotransmitters, are involved in contraction of airway smooth muscle [1, 2]. However, while in guinea pigs both adrenergic nerves and inhibitory nonadrenergic, non-cholinergic (i-NANC) nerves are responsible for relaxation of airway smooth muscle [3, 4], it appears that in human airway smooth muscle the only neuronal bronchodilator pathway consists of the i-NANC system which uses vasoactive intestinal peptide (VIP) and nitric oxide (NO) as neurotransmitters [5–7]. The interaction between these separate neuronal pathways and the modulation of neurotransmitter release from airway nerves by prejunctional auto- and heteroreceptors and, additionally, by complementary or opposing effects on postjunctional receptors, serve as important physiological mechanisms for controlling airway calibre and function [8].

Although there exist marked differences between species with respect to innervation, receptors and neuromodulatory mechanisms, dissected guinea pig tracheal tissue immersed or superfused by isolated-tissue bath techniques provides an important way of studying the effects of drugs either to influence these neuronal pathways or to act directly on respiratory smooth muscle. The guinea pig trachea is generally accepted as a relevant and sensitive model of human large and central airways which enables to screen new compounds with potential therapeutic efficacy in disorders of the respiratory tract, such as airway obstruction [9]. Since most researchers lack access to human lung tissue, this chapter is confined to describing isolated tracheal preparations of the guinea pig, thereby emphasizing that most of the mechanisms found in this species are also operative in human airways, for example i-NANC responses [10–12], e-NANC responses [13–16], $\beta_2$ adrenoceptors [17–20], cholinergic mechanisms [21, 22], phosphodiesterase (PDE) isoenzyme composition [23–27] and role of airway epithelium [28–30].

# Methods

## Guinea pig tracheal preparations

Several methodical variations of the isolated guinea pig trachea have been described in the literature demonstrating the usefulness and remarkable versatility of this tissue in pulmonary research. This chapter deals with the most frequently employed tracheal preparations and discusses their possible advantages, however, the choice of the most suitable technique depends on the type of information required in a particular case.

### Immersion techniques

In most cases, the isolated tracheal tissue is immersed in an isolated tissue bath warmed by water of 37 °C from a constant-temperature circulator. The tissue is suspended in Krebs-Henseleit (KH) solution and fixed to the bottom of the bath chamber on one side and to an isometric transducer for measurement of change in developed force on the other. A mixture of 95 % $O_2$/5 % $CO_2$ is continuously bubbled from the bottom of the bath chamber for oxygenation, mixing and pH maintenance.

### Tracheal chain

The tracheal chain preparation was introduced by Castillo and De Beer [31] and initially used to study the effects of relaxant drugs, especially those acting on $\beta_2$ adrenoceptors, in tracheal tissues with spontaneously developed intrinsic tone [32]. Guinea pigs (both sexes, 430–600 g) are killed by cervical dislocation and bleeding. The trachea is excised, separated from surrounding connective tissue and then divided into rings.

Four to six alternately allocated tracheal rings are tied together by means of cotton thread forming up to six chains from one animal. After securing the tracheal chain at both ends with cotton thread it is mounted in a 10 ml organ bath containing KH solution and fixed on a rod at the bottom of the bath and connected to a force-displacement transducer (for example HSE, type K 30; Grass, type FT03) coupled to multi-channel recorders. Tension of the tracheal chains is adjusted until a constant baseline of approximately 2 g is reached after 45 min. The degree of spontaneous tone, generally amounting to 60–70% of the whole contraction-relaxation amplitude, can be ascertained by adding histamine ($10^{-4}$ M) followed by isoprenaline ($10^{-5}$ M) for defining this range, which also assesses the viability of each preparation. Cumulative concentration-response curves [33] of isometric tension changes either to contractile agents (such as histamine, acetylcholine, carbachol, methacholine, $LTC_4$, serotonin, thromboxane $A_2$ mimetic U-46.619, KCl) or to relaxant drugs (such as $\beta_2$ adrenoceptor agonists, methylxanthines, papaverine, sodium nitroprusside) are obtained by increasing drug concentrations in 0.5 log unit increments. Contractile or relaxant responses are expressed as percentage values in comparison with the maximum response caused by a reference standard, for example 50 mM KCl or by the agent alone, or in case of relaxation, with that induced by isoprenaline ($10^{-5}$ M) or papaverine ($10^{-3}$ M). Disadvantages of the tracheal chain are the tedious process of tying the rings together and the small maximum responses often observed as compared to other tracheal preparations.

The tracheal chain can also be used to study the relaxant effects of $\beta_2$ adrenoceptor agonists on preparations with tone raised by carbachol [34] and by KCl [35]. The potencies of $\beta_2$ adrenoceptor agonists are significantly reduced in tissues precontracted by either carbachol or KCl, however, due to its lower receptor reserve, one advantage of the KCl-depolarized trachea may be its ability for identifying $\beta_2$ adrenoceptor agonists with low intrinsic activities. In this case, the partial relaxation reached by the test compound is related to the maximal relaxation of the tissue by a high concentration of papaverine. The assessment of a possible partial agonist activity cannot be done on the spontaneously contracted trachea, where drugs with different intrinsic activities often achieve the same maximum relaxation because of the large receptor reserve present under intrinsic tone conditions [36]. Conversely, for the assessment of affinity values for antagonists at tracheal $\beta_2$ adrenoceptors (pA$_2$), it is recommended to use the spontaneously contracted tissue [37], thereby circumventing the interfering functional antagonism observed in carbachol- or methacholine-contracted tissue [36, 38]. Generally, for studying $\beta_2$ adrenoceptor interactions, the KH solution may also contain ascorbic acid to prevent oxidation of added catecholamines, phentolamine to block $\alpha$ adrenoceptors, and corticosterone to prevent extraneuronal uptake of catecholamines [35, 36].

Often the guinea pig trachea requires an exceptionally long equilibration time to permit optimal agonist-induced contractions. Inhibition of cyclooxygenase by indomethacin, which abolishes spontaneous active tension generation [39], putatively because of the decreased production of bronchodilator prostaglandin E$_2$, serves to reduce the time necessary to obtain reproducible and optimal contractile responses to spasmogens [40].

### Spirally cut trachea

A modified and improved method, which eliminates the time consuming process of tying the tracheal rings together and which has the additional advantage of greater force development, is the spirally cut trachea [41, 42]. The trachea is cut diagonally to produce several segments each containing up to five rings. By means of a stainless steel wire introduced into the tracheal lumen, spirally formed strips can be prepared within a short time by cutting the connective tissue to separate the rings in a manner that they are still held together by a small portion of the connective ligament between each single ring. After mounting the spiral strips in tissue baths containing KH solution under a resting tension of 2 g and development of spontaneous tone, isometric contractions to cumulatively added spasmogens (acetylcholine, histamine, 5-hydroxytryptamine, carbachol and bradykinin), can be reproducibly evoked for 6 h. Maximal tension responses to these spasmogens are between 0.6 and 2.3 g. Less potent acetylcholine responses approach those of carbachol when acetylcholine esterase is blocked by eserine [43]. By using the spirally cut trachea from chronically pretreated guinea pigs, Anderson and Lee [44] demonstrated tolerance to bronchodilator drugs *in vitro*. For testing contractile responses to $LTC_4$ the l-glutamyl transpeptitase inhibitor, l-serine borate, is added to the nutrient solution to prevent the conversion of $LTC_4$ to $LTD_4$ [9].

*Antigen-evoked mediator release:* Various pathophysiologic manifestations of allergic asthma are produced by the effects of mediators released from mast cells upon contact with antigen [45]. For studying smooth muscle contraction resulting from generation and release of a mixture of inflammatory mediators, prostaglandins and NO, spirally cut tracheae prepared from actively sensitized guinea pigs are exposed to specific antigen [9, 46]. For this purpose, guinea pigs are sensitized by i.p. injections of ovalbumin-saline solution on days 1 and 4 and are used after day 25. Contractions of the dissected trachea in response to added ovalbumin consist of two components, a fast developing phasic component (within 2 min) and a later tonic component (10–15 min), which have been correlated with histamine (preformed mediator) release and eicosanoid synthesis and release, respectively [30]. To study exclusively the effects of lipoxygenase-derived mediators of contraction, tissues are pretreated with indomethacin to inhibit the formation of cyclooxygenase-derived bronchoactive prostaglandins, thus increasing the amounts of leukotrienes produced [9, 39, 45, 47]. The initial phase of antigen-evoked contraction, but not the secondary response, can be significantly reduced by the histamine $H_1$ receptor antagonist, mepyramine, or by mast cell stabilization by disodium cromoglycate, confirming its dependence on the release of histamine [45]. The second phase of contraction is susceptible to inhibition by FPL 55712 (a leukotriene receptor antagonist), nordihydroguaiaretic acid (a lipoxygenase inhibitor), p-bromophenacyl bromide (a phospholipase $A_2$ inhibitor) and BW 755c (a dual inhibitor of lipoxygenase and cyclooxygenase)[47]. Also the selective PDE 4 inhibitor, rolipram, markedly suppresses the second phase of trachea contraction, suggesting that PDE 4 inhibitors are more effective in inhibiting the formation and release of newly formed and released lipid mediators ($LTC_4$ and $PGD_2$) than histamine release in the airways [46].

## Zig-zag tracheal strip

A similar preparation to the spirally cut trachea is the quickly prepared zig-zag strip described by Emmerson and Mackay [48]. The trachea is opened by cutting longitudinally through the cartilage rings diametrically opposite the trachealis muscle, then pinned open on a cork board to cut transverse slits into the connective tissue at equally spaced intervals, first on one side of the preparation and then on the other, thus resulting in two strip preparations from one animal. Threads are tied to the ends of each zig-zag strip which are set up in organ baths in the usual way under a resting tension of 0.5–1.0 g. Vitality of the preparation is determined by adding 50 mM KCl for 10 min, during which time approximately 1.8 g of force should be attained. Some representative applications of this often employed tracheal preparation are described in the following.

Cyclic nucleotides, predominantly cAMP and less cGMP, play an important role in the regulation of guinea pig tracheal smooth muscle tone [49, 50]. $\beta_2$ Adrenoceptor agonists evoke relaxation of the trachea by stimulating the formation of cAMP via activation of adenylate cyclase, and agents that inhibit cyclic nucleotide phosphodiesterase (PDE) have been proposed to exert a major part of their tracheal relaxant effect by increasing the intracellular levels of cAMP [49]. Mainly two isoenzymes, PDE 3 and PDE 4, have been found in guinea pig trachea which selectively hydrolyse cAMP with a high affinity [23]. Rolipram and CI-930, selective inhibitors for PDE 4 and 3, respectively, exhibit biphasic concentration-response curves of relaxation of the spontaneously or precontracted zig-zag strip, whereas the unselective PDE inhibitors, theophylline and papaverine, produce sigmoidal monophasic curves [23]. To explore the inhibition of tracheal smooth muscle PDE 3 or PDE 4, tracheal preparations were pretreated with either rolipram or CI-930, thus inhibiting PDE 4 and PDE 3 activity, respectively, and sensitizing the preparation to the relaxant effects of either PDE 3 or PDE 4 inhibitors. Selective PDE 4 inhibitors, for example Ro 20-1724, synergistically increase the relaxant effect of $\beta_2$ adrenoceptor agonists, for example salbutamol, of methacholine-precontracted guinea pig trachea [51], suggesting that the PDE 4 isoenzyme is functionally associated with $\beta_2$ adrenoceptor responses in this tissue [52].

As a further example, the zig-zag preparation has been used to demonstrate the participation of $Ca^{2+}$-activated $K^+$ channels ($BK_{Ca}$) in trachea relaxation by $\beta_2$ adrenoceptor agonists [53], the mode of action of which has until recently been thought to be solely due to cAMP-dependent increase in the sequestation of intracellular $Ca^{2+}$ and/or extrusion from the cell [54]. Tracheal smooth muscle contains a variety of distinct $K^+$ channels, which include voltage-dependent $K^+$ channels [55], a high density of $Ca^{2+}$-activated $K^+$ channels [55], and possibly ATP-dependent $K^+$ channels [56] which play an important role in regulating membrane potential and thus the contractile state of airway smooth muscle [57]. Drugs such as cromakalim, acting as openers of ATP-dependent $K^+$ channels [58], or isoprenaline and salbutamol [59], acting on the other more prevalent high-conductance $Ca^{2+}$-activated $K^+$ channel, relax airway smooth muscle via membrane hyperpolarization. For studying these two latter $K^+$ channels, carbachol-precontracted zig-zag strips are set up for isometric tension recording in the presence of indomethacin and exposed to increasing concentrations of salbutamol or theophylline to obtain cumulative concentration-response curves which are then repeated in the presence of the $BK_{Ca}$ antagonists, charybdotoxin and iberiotoxin [53].

These antagonists also produce a further contraction of the precontracted tracheal tissue by causing smooth muscle membrane depolarization via opening voltage-dependent $Ca^{2+}$ channels and enhancement of $Ca^{2+}$ influx [53]. In contrast, activation of the $BK_{Ca}$ channel pathway does not contribute to the relaxant response produced by cromakalim and pinacidil, the effect of which are not blocked by charybdotoxin, but by the ATP-dependent $K^+$ channel blocker, glibenclamide [59]. Conversely, tracheal smooth muscle relaxation following hyperpolarization evoked by $\beta_2$ adrenoceptor agonists and methylxanthines are not sensitive to apamin or other ATP-dependent $K^+$ channel blockers [60, 61].

*Nonadrenergic, noncholinergic responses:* The electrically stimulated version of the zig-zag strip has frequently been used to investigate the nonadrenergic, noncholinergic (NANC) innnervation and neurotransmission of the guinea pig trachea. In addition to its predominant parasympathetic [62, 63] and the relatively minor sympathetic innervation [64], additional nonadrenergic, noncholinergic (NANC) components in

the innervation of tracheal smooth muscle result in either bronchodilation or bronchoconstriction, depending on whether inhibitory (i-NANC)
or excitatory (e-NANC) nerves are activated [7, 62, 65, 66]. Current evidence suggests that both vasoactive intestinal peptide (VIP) and nitric
oxide (NO) are involved in propranolol-resistant i-NANC responses and
may be co-released with acetylcholine from cholinergic nerve terminals
[3, 5, 67]. Vagus nerve stimulation also produces a component of bronchoconstriction that is resistant to blockade by atropine which has been
termed excitatory NANC (e-NANC) response mediated by neuropeptides released retrogradely from a certain population of unmyelinated
sensory nerves [68].

Both responses, i-NANC and e-NANC, can be demonstrated in zig-
zag strips suspended in organ baths between parallel platinum wire electrodes on either side of the strip for electrical field stimulation (EFS).
EFS, applied in close proximity of tracheal preparations, is generally
used to stimulate postganglionic cholinergic nerve endings, but inevitably also stimulates adrenergic and i-NANC nerves. For this purpose,
the KH solution additionally contains atropine and guanethidine to
block a possible cholinergic and adrenergic involvement in the response,
respectively, and histamine to raise the tone of the smooth muscle [3, 69].
i-NANC-mediated relaxations are then elicited by stimulation of the in-
tramural nerves (40 V, 1 ms, 5 Hz, for 1 min every 5–10 min) delivered
from a stimulator (for example Grass, type S9 or S88; HSE, type 215],
which should be completely blockable by the $Na^+$ channel blocker tetro-
dotoxin (TTX) confirming their neuronal origin. The relaxations are reduced after inhibition of NO synthesis by L-nitroarginine methylester
(L-NAME), VIP antibody and α-chymotrypsin, a proteolytic enzyme
which degrades VIP, indicating that NO as well as VIP mediate i-NANC
responses of guinea pig tracheal smooth muscle [3, 5]. To further reduce
the potential influence of a tachykinergic e-NANC contractile response,
the tissue can additionally be treated with CP 96.345 and SR 48.968 to
block neurokinin NK-1 and NK-2 receptors, respectively [70].

The e-NANC constrictor response is more difficult to demonstrate in
guinea pig trachea. However, in the presence of atropine, propranolol
and indomethacin, to eliminate a contribution of cholinergic and adrenergic neurotransmission and to reduce spontaneous tone of the prepara-

tion, respectively, e-NANC responses can be evoked by EFS (40 V, 0.5 ms, 4–8 Hz, for 15–20 s every 4 min) [67]. Since the concomitant i-NANC relaxant component, which functionally counteracts e-NANC constrictor responses to EFS, is less prevalent in the distal portion of the guinea pig trachea, experiments to detect the capsaicin-sensitive e-NANC responses can especially be performed in distal portions of the trachea [14] but also in main bronchi [71].

*Modulation of transmitter release:* The field-stimulated guinea pig trachea has frequently been used to study indirectly the modulation of neurotransmitter release from airway nerves by measuring the post-junctional response which often overcomes some of the problems associated with the direct measurement of transmitter overflow. For this purpose, the effect of an agent to potentially modulate the response of the trachea to endogenous transmitter released by EFS is compared to equivalent responses to the neurotransmitter administered exogenously. Any difference in these responses can be interpreted as a modulatory effect on the nerve, in a way that neurotransmitter release may either be facilitated or inhibited by the agent interacting with prejunctional (or presynaptic) receptors which are subdivided into autoreceptors and heteroceptors, depending upon which neurotransmitter, their own, a co-transmitter, or even that from neighboring and normally opposing airway nerves, respectively, mediates the effect. Muscarinic receptors located on post-ganglionic cholinergic nerve endings [72] and sympathetic nerve endings [73], providing a functional negative feedback modulation of acetylcholine and noradrenaline release, are examples of autoreceptors and heteroreceptors, respectively.

Contractile responses of the isolated guinea pig trachea to EFS should be sensitive to TTX, confirming their neuronal origin. In case of a residual and TTX-resistant component of response, this may occur either due to direct stimulation of airway smooth muscle or due to the possible release of arachidonic acid products formed by the epithelium [74]. Often, a change in the stimulation parameters to lower voltage strength and to low frequencies, when modulation is more pronounced than at high frequencies of nerve stimulation [75, 76], may overcome these problems.

EFS-evoked release of acetylcholine from cholinergic nerve endings, which leads to contraction of the isolated guinea pig trachea, can be influenced by a variety of prejunctional mechanisms such as inhibitory $\alpha_2$ adrenoceptors [77]. Stimulation by platinum electrodes (supramaximal voltage, 20 monophasic pulses of 1 ms, 20 Hz, for every 1 min) of organ bath-suspended zig-zag strips prepared from reserpinized guinea pigs, evokes rapid contractions blockable by atropine and TTX indicating that they were induced by activation of cholinergic neurons. In these experiments, the KH solution should also contain propranolol to block $\beta_2$ adrenoceptors and choline chloride in order to "feed" the cholinergic neurons and preserve their acetylcholine stores. For the elimination of possible occurring sympathetic components and endogenous prostaglandin biosynthesis in response to EFS, the nutrient solution can also contain guanethidine and indomethacin. Selective $\alpha_2$ adrenoceptor agonists, such as clonidine and B-HT 920, inhibit EFS-induced contractions, but not those to added acetylcholine in unstimulated preparations [78]. An example of facilitatory $5\text{-}HT_3$ receptors present on cholinergic nerve terminals in guinea pig trachea, which upon stimulation by the selective agonist, 2-methyl-serotonin, augment neuronal contractions to EFS (4–15 V, 8 Hz. 0.5 ms for 5 s each min), has been reported by Rizzo et al. [79].

Prejunctional muscarinic $M_2$ receptors, which inhibit the release of acetylcholine, and postjunctional muscarinic $M_3$ receptors mediating smooth muscle contraction can be studied on contractions elicited either by EFS or by methacholine of the guinea pig trachea [80]. Stimulation of single ring preparations by EFS (8 V, 0.5 ms, 30 Hz, for 5 s at 1 min intervals) produces rapid monophasic contractions which can be increased by low concentrations of selective muscarinic $M_2$ receptor antagonists, for example gallamine and AQ-RA 741, followed gradually by a complete blockade of contractions at higher concentrations thereby yielding information about the difference between the prejunctional $M_2$ and postjunctional $M_3$ receptor affinity of a particular muscarinic antagonist within the same experiment. The affinity constant ($pA_2$ value) of the antagonist at smooth muscle muscarinic $M_3$ receptors can be determined by using cumulatively administered methacholine as the agonist in the absence and 30-min presence of the antagonist in unstimulated preparations.

An example for the modulation of e-NANC neurotransmission in guinea pig airways via different prejunctional mechanisms is given in the following. Small pieces of the bronchial tree are prepared from the hilus region of the lower lung lobes, preferably containing bronchi with inner diameter of approximately 0.5 mm [81], are mounted in organ baths in the presence of atropine and guanethidine. Isometric contractions in response to EFS (supramaximal voltage, 1 ms, 5 Hz, for 10 s) reflecting e-NANC responses can be inhibited by neuropeptide Y, by the selective $\alpha_2$ adrenoceptor agonists UK 14.304, and by morphine. These agents do not attenuate contractions of the unstimulated tissue evoked by neurokinin A, suggesting a prejunctionally located inhibition by these agents via different receptors.

Generally, EFS-induced contractile responses of isolated guinea pig airways are considered to be an indirect but reliable measure of neurotransmitter release. However, by using mechanical changes of the smooth muscle alone, it is not always possible to unambiguously differentiate a prejunctionally inhibitory action of a compound to inhibit acetylcholine release from a direct relaxant effect on airway smooth muscle. As an example, in guinea pig zig-zag tracheal strips, isoprenaline inhibits the contractile response evoked by EFS at a similar extent to that evoked by exogenous acetylcholine, which may indicate that isoprenaline inhibits EFS-induced contractile responses by interacting with $\beta_2$ adrenoceptors located on smooth muscle [82]. To elucidate unequivocally the additional existence of $\beta_2$ adrenoceptors on cholinergic nerve terminals, the direct measurement of neurotransmitter release following EFS, in this case [$^3$H]-acetylcholine, from tracheal tissue previously labeled with the precursor [$^3$H]-choline, is needed when examining the effects of agents that are purported to act prejunctionally [82, 83].

## Tracheal tube preparations
*Unstimulated, perfused tracheal tube:* Dissected tracheal preparations usually suspended in organ baths constantly exposed to drugs added to the nutrient solution, lack a lumen-epithelium interface which represents a significant departure from the normal respiratory tract physiology. Since the epithelium can release relaxing factors like cyclooxygenase products or NO [3, 71, 84] and has an important passive barrier

function for drugs and antigens [28, 85], an appropriate model which more closely simulates conditions *in vivo*, is the lumen-perfused tracheal tube in which the orientation of the epithelium on the underlying lamia propia and submucosa is preserved. For this purpose, the trachea is perfused in an organ bath according to the method described by Pavlovic et al. [86]. Two steel hooks are inserted through opposite sides of the tracheal wall with the smooth muscle between them, one attached to a fixed point in the organ bath, the other being connected to a force-displacement transducer. The inside of the trachea is then perfused independently of the outside at a constant flow of 2 ml/min with a peristaltic pump. This method enables, for example, studies to detect airway hyperresponsiveness to luminally administered carbachol, histamine [87] and bradykinin [88] following nitric oxide synthesis inhibition and/or epithelium removal.

*Transmural stimulation:* Another version of the intact tracheal tube that is not perfused but can be subjected to EFS, has been introduced by Farmer and Coleman [89], which offers the possibility to measure both adrenergic and cholinergic responses due to simultaneous stimulation of postganglionic sympathetic and vagal nerve endings. By dividing the trachea halfway along its length, two preparations can be made from one animal. The tracheal tubes are tied over vertically located mounting blocks, the lower one containing a platinum electrode, the upper one being supplied with an outlet for the continuous measurement of intraluminal pressure recorded with a pressure transducer (for example, Statham, type P23AC; Gould, type P50; Grass, type 7D). The closed tracheal tube is then suspended in a jacketed organ bath containing KH solution which is allowed to have contact with the inner and outer surface of the trachea. After setting the intraluminal pressure of 10 cm $H_2O$ by means of a syringe, EFS (supramaximal voltage, 1 ms, 20 Hz, for 7 s every 1 min) applied by the intraluminally located platinum electrode and a second one placed outside, but in close proximity to the tube, evokes a biphasic response consisting of a rapid increase in intraluminal pressure followed by a decrease and a slow return to baseline. In the presence of propranolol, a vagally mediated monophasic response can be generated which is sensitive to atropine. Additionally, the lumen of the tracheal tube can separately be perfused under constant-pressure conditions provided that a flow reduction system (thin tubing) prevents the impairment of pressure recording during EFS.

*Sympathetic and vagus nerve stimulation:* A disadvantage of the transmurally stimulated tracheal tube by EFS is that all postganglionic intrinsic nerves, including the i-NANC nerves, within the tissue are stimulated simultaneously and the different components of the response may be distinguished only by the use of appropriate antagonists [90]. A closed tube preparation in which sympathetic and pre- and postganglionic parasympathetic tracheal responses can be evoked separately was introduced by Blackman and McCaig [91], who provided a method of assessing transmission through the parasympathetic airway ganglia and, additionally, enabled the study of the interaction between the sympathetic and parasympathetic nerves for mutual modulation of transmitter release [92, 93]. For this purpose, the cervical trachea with the right recurrent laryngeal nerve carefully maintained intact, is exposed and freed along with the right vagal and sympathetic trunks intact and cannulated below the cricoid cartilage. The vagus is freed and cut below the recurrent laryngeal branch and the sympathetic system dissected down to the stellate ganglion. The trachea is then removed with the sympathetic and vagus nerves attached and cannulated at both ends and mounted horizontally in an organ bath. The lumen of the trachea is filled with nutrient solution to form a fluid-filled tube which is closed at one end with a clamp and the other connected to a transducer for measurement of intraluminal pressure.

In order to observe a relaxation by sympathetic nerve stimulation, the intraluminal pressure must be raised, for example with the stable thromboxane $A_2$ mimetic, U-46.619. Stimulation of the stellate ganglion (supramaximal voltage, 0.2 ms, 40 Hz, for 5 s every 90 s) which is placed on bipolar platinum electrodes, induces relaxation of the trachea that causes a rapid and nearly complete fall in the intraluminal pressure [93]. The pressure fall is abolished by propranolol and TTX, but not by hexamethonium, confirming a postganglionic sympathetic nerve stimulation that releases noradrenaline onto $\beta_2$ adrenoceptors on airway smooth muscle. By using this method, for example inhibitory prejunctional muscarinic

$M_3$ receptors on sympathetic nerves in guinea pig trachea have been characterized [93].

In this preparation, preganglionic vagus nerve stimulation (30 V, 0.2 ms, 30 Hz, for 5 s every 40 s) by suction electrodes produces a rapid increase in intraluminal pressure of about 200 cm $H_2O$, which is sensitive to blockade by atropine, TTX and hexamethonium, indicating preganglionic vagal nerve stimulation [94]. This is also underlined by the markedly increased response observed after acetylcholine esterase inhibition by physostigmine [95]. Postganglionic vagal nerve stimulation can be achieved by bipolar platinum electrodes using the same stimulation parameters, but in the presence of indomethacin, propranolol, and hexamethonium to eliminate prostanoid-induced tone, and interference of the contraction due to possible stimulation of sympathetic and preganglionic vagal nerve fibers, respectively. The pre- and postganglionically stimulated guinea pig tracheal tube preparation for example enabled the location and characterization of muscarinic $M_2$ receptors mediating autoinhibition of acetylcholine release on cholinergic nerve terminals [94].

## Superfusion techniques

The most commonly employed technique for studying the effects of drugs on isolated tracheal smooth muscle is that of immersion of the preparation in an organ bath. However, there are some applications for which superfusion is more appropriate, for example bioassay of perfusates and evalution of potency of labile substances or those of extremely low quantity. An apparent beneficial effect of this technique may also result from the rapid removal of potentially toxic metabolites, which thus have no chance to accumulate within the tissue and the organ bath, thus obviating the necessity for repeated washings required in bath technique.

### Electrically stimulated trachea

An eight-chamber superfusion system of the tracheal zig-zag strip suitable for a variety of applications has been described by Coleman and Nials [96], which additionally allows electrical stimulation of the preparation and thus can be used to study drugs that interfere with neurotransmission. Particularly, by using this technique, the potencies and the times required for onset and offset of actions of spasmogens, such as acetylcholine, histamine, and $PGF_{2\alpha}$, or those of relaxants, such as $\beta_2$ adrenoceptor agonists, papaverine, theophylline, verapamil and the adenosine receptor agonist, 5'-N-ethylcarboxamidoadenosine (NECA), have been determined. The spasmolytics can either be tested against a raised smooth muscle tone induced by $PGF_{2\alpha}$ or against electrically evoked phasic contractions evoked by EFS (8–16 V, 0.1 ms, 5 Hz, for 10 s every 2 min).

For the continuous study of the time-course of reversal and reassertation of trachea relaxant drugs, especially those of long acting $\beta_2$ adrenoceptor agonists, the electrically stimulated, superfused zig-zag strip prepared from guinea pigs pretreated with 6-hydroxydopamine, in order to eliminate any adrenergic component in the electrically evoked response, has been applied [17]. Tissues are mounted into a superfusion chamber and superfused at a rate of 2 ml/min. Bipolar platinum electrodes are positioned parallel with, and in close proximity to the superfused tissue. To measure the relaxant activity of superfused $\beta_2$ adrenoceptor agonists and their reversal by $\beta$ adrenoceptor blocking drugs, for example the rapidly acting $\beta$ blockers atenolol and sotalol, phasic contractile responses are evoked by EFS (8–16 V, 0.1 ms, 5 Hz, for 10 s every 2 min). Cumulatively increased $\beta_2$ adrenoceptor agonist concentrations can be used to calculate their potency of trachea relaxation ($EC_{50}$). In case of long acting $\beta_2$ adrenoceptor agonists, the time for onset of action is defined as the time from starting the administration of test compound to attainment of 50% of the response maximum at an $EC_{50}$ concentration, whereas the offset time is defined as the time from stopping administration of the agent to attainment of 50% recovery at an $EC_{50}$ concentration. Thus, for the short acting salbutamol and the long acting salmeterol, onset times of 3 *versus* 28 min and offset times of 6 *versus* >470 min, respectively, could be calculated [17].

### Epithelium-denuded trachea
Since chronic airway inflammation leads to progressive epithelium damage [97], the role of airway epithelium has been subject to a great num-

ber of studies on the isolated guinea pig trachea demonstrating its important role in modulating the responsiveness of the airway smooth muscle to drugs [28, 71, 98]. Removal of the epithelium augments contraction and reduces relaxation to several bronchoactive agents, and bioassay experiments have demonstrated that the protective effect of the epithelium can be transferred to denuded preparations. Airway epithelial cells can generate significant quantities of arachidonic acid metabolites, such as $PGE_2$ and prostacyclin, which modulate airway smooth muscle contraction [29, 30, 84]. Furthermore, NO and VIP are postulated to act as epithelium-derived relaxing factors (EpDRF) that regulate the tracheal responsiveness to various agonists [3, 99]. Additionally, the tracheal epithelium can partially act as a permeability barrier, influencing the concentration of drug to act at the level of the underlying smooth muscle [28].

For studying the effects of drugs on the epithelium-denuded trachea in comparison with the intact tissue, the epithelium is removed by gently rubbing the lumen with a cotton-covered wire saturated with KH solution. Microscopic examination of control tissue fixed with formalin and stained with hematoxylin and eosin can be used to verify that the rubbing procedure removed the epithelium without damaging the submucosa or trachealis. Control and epithelium-denuded tracheal halves are cut into spirals or zig-zag strips and superfused with KH solution at a rate of 1.5 ml for at least 60 min, before antigen challenge with ovalbumin and mediator release studies are started [30]. The superfusate can either be collected for measurement of histamine, immunoreactive prostaglandin and sulfidopeptide leukotriene release, or directed to an acceptor trachea which serves as a detector organ in a cascade superfusion technique to determine if antigen challenge or other spasmogens evoke the release of an epithelium-derived relaxing substance [30]. For this purpose, donor and acceptor trachea are suspended in a single superfusion chamber. The donor trachea (with or without epithelium) is loosely fixed longitudinally on the thread suspending the acceptor trachea (without epithelium), so that the distal end of the donor trachea is 5 mm from the proximal end of the acceptor trachea. In this way, the dead space between the donor and acceptor tissue is minimized and tension changes of the smooth muscle of the donor trachea does not influence the tension recording of the acceptor trachea.

# Conclusion

Several modifications of the isolated guinea pig trachea have been described in the literature from which an appropriate method can be chosen for investigating drugs that may act directly on respiratory smooth muscle and/or modulate neurotransmission in airways. Moreover, the role of various mediators released by nerve stimulation or from mast cells and their influence on airways smooth muscle tone can be selectively assessed by using isolated tracheal tissue. However, due to the complex regulation of airways smooth muscle tone, the characterization of a drug's action often requires the use of more than mechanical experiments on isolated tracheal tissue alone. Thus, such refined techniques as transmitter release and electrophysiological studies may help to elucidate its mode of action and potential therapeutic value in airways obstruction.

# References

1  Lundberg JM, Hökfelt T, Martling CR, Saria A and Cuello C (1984) *Cell Tissue Res.* **235**: 251

2  Hua X-T, Theodorsson-Norheim E, Brodin E, Lundberg JM and Hökfelt T (1985) *Regul. Pep.* **13**: 1

3  Li CG and Rand MJ (1991) *Br. J. Pharmacol.* **102**: 91

4  Matsuzaki Y, Hamasaki Y and Said SI (1980) *Science* **210**: 1252

5  Tucker JF, Brave SR, Charalambous L, Hobbs AJ and Gibson A (1990) *Br. J. Pharmacol.* **100**: 663

6  Belvisi MG, Stretton D, Yacoub M and Barnes PJ (1992) *Eur. J. Pharmacol.* **210**: 221

7  Barnes PJ (1986) *Arch. Int. Pharmacodyn. Ther.* **280**: 208

8  Barnes PJ (1994) Modulation of Neurotransmitter Release from Airways Nerves. In: *Airways Smooth Muscle: Structure,* *Innervation and Neurotransmission,* Raeburn D and Giembycz MA (eds), p. 209, Birkhäuser Verlag Basel

9  Muccitelli RM, Tucker SS, Hay DWP, Torphy TJ and Wasserman MA (1987) *J. Pharmacol. Exp. Ther.* **243**: 467

10  Ward JK, Barnes PJ, Tadjkarini S, Yacoub MH and Belvisi MG (1995) *J. Physiol. (London)* **483** (Part 2): 525

11  Belvisi MG, Ward JK, Mitchell JA and Barnes PJ (1995) *Arch. Int. Pharmacodyn. Ther.* **329**: 97

12  Ellis JL and Conanan N (1994) *J. Pharmacol. Exp. Ther.* **266**: 1073

13  Belvisi MG, Stretton CD, Verleden GM, Yacoub MH and Barnes PJ (1991) *Am. Rev. Respir. Dis.* **143**: A355

14  Ellis JL and Undem BJ (1990) *Br. J. Pharmacol.* **101**: 875

15  Aizawa H, Inoue H, Shigyo M, Takata S, Kato H, Matsumoto K and Hara N (1994)

*Lung* **172**: 159

16 Lundberg JM, Martling CR and Saria A (1983) *Acta Physiol. Scand.* **119**: 49

17 Nials AT, Sumner MJ, Johnson M and Coleman RA (1993) *Br. J. Pharmacol.* **108**: 507

18 Nials AT, Coleman RA, Johnson M, Magnussen H, Rabe KF and Vardey CJ (1993) *Br. J. Pharmacol.* **110**: 1112

19 Kallstrom BJ, Sjoberg J and Waldeck B (1994) *Br. J. Pharmacol.* **113**: 687

20 Naline E, Zhang Y, Qian Y, Mairon N, Anderson GP, Grandordy B and Advenier C (1994) *Eur. Respir. J.* **7**: 914

21 del Monte M, Omini C and Subissi A (1990) *Br. J. Pharmacol.* **99**: 582

22 Minette PA and Barnes PJ (1990) *Am. Rev. Respir. Dis.* **141**: S162

23 Harris AL, Connell MJ, Ferguson EW, Wallace AM, Gordon RJ, Pagani ED and Silver PJ (1989) *J. Pharmacol. Exp. Ther.* **251**: 199

24 Cortijo J, Bou J, Beleta J, Cardelus I, Llenas J, Morcillo E and Gristwood RW (1993) *Br. J. Pharmacol.* **108**: 562

25 Rabe KH, Tenor H, Dent G, Schudt C, Liebig S and Magnussen H (1993) *Am. J. Physiol. (Lung Cell Mol. Physiol. 8)* **264**: L458

26 Rabe KH, Magnussen H and Dent G (1995) *Eur. Respir. J.* **8**: 637

27 Torphy TJ, Undem BJ, Cielinski LB, Luttmann MA, Reeves ML and Hay DW (1993) *J. Pharmacol. Exp. Ther.* **265**: 1213

28 Holroyde MC (1986) *Br. J. Pharmacol.* **87**: 501

29 Raeburn D (1990) *Agents Actions* (Suppl) **31**: 259

30 Undem BJ, Raible DG, Atkinson NF and Adams GK (1988) *J. Pharmacol. Exp. Ther.* **244**: 659

31 Castillo JC and De Beer EJ (1947) *J. Pharmacol. Exp. Ther.* **90**: 104

32 O'Donnell SR and Wanstall JC (1974) *Br. J. Pharmacol.* **52**: 407

33 Van Rossum JM (1963) *Arch. Int. Pharmacodyn. Ther.* **143**: 299

34 O'Donnell SR (1976) *Arch. Int. Pharmacodyn. Ther.* **244**: 190

35 O'Donnell SR and Wanstall JC (1980) *J. Pharmacol. Meth.* **4**: 43

36 Buckner CK and Saini RK (1975) *J. Pharmacol. Exp. Ther.* **194**: 565

37 O'Donnell SR and Wanstall JC (1980) *J. Pharm. Pharmacol.* **32**: 413

38 Patil PN (1967) *J. Pharmacol. Exp. Ther.* **160**: 308

39 Orehek J, Douglas JS and Bouhys A (1975) *J. Pharmacol. Exp. Ther.* **194**: 554

40 Watts SW and Cohen ML (1993) *J. Pharmacol. Exp. Ther.* **266**: 950

41 Constantine JW (1965) *J. Pharm. Pharmacol.* **17**: 384

42 Timmerman H and Scheffer NG (1968) *J. Pharm. Pharmacol.* **20**: 78

43 Hanna CJ and Roth SH (1978) *Can. J. Physiol. Pharmacol.* **56**: 823

44 Anderson AA and Lee GM (1976) *Br. J. Pharmacol.* **56**: 331

45 Adams GK and Lichtenstein L (1979) *J. Immunol.* **122**: 555

46 Underwood DC, Osborn RR, Novak LB, Metthews JK, Newsholme SJ, Undem BJ, Hand JM and Torphy T (1993) *J. Pharmacol. Exp. Ther.* **266**: 306

47 Chand N, Diamantis W and Sofia RD (1986) *Br. J. Pharmacol.* **87**: 443

48 Emmerson J and Mackay D (1979) *J. Pharm. Pharmacol.* **31**: 798

49 Chu SS (1984) *Drugs Today* **20**: 509

50 Sadeghi-Hashjin G, Folkerts G, Henricks PAJ, van de Loo PGF, Dik IEM and Nijkamp FP (1996) *Br. J. Pharmacol.* **118**: 466

51 Miyamoto KI, Kurita M, Sakai R, Sanae F, Wakusawa S and Takagi K (1994) *Biochem. Pharmacol.* **48**: 1219

52 Tomkinson A, Karlsson JA and Raeburn D (1993) *Br. J. Pharmacol.* **108**: 57

53 Huang JC, Garcia ML, Reuben PP and

Kacsorowski GJ (1993) *Eur. J. Pharmacol.* **235**: 37

54  Giembycz MA and Raeburn D (1991) *J. Auton. Pharmacol.* **11**: 345

55  McCann JD and Welsh MJ (1986) *J. Physiol.* **372**: 113

56  Weston AH (1989) *Pflügers Arch.* **414** (Suppl 1): S99

57  Kotlikoff MI (1989) Ion Channels in Airway Smooth Muscle. In: *Airway Smooth Muscle in Health and Disease*, Coburn RF (ed.), p. 169, Plenum Press New York

58  Allen SL, Boyle JP, Cortijo RW, Foster RW, Morgan GP and Small RC (1986) *Br. J. Pharmacol.* **89**: 395

59  Jones TR, Charette L, Garcia ML and Kaczorowski GJ (1990) *J. Pharmacol. Exp. Ther.* **255**: 697

60  Allen SL, Beech DJ, Foster RW, Morgan GP and Small RC (1985) *Br. J. Pharmacol.* **86**: 843

61  Allen SL, Cortijo RW, Foster RW, Morgan GP, Small RC and Weston AH (1986) *Br. J. Pharmacol.* **88**: 473

62  Richardson JB (1979) *Am. Rev. Respir. Dis.* **119**: 785

63  Canning BJ and Undem BJ (1994) Parasympathetic Innervation of Airways Smooth Muscle. In: *Airways Smooth Muscle: Structure, Innervation and Neurotransmission*, Raeburn D and Giembycz MA (eds), p. 43, Birkhäuser Verlag Basel

64  Ind PW (1994) Role of the Sympathetic Nervous System and Endogenous Catecholamines in the Regulation of Airways Smooth Muscle Tone. In: *Airways Smooth Muscle: Structure, Innervation and Neurotransmission*, Raeburn D and Giembycz MA (eds), p. 29, Birkhäuser Verlag Basel

65  Belvisi MG and Bai TR (1994) Inhibitory Nonadrenergic, Noncholinergic Innervation of Airways Smooth Muscle: Role of Nitric Oxide. In: *Airways Smooth Muscle: Structure, Innervation and Neurotransmission*,

Raeburn D and Giembycz MA (eds), p. 157, Birkhäuser Verlag Basel

66  Karlsson J-A (1994) Excitatory Nonadrenergic, Noncholinergic Innervation of Airways Smooth Muscle: Role of Peptides. In: *Airways Smooth Muscle: Structure, Innervation and Neurotransmission*, Raeburn D and Giembycz MA (eds), p. 103, Birkhäuser Verlag Basel

67  Belvisi MG, Stretton D and Barnes PJ (1991) *Eur. J. Pharmacol.* **198**: 221

68  Grundström N, Andersson RGG and Wikberg JES (1981) *Acta Pharmacol. Toxicol.* **49**: 150

69  Burka JF, Berry JL, Foster RW, Small RC and Watt AJ (1991) *Br. J. Pharmacol.* **104**: 263

70  Undem BJ, Meeker SN and Chen J (1994) *J. Pharmacol. Exp. Ther.* **271**: 811

71  Johansson-Rydberg IGM, Andersson RGG and Grundström N (1992) *Acta Physiol. Scand.* **144**: 439

72  Minette PA and Barnes PJ (1988) *J. Appl. Physiol.* **64**: 2532

73  Racké K, Hey C and Wessler I (1992) *Br. J. Pharmacol.* **107**: 3

74  de Jongste JC, Mons H, Bonta IL and Kerrebijn KF (1987) *J. Appl. Physiol.* **63**: 1558

75  Belvisi MG, Stretton CD and Barnes PJ (1990) *Br. J. Pharmacol.* **100**: 131

76  Eltze M and Galvan M (1994) *Pulm. Pharmacol.* **7**: 109

77  Grundström N, Andersson RGG and Wikberg JES (1981) *Life Sci.* **28**: 2981

78  Kamikawa Y and Shimo Y (1986) *J. Pharm. Pharmacol.* **38**: 742

79  Rizzo CA, Kreutner W and Chapman RW (1993) *Eur. J. Pharmacol.* **234**: 109

80  Ten Berge REJ, Roffel AF and Zaagsma J (1993) *Eur. J. Pharmacol.* **233**: 279

81  Matran R, Martling CR and Lundberg JM (1989) *Eur. J. Pharmacol.* **163**: 15

82  Belvisi MG, Patel HJ, Takahashi T, Barnes PJ and Giembycz MA (1996) *Br. J.*

*Pharmacol.* **117**: 1413

83 Wessler I, Reinheimer T, Brunn G, Anderson GP, Maclagan J and Racké K (1994) *Br. J. Pharmacol.* **113**: 1221

84 Butler BG, Adler KB, Evans JN, Morgan DW and Szarek JL (1987) *Am. Rev. Respir. Dis.* **135**: 1099

85 Grundström N, Lindstrom EG, Axelsson KL and Andersson RGG (1992) *J. Appl. Physiol.* **72**: 1953

86 Pavlovic D, Fournier M, Aubier M and Pariente R (1989) *J. Appl. Physiol.* **67**: 2522

87 Nijkamp FP, van der Linde HJ and Folkerts G (1993) *Am. Rev. Respir. Dis.* **148**: 727

88 Figini M, Ricciardolo FLM, Javda P, Nijkamp FP, Emanueli C, Pradelles P, Folkerts G and Geppetti P (1996) *Am. J. Respir. Crit. Care Med.* **153**: 918

89 Farmer JB and Coleman RA (1970) *J. Pharm. Pharmacol.* **22**: 46

90 Watson N, Maclagan J and Barnes PJ (1993) *J. Appl. Physiol.* **74**: 1964

91 Blackman G and McCaig DJ (1983) *Br. J. Pharmacol.* **80**: 703

92 McCaig DJ (1987) *Br. J. Pharmacol.* **91**: 385

93 Pendry YD and Maclagan J (1991) *Br. J. Pharmacol.* **103**: 1165

94 Watson N, Barnes PJ and Maclagan J (1992) *Br. J. Pharmacol.* **105**: 107

95 Widmark E and Waldeck B (1986) *J. Auton. Pharmacol.* **6**: 187

96 Coleman RA and Nials AT (1989) *J. Pharmacol. Meth.* **21**: 71

97 Laitinen LA, Heino M, Kava T and Haahtela T (1985) *Am. Rev. Respir. Dis.* **131**: 599

98 Hay D, Farmer SG, Raeburn D, Robinson VA, Fleming W and Fedan JS (1986) *Eur. J. Pharmacol.* **129**: 11

99 Lei Y-H, Barnes PJ. and Rogers DF (1993) *Br. J. Pharmacol.* **108**: 228

# Vessels

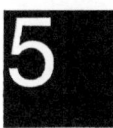

# Intravital microscopy: Airway circulation

M.R. Corboz and
S.T. Ballard

Tracheobronchial circulation provides many important physiological functions including delivery of blood-borne nutrients and hormones, removal of waste products, conditioning of inspired air, and maintenance of interstitial fluid volume. Blood flow to the airways must be closely regulated to maintain these critical functions in the face of continually changing metabolic and respiratory demands. Study of the mechanisms which regulate blood flow to the airways is unfortunately problematic due to the complex morphology of this vascular bed. The tracheobronchial circulation receives inputs from the intrathoracic bronchial artery, the inferior and superior thyroid arteries, and anastomoses with the esophageal circulation. Venous blood may leave the airway tissue via the superior and inferior thyroid veins, the intrathoracic bronchial vein, or through bronchopulmonary and esophageal anastomoses. Therefore, it is problematic to isolate and study the airway vasculature by traditional methods that have been applied with great success to other vascular systems, such as the pulmonary, mesenteric, and skeletal muscle circulations.

Despite these difficulties, a great deal of information about airway vascular responses can be obtained using intravital microscopy. In this chapter, we describe a microscopy technique that we recently developed to study constrictor and dilator responses of the airway microvessels *in vivo* [3–5]. Regional differences in airway microvessel responses can be determined with this method providing important clues toward understanding the physiologic roles of these mechanisms. In our model, we study the microvessels of the adventitial surface of the trachea in anesthetized rats.

---

## Materials and equipment

### Microscope

For intravital microscopic study of tracheal microvessels, the rat is placed in a supine position on the microscope stage directly underneath the microscope objective; consequently, the distance between the objective and the microscope stage is typically greater than required for most conventional microscopic work. Many mineralogical and industrial microscopes can be easily adapted for this application because the distance between the objectives and the stage of these microscopes can be adjusted through a wide range. The microscope stage should be rigid and as large as possible to support the weight of the animal. Microscopes with a nosepiece focusing mechanism located above the stage are preferred for this application. For our studies, we use a Zeiss ACM microscope equipped with a 10.5 in × 14.0 in stage (Fig. 5.1). Because the objectives must be placed in physiological saline suffusion solution to visualize the tracheal vessels, water immersion objectives must be used. While cheaper conventional objectives are sometimes substituted for this work, the investigator should be aware that such objectives are not watertight and, because they are not designed for water immersion, magnification may be significantly altered.

Because tracheal vessels *in situ* obviously cannot be transilluminated by conventional means, epi-illumination must be used. Illumination is provided by a flexible fiber optic light guide attached to a low noise illuminator (Cole-Parmer). The light guide is held 0.5 cm from the visual field at about 20 degrees above horizontal. This lighting angle provides a good combination of illumination and shadowing of tissue structures. Vessel walls of both arterioles and venules are thus well-defined in this preparation (Fig. 5.2).

### Video equipment

The microscope is equipped with a black and white Hamamatsu XC-77 CCD video camera and a detachable Hamamatsu image intensifier for

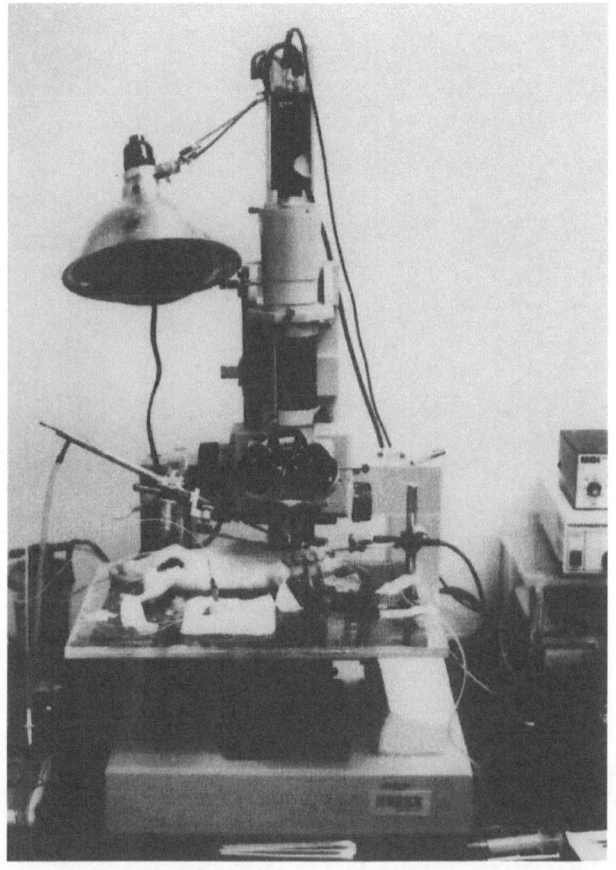

**Figure 5.1. Videomicroscope for study of tracheal microvessels**
*Zeiss ACM microscope equipped for video recording is shown. Note the large (10.5 in × 14.0 in) stage, the nosepiece focusing mechanism, and the capability to adjust the working distance between objective and stage through a wide range.*

low-light and fluorescence work. The video signal is passed in series through a Panasonic time-date generator (model WJ-810), a video caliper (Microcirculation Research Institute, Texas A&M University) for

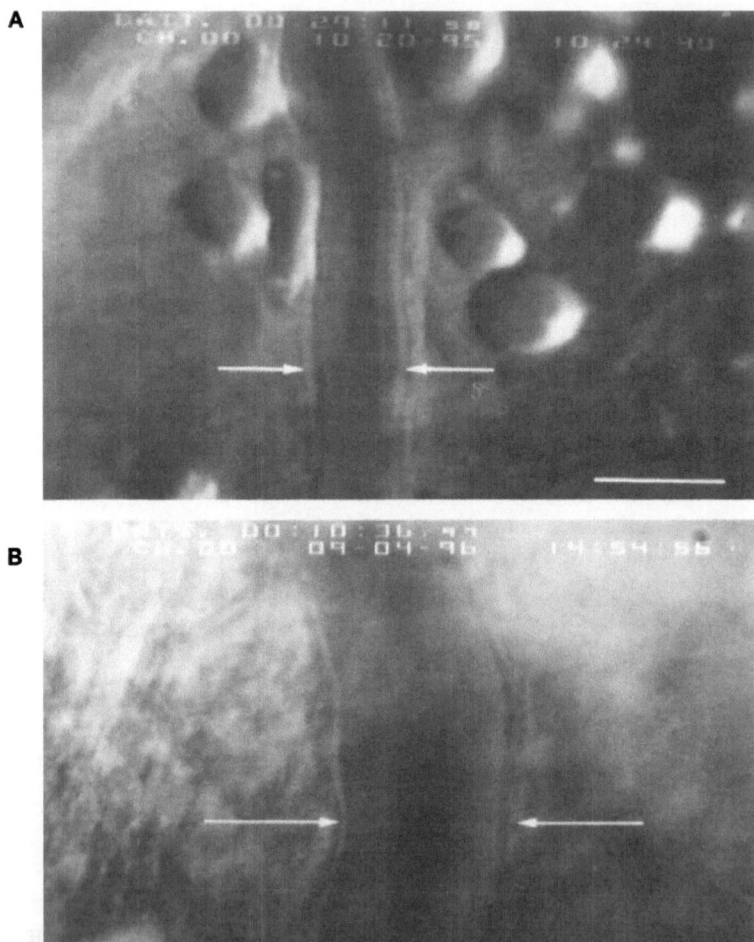

**Figure 5.2. Video images of tracheal vessels**

*Arteriole is shown in (A), venule is shown in (B). Vessel walls are indicated by the arrows. Bars are 50 μm.*

measuring vessel diameter, a JVC video cassette recorder (model HR-D670U), and a Panasonic video monitor (model WV-5490). Video images may also be directly acquired from the video camera and digitized using a Dell 486 microcomputer equipped with a Data Translation 2867LC frame grabber board and Global Lab Image analysis software (Data Translation).

## Peripheral equipment

Suffusion solutions are warmed to 37 °C in a heated water bath and gassed with a mixture of $N_2$ and $CO_2$ to yield a $pO_2$ of 25–45 mmHg, a $pCO_2$ of 30–40 mmHg, and a pH of 7.35–7.45, the approximate values of these parameters in interstitial fluid. A Masterflex peristaltic pump (Cole-Parmer) is used to deliver the suffusate to the exposed trachea at a rate of approximately 10 ml/min. Suffusate overflow is continuously siphoned away from the tracheal surface. An in-line heat exchanger maintains the suffusate temperature at 37 °C as it flows through the tubing and onto the tracheal surface. An infrared heat lamp is used to maintain animal body temperature which is monitored with an anal temperature probe (Cole-Parmer Digi-Sense thermometer).

## Ventilation

The rats are ventilated through an uncuffed polyethylene endotracheal tube with a gas mixture of 40% $O_2$ (balance $N_2$) to maintain blood gases in the physiologic range. Ventilation gas is humidified with a gas washer and conducted through the endotracheal tube via a rodent ventilator (MD Industries, Mobile, AL) which is set to a 1-s cycle, 50% duration positive pressure ventilation. Ventilation gas flow rate is adjusted as necessary to maintain blood pH at 7.35–7.45, $pCO_2$ at 40–50 mmHg, and $pO_2$ at 140–160 mmHg.

## Solutions

Krebs Ringer bicarbonate is used as the suffusion solution and is composed of 112.0 mM NaCl, 4.7 mM KCl, 2.5 mM $CaCl_2$, 2.5 mM $MgSO_4$, 1.2 mM $KH_2PO_4$, 25.0 mM $NaHCO_3$, and 11.6 mM glucose.

*Table 5.1. Summary: Materials and equipment*

| Conditions, media, species, cell types, etc. | Facts |
| --- | --- |
| Species | Rats, 200–550 g |
| Suffusate | Krebs Ringer |
|    Temperature | 37 °C |
|    $pO_2$ | 25–45 mmHg |
|    $pCO_2$ | 30–40 mmHg |
|    Flow rate | 10 ml/min |
|    pH | 7.35–7.45 |
| Ventilation | |
|    Inspiration | Constant pressure |
|    Expiration | Passive deflation |
| Arterial blood gases | |
|    $pO_2$ | 140–160 mmHg |
|    $pCO_2$ | 40–50 mmHg |
|    pH | 7.35–7.45 |
| Criteria for quality of preparation | Mean arterial pressure ≥80 mmHg |
| | Blood pH of 7.35–7.45 |
| | No visible tracheal hemorrhage |
| Time to set up experiment | Surgery: 30–40 min |
| | Stabilization: 60 min |
| Typical duration of experimental protocol | 50–60 min |
| Papers that exemplify usage of this technique | [1, 3, 4, 5, 7, 12] |
| Approximate cost per unit | $55 000 |
| Experiments/day/unit | 1–2 |

# Methods

## Surgery

Experiments are performed on rats (250–550 g) as this species is of convenient size to place on the microscope stage. Rats are anesthetized initially by intraperitoneal injection of pentobarbital sodium (50 mg/kg). The left femoral artery is then cannulated with polyethylene tubing for the measurement of systemic arterial blood pressure and blood gases. A polyethylene cannula is also inserted in the left femoral vein for the administration of supplemental anesthetic and paralytic drugs.

Rats are then placed in the supine position and the head is secured in a stereotaxic device. A midline incision from the mandible to the most cephalad portion of the sternum was made, and the skin and musculature are retracted with suture to expose the trachea (Fig. 5.3). The rat is then placed onto the microscope stage, and the polyethylene endotracheal tube is inserted into the trachea. When ventilation is initiated, pancuronium sodium (2 mg/kg) is administered intravenously to paralyze the musculature and reduce the movement associated with voluntary breathing. Arterial blood samples are withdrawn periodically for measurement of blood gasses and pH, and ventilation flow rate is adjusted to maintain these parameters at physiological levels.

To visualize the tracheal microvessels, the anesthetized and ventilated rat is placed on the stage of the microscope. The exposed trachea is continuously suffused with Krebs buffer, and tracheal microvessels are epi-illuminated as described above. The animal is allowed to stabilize for approximately 1 h before the experimental protocol is initiated. The preparation is considered acceptable if (i) mean arterial pressure is ≥80 mmHg and stable, (ii) blood pH is 7.35–7.45, and (iii) no visible hemorrhages are present in the tracheae. If any of these criteria are not achieved, the experiment is terminated. The preparation should be stable for approximately 2–3 h. The stability of the preparation is usually dictated by the ability to maintain arterial pressure and blood gases and pH within acceptable limits. A summary of experimental conditions of materials is shown in Table 5.1.

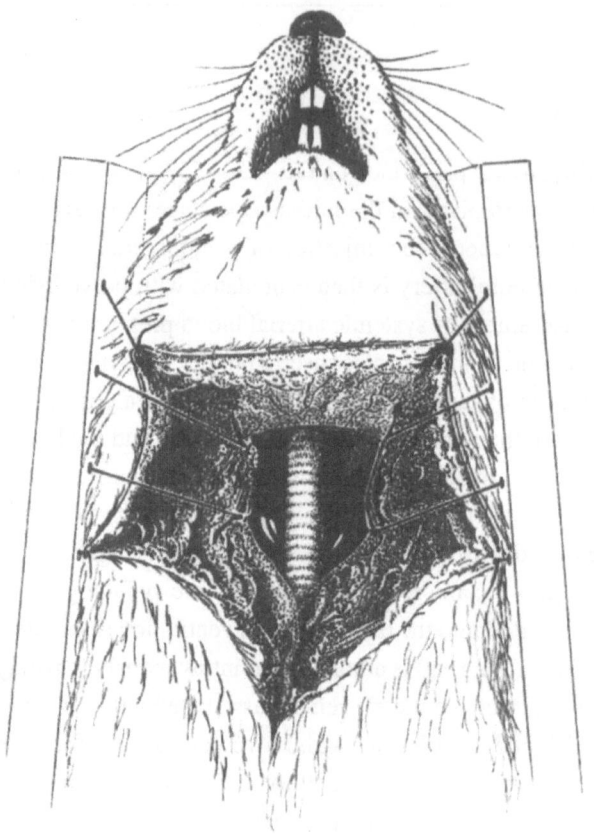

**Figure 5.3. Schematic representation of rat trachea preparation**
*The head of the animal is secured in a stereotaxic device, and the skin and musculature is retracted with sutures to expose the ventral adventitial surface of the trachea. The retracted tissue forms a cavity which permits suffusion of Krebs solution over the trachea.*

## Experimental procedure

The tracheal circulation of many species is organized as distinct mucosal and adventitial plexuses [13]. The rat trachea is sufficiently thin so that no such distinction exists [3]. In our studies, we have chosen to study the tracheal adventitial vessels because these vessels can be accessed without tracheal resection which induces inflammation and edema formation in this tissue [9]. The adventitial vasculature of the rat trachea is not organized in the ordered fashion of other tissues such as mesentery, skeletal muscle, and heart [3]. The area overlying the cartilage is relatively avascular in contrast to the intercartilaginous regions which are highly vascularized. Both arterioles and venules are found in this space although venules are much more numerous. Arterioles (Fig. 5.2) are approximately 10–50 µm diameter and can be identified by the presence of rapid blood flow which moves from large vessels into progressively smaller vessels. The venules (Fig. 5.2) form extensive networks and arcades and vary in size from the 10 µm diameter post-capillary venules to the 60–100 µm diameter collecting venules. Venules can be identified by relatively sluggish blood flow which moves from small branched vessels into progressively larger vessels. Adherent leukocytes are sometimes observed in venules but never in arterioles. These distinguishing criteria between arterioles and venules have been confirmed in a previous study where intravascular pressures in individual arterioles and venules were measured [1].

Once a vessel has been selected for study, it is viewed for an appropriate control period (approximately 20 min). Then, vasoconstrictor substances may be added to the suffusate, and their effect on vessel diameter can be measured after allowing a suitable period for the maximum response to develop. Figure 5.4 shows the effect of serial increases in concentration of the α-adrenergic receptor agonist norepinephrine in the presence of propranolol on the diameter of tracheal arterioles (13–27 µm dia.), medium-size venules (35–59 µm dia.), and large collecting venules (61–96 µm dia.). From these data, concentration-response curves to the constrictor effects of norepinephrine in the presence of propranolol can be constructed (Fig. 5.5). Prazosin, a selective $\alpha_1$-adrenergic receptor antagonist, caused a rightward shift in the concentration-response curve confirming that the constriction response was mediated, at least in part, by activation of $\alpha_1$-adrenergic receptors.

This system can also be used to evaluate the actions of vasodilators [4]. However, to ensure that a measurable dilatory response can be achieved, it is usually necessary to preconstrict the vessels prior to the addition of the dilator. Because $\alpha_1$-adrenergic receptors mediate constriction in all

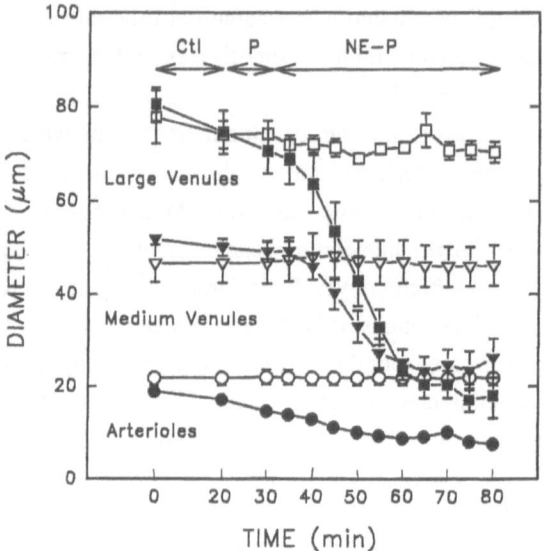

**Figure 5.4 Time-course of microvessel diameter changes in the absence or presence of nor-epinephrine (NE) and propranolol (P) in rat trachea**

*Ctl indicates control period. Constriction responses to increasing NE concentrations ($10^{-8}$ M to $10^{-3}$ M) were measured in the presence of propranolol ($10^{-6}$ M). Sham control diameters are indicated by open symbols while experimental conditions are indicated by filled symbols. Circles are 13–27 µm diameter arterioles, triangles are 35–59 µm diameter (medium) venules, and squares are 61–96 µm diameter (large) venules. Values are means ± SEM. Note that the greatest response to NE was in the large venules and the lack of an effect of protocol duration on measured diameters in the absence of drug treatment. (Reproduced from [3] with permission from* Am. J. Respir. Crit. Care Med.*)*

classes of tracheal microvessels except the smallest (<25 µm dia.) venules [3], phenylephrine is an effective preconstrictor substance. Other effective means of preconstricting tracheal microvessels include suffusion with high $K^+$ Krebs (unpublished observations) or a nitric oxide synthase (NOS) inhibitor [5]. The choice of preconstricting agent can, in fact, provide an important means by which to dissect the mechanism of dilation of a particular substance. For instance, if a dilation response to an agent was mediated through nitric oxide release or by a membrane potential-dependent mechanism, the response would be attenuated by the respective use of an NOS inhibitor or high $K^+$ suffusate to preconstrict the vessels.

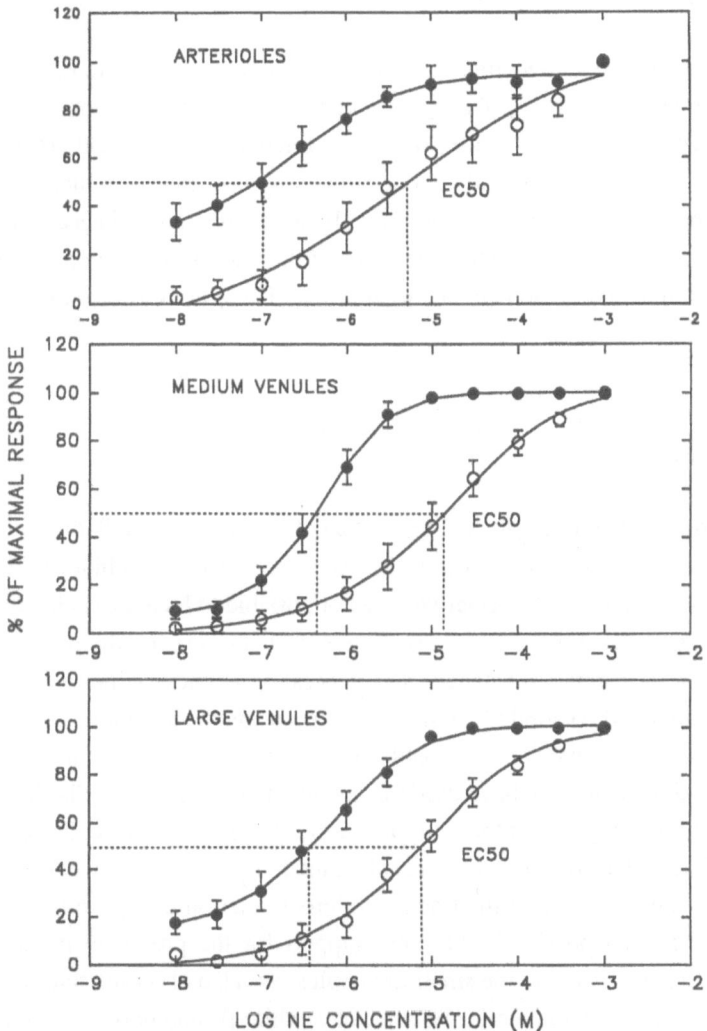

**Figure 5.5. Effect of prazosin on norepinephrine-propranolol induced constriction response in tracheal vessels**

Concentration-response curves for 16–30 µm diameter arterioles (upper panel), 28–60 µm diameter venules (middle panel), and 65–99 µm diameter venules (lower panel) are shown for norepinephrine (NE) with propranolol (filled circles) and NE with prazosin and propranolol (open circles). Data are normalized to the maximum constriction response. The concentration-response curves to NE in the presence of $10^{-6}$ M propranolol were shifted significantly to the right in all three vessel groups by $10^{-6}$ M prazosin. Values are means ± SEM. (Reproduced from [3] with permission from Am. J. Respir. Crit. Care Med.)

## Species differences

To our knowledge, this technique has only been used with rats [3–5, 12] and guinea pigs [7]. These species are of a convenient size for study since they can be easily placed on a large microscope stage. Other rodents of comparable size could also be studied by this approach including mice and rabbits. Adaptation for use with much larger animal species is possible but the stage and the nosepiece of the microscope may have to be altered to accommodate the larger size and weight of the animal.

# Discussion

Most studies of the reactivity and regulation of the airway vasculature rely upon measurements of pressure and flow in large tracheal or bronchial arteries. Although such studies are informative, it is not possible to localize such activity to specific segments of the airway vasculature. To better predict the physiological effects of a vasoactive substance, it is necessary to know which vessels of a microvascular bed respond to the substance. By using the technique described in this chapter, the researcher is capable of directly measuring local changes in microvessel diameter. We have used this method to determine the distribution of functional adrenergic receptor subtypes in the tracheal microcirculation of rats [3, 4]. We find that $\alpha_1$-adrenergic receptors mediate constriction when activated and are located throughout the tracheal microcirculation except in the smallest venules. Our data provided additional support for the presence of functional $\alpha_2$-adrenergic receptors in the smallest venules. We also observed that $\beta_2$-adrenergic receptors predominate in the arterioles while $\beta_1$-adrenergic receptors are preferentially localized to the large collecting venules [4]. Both $\beta$ receptor subtypes mediate dilation of these vessels. Studies from our laboratory [5] and others using a similar technique [12] suggest that basally released nitric oxide has a substantial vasodilatory influence on tracheal microvessels.

This technique can be easily adapted to make other physiologically important measures and observations. Using the servo-null technique of Wiederhielm [14], microvascular pressures in rat tracheal arterioles and venules have been measured [1]. Future study of the effects of vasoactive substance on microvascular pressures would provide further important information as to how local fluid balance is affected by such agents. Other potential uses for this technique could be the study of leukocyte kinetics and their role in airway inflammation. In our preparation, leukocytes can be clearly seen adhering to and rolling along the venular endothelium of the rat tracheal vessels. Quantitation of this behavior could be easily accomplished.

One limitation of our technique is that surgery in and around the trachea stimulates local sensory afferents which release neuropeptides such as substance P and calcitonin gene-related peptide [11]. These substances are proinflammatory and cause vasodilation and increases in vascular permeability in airways [8]. Although our technique can provide investigators with a great deal of useful information about the vasculature of the trachea, they should be aware that vessel reactivity may not reflect solely the activity of the applied substance, but rather a summation response to both exogenous and locally released substances.

Because intraluminal pressures in venules could be altered by arterial constriction or dilation, one could argue that venular diameter responses to a putative vasoactive substance reflects passive pressure changes and not changes in venular smooth muscle tone. However, this is unlikely to be the case based on numerous observations of differential reactivity by our laboratory and others. We have shown that large collecting venules are almost 10-fold less sensitive to norepinephrine than either smaller venules or arterioles [3]. We have also shown differential reactivity between arterioles and venules to $\beta_1$ and $\beta_2$ adrenoceptor stimulation [4]. Other investigators using intravital microscopic techniques to study cremaster muscle [6, 10] and coronary [2] microcirculations also report differential arteriolar and venular reactivity. Consequently, it is likely that venular diameter changes truly reflect active changes in vascular smooth muscle tone.

In summary, we describe an intravital microscopy technique that has many potential applications for study of the airway microcirculation. This technique has proven useful to evaluate the *in vivo* activity of vasodilator and vasoconstrictor substances as well as for measurement of microvascular pressure. This method could be easily adapted to document leukocyte-endothelial cell interactions and macromolecule leakage in these vessels as a means for study of airway inflammatory processes. We believe that appropriate application of this methodology could provide important insight into the regulatory mechanism of airway blood flow both in health and disease.

# References

1   Ballard ST, Nations RH and Taylor AE (1992) *Am. J. Physiol.* **262**: H1303
2   Chilian WM, Layne SM, Eastham CL and Marcus ML (1989) *Circ. Res.* **64**: 376
3   Corboz MR, Ballard ST, Boyette ST and Taylor AE (1995) *Am. J. Resp. Crit. Care Med.* **151**: 1589
4   Corboz MR, Ballard ST, Inglis SK and Taylor AE (1996) *Am. J. Resp. Crit. Care Med.* **153**: 1093
5   Corboz MR, Ballard ST, Inglis SK and Taylor AE (1997) *Am. J. Resp. Crit. Care Med.* **156**: 478
6   Faber JE (1988) *Circ. Res.* **62**: 37
7   Kern DF (1994) *FASEB J.* **8**: A538
8   MacDonald DM (1988) *J. Neurocytol.* **17**: 583
9   Nordin U, Kallskog O, Lindholm CE and Wolgast M (1978) *Microvasc. Res.* **15**: 287
10  Ohyanagi M, Faber JE and Nishigaki K (1991) *Circ. Res.* **68**: 232
11. Salonen RO, Webber SE and Widdicomb JG (1988) *Br. J. Pharmacol.* **95**: 1262
12  Smith TL, Prazma J, Coleman CC, Drake AF and Boucher RC (1993) *Otolaryngol. Head Neck Surg.* **109**: 646
13  Widdicombe JG (1993) *Exp. Physiol.* **78**: 433
14  Wiederhielm CA, Woodbury JW, Kirk S and Rushmer RF (1964) *Am. J. Physiol.* **207**: 173

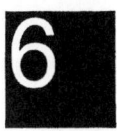

# 6 The bronchial circulation

*R.P. Michel*

---

The bronchial circulation provides the second vital vascular supply to the lung, complementary to that provided by the pulmonary circulation. Although its flow rate is only about 1% of cardiac output, it nourishes the larger airways, pulmonary arteries and veins, hilar structures and parts of the parenchyma and of the visceral pleura. From a historical perspective, although the claim that Leonardo da Vinci actually described the anatomy of the bronchial circulation approximately 500 years ago has been recently disputed [62] and remains controversial [16, 63], it is particularly its functional importance that he first recognized, as evident in his statement: "nature gave a vein and artery to the trachea ... for its life and nourishment, and ... to nourish the substance of the lung with greater convenience" [18, 20]. This prime directive of the bronchial circulation is manifest through its prominence in several diseases and conditions both in humans and animal models, which arises from its ability to proliferate and undergo angiogenesis, a process that occurs to a very limited degree if at all, in the pulmonary circulation.

## Importance and role of the bronchial circulation

The conditions in which the bronchial circulation plays a major role are listed in Table 6.1. The disorders in the first group, associated with edema and inflammation are devoid of significant bronchial vascular proliferation, and invoke the role of the bronchial circulation in fluid accumulation and altered permeability. In pulmonary edema, the bronchial circulation has been shown to be important in the clearance of lung fluid, and more recently to have either protective or detrimental effects in its accumulation depending on the experimental model. In support of its role in fluid clearance, Jayr and Matthay [42] showed that in the absence of pulmonary arterial flow, the bronchial circulation cleared about 50%

*Table 6.1. Role and importance of the bronchial circulation in disease*

| Conditions/diseases | References |
|---|---|
| A. Pulmonary edema and inflammation | |
|   1. Pulmonary edema | |
|     a. Clearance | [42] |
|     b. Protective | [6, 68] |
|     c. Deleterious | [1] |
|   2. Asthma: edema and congestion of the mucosa | [50, 85, 87] |
| B. Proliferation and angiogenesis | |
|   1. Across bronchial anastomosis in lung transplantation | [19, 23, 53, 73] |
|   2. Chronic inflammatory and infectious processes | [20] |
|     a. Bronchiectasis and chronic bronchitis | [15, 49, 85] |
|     b. Chronic tuberculosis | |
|     c. Lung abscesses and empyema | |
|     d. Intralobar pulmonary sequestration | [79] |
|     e. Exercise-induced hemorrhage in the horse | [65, 66] |
|   3. Pulmonary neoplasms | [37] |
|   4. Pulmonary vascular obstruction | |
|     a. Congenital cardiac anomalies with reduced pulmonary perfusion | [25, 70] |
|     b. Chronic pulmonary thromboembolism | [20, 41, 43, 52, 64] |
|     c. Postobstructive pulmonary vasculopathy | [24, 31, 45–48, 58, 60, 61, 86] |

of interstitial edema in sheep. Agostoni et al. [6] reported that in humans with heart failure for over 6 months, bronchial collateral blood flow increased, suggesting that the bronchial circulation thus contributed to reduce fluid overload. Invoking a protective role for this circulation, Pearse and Wagner [69] found, in isolated sheep lungs subjected to 30 min of pulmonary artery ischemia and 180 min of reperfusion, that bronchial artery perfusion reduced reperfusion edema by attenuating the increase in pulmonary vascular permeability caused by the injury, and surmised that the ameliorating effect was mediated principally by perfusion of the vasa vasorum of the pulmonary vessels. In contrast, a detrimental effect was shown by Abdi et al. [1] in a model of smoke-induced injury in sheep: maintaining bronchial artery perfusion for 24 h augmented lung lymph flow and extravascular water compared with its interruption, implicating the bronchial circulation as a significant source of edema fluid, or in the delivery of chemotactic substances to the parenchyma of the lung. A discussion of the role of the bronchial circulation in asthma is beyond the scope of this chapter, but comprehensive overviews are available [50, 85, 87].

The conditions in the second group of Table 6.1 involve proliferation and angiogenesis of the bronchial circulation. In lung transplantation, the reestablishment of vascular supply to the airways across the bronchial anastomosis via the bronchial circulation is pivotal to graft and patient survival. Very good results have been obtained with direct bronchial revascularization in single lung transplants (although not as critical as in double lung transplants), and procedures such as omental, pleural or pericardial wrap have also been advocated to supply the lung with bronchial blood flow [19, 23, 51, 53, 74].

Under the heading of chronic inflammatory and infectious processes (Tab. 6.1) are several conditions that produce hypertrophy and angiogenesis of the bronchial circulation. In these, abnormal vessels are demonstrated by macroscopic (including angiographic) and microscopic examination. Increased bronchial blood flow rising to 20–30% of cardiac output or greater may be seen in bronchiectasis [15, 49]. The mechanism of the bronchial angiogenesis in this instance is unclear although presumably due to the elaboration of cytokines and growth factors by the diverse cells participating in the inflammation. Bronchopulmonary sequestration, specifically the intralobar variety, is believed to be acquired as a result of chronic inflammation in a lung segment, with secondary bronchial vascular proliferation [79].

An unusual model of bronchial vascular proliferation in racehorses with exercise-induced pulmonary hemorrhage was reported by O'Callaghan and his colleagues [65, 66]. By light microscopy, lesions are reminiscent of a severe postbronchiolitic state with fibrosis and dense plexuses of hypertrophied and branched bronchial arterial networks centered around small airways. The authors suggest that the bronchial vascular lesions are the source of the hemorrhage and that the airway disease stimulates the bronchial vascular proliferation.

The complex issue of the origin of the vascular supply of lung neoplasms is elegantly summarized by Hyde [37] who emphasizes some of the technical difficulties: most studies have utilized injection of colored substances or angiographic media, and perfusion pressures must be weighed in the interpretation of the data. Although the results of the studies to date are conflicting, some conclusions emerge: 1) The bronchial circulation has the ability to proliferate in response to pulmonary neoplasms, particularly primary ones, whereas, for reasons unclear, the pulmonary vasculature does not; 2) Most primary lung cancers are indeed supplied by bronchial vessels; 3) Metastatic lesions to the lung may be supplied by either the bronchial or the pulmonary circulation. Despite a waning interest in regional perfusion of pulmonary malignancies since its peak in the 1960s, there has been a rising enthusiasm in angiogenesis and in antiangiogenesis in neoplasms in the last 25 years [29, 30]: thus it appears to this author that a fresh approach is required to answer the question of the vascular supply to lung neoplasms on one hand, and to elucidate the reasons for which only the bronchial, not the pulmonary vessels undergo angiogenesis *in vivo* on the other; indeed, pulmonary endothelial (and smooth muscle) cells readily multiply *in vitro* [38].

Proliferation and angiogenesis of the bronchial vasculature also follows interruption of the pulmonary artery, either in cyanotic congenital cardiac diseases with reduced or absent pulmonary flow, in pulmonary thromboembolic disease, or in the experimental model termed postobstructive pulmonary vasculopathy (POPV), produced by chronic ligation of one pulmonary artery (*see* below). The role of the bronchial circulation in congenital cardiac diseases is reviewed in detail by others [25, 70] and not elaborated further here. Increased bronchial collateral circulation is an integral part of chronic pulmonary thromboembolism [20, 44, 52, 64]. Although Jandik et al. [41] failed to relate expansion of the bronchial vasculature and prevention of infarction in experimentally embolized canine lungs, rather relating infarction to venous obstruction, recently Kauzcor et al. [43] determined with spiral CT scanning that dilated bronchial arteries are a positive predictor of survival after thromboendarterectomy. Thus, the bronchial circulation may have a protective effect in pulmonary thromboembolic disease. Another protective factor was promulgated by Butler's group [67] who found that after pulmonary artery ligation, left atrial blood refluxes via the pulmonary veins to the gas-exchanging portions of the lung, an effect augmented by positive end-expiratory pressure (PEEP).

## Postobstructive pulmonary vasculopathy (POPV) and principles of the techniques

This experimental model of chronic pulmonary artery occlusion is used to illustrate the methods dealing with the bronchial circulation presented in this chapter. First studied by Kuttner in 1878 (quoted in [73]), POPV is produced by chronic unilateral pulmonary artery ligation and provides a unique opportunity to study the relationships between the bronchial and pulmonary circulations. Based on older studies in the literature [24, 48, 86] and our own findings [31, 45, 46, 47, 58, 60, 61], the principal characteristics of the lung or lobe with POPV are: 1) a marked rise in bronchial blood flow associated with proliferation of new bronchial collaterals around pulmonary vessels and airways, and in the pleura, 2) precapillary anastomoses between the bronchial collaterals and pulmonary vessels, 3) a doubling of total pulmonary vascular resistance due to a three-fold rise in resistance of the arterial segment and a 65% rise in venous resistance measured by arterial and venous occlusion, and correlating with peripheral muscularization and increased medial thickness in pulmonary arteries, 4) increased reactivity of pulmonary arteries to serotonin and of pulmonary veins to histamine, 5) augmented expression of the endothelium-derived vasoconstrictor endothelin demonstrated by immunohistochemistry, 6) an elevated number of myoendothelial junctions, compared with control contralateral lungs, and 7) a reduced minute ventilation and increased lung resistance and elastance.

The methods detailed herein have been devised or adapted to study the bronchial circulation and its relationship with the pulmonary circulation in POPV, but also apply to other models and experiments. Comprehensive references for the bronchial circulation include volume 21 of the Lung Biology in Health and Disease series, edited by John Butler [13] and the review article of which he is senior author [20]. In addition, there is a recent review by Charan et al. [14]. The plan of the chapter is as follows.

First, the technique of left pulmonary artery ligation for survival studies in dogs and smaller species (rats and guinea pigs) is detailed. In dogs, the left pulmonary artery is ligated because 1) it is most amenable to later *in situ* perfused lobe studies than the right side, and 2) ligating the artery to the smaller left lung leads to less overall perturbation.

Second, physiological methods in *in situ* perfused left lower lobes (LLL) to measure bronchial blood flow, bronchial microvascular pressures, segmental

pulmonary vascular pressures and resistances by arterial (AO) and venous occlusion (VO) (*see* also Chapter 7), are presented here in the context of elevated
bronchial blood flow, to determine the site of bronchopulmonary anastomoses,
and the effect of bronchial blood flow on calculations of pulmonary vascular resistance [47, 58, 60]. In addition, the measurement of microvascular pressure in
bronchial collateral vessels on the pleural surface by micropuncture is described.

Third, morphological methods, primarily morphometric, are discussed to assess 1) pulmonary vascular medial thickness and peripheral muscularization,
which can be correlated with functional parameters in various physiological and
pathological processes [56–59], and 2) proliferation of the bronchial vasculature
using direct vessel counting and bromodeoxyuridine (BrdU) incorporation into
endothelial cells.

For the physiological studies presented below, we utilize assumptions provided by the simple model of the pulmonary circulation initially put forth by
Hakim, Dawson and Linehan [32], and further expanded by Hakim et al. [34], in
which an upstream arterial segment and a downstream venous segment, each
with a relatively high resistance, flank a compliant middle segment. The pressure
drops and resistances of each segment are obtained by AO and VO. Although this
model may lack the sophistication of some subsequent models (Chapter 7), it retains a simplicity that has made it amenable to physiological, pharmacological
and pathological manipulation [34, 35, 56–59], including in POPV. Regarding
the anatomical limits of each of the segments defined physiologically by AO and
VO, morphological and physiological clues suggest they lie in arteries and veins
respectively of about 100 µm diameter [57, 58, 60], consistent with the notion
that the middle segment includes extraalveolar as well as alveolar vessels [35].

# Material and equipment

## Production of POPV in dogs, rats and guinea pigs: Ligation of the left main pulmonary artery

Table 6.2 lists the materials and supplies. The canine ligation requires a
sterile operating room environment. Instruments are sterilized by autoclaving. For further details see [39, 45, 47, 60, 76, 77, 81].

*Table 6.2. Material and equipment for ligation of left pulmonary artery*

| Parameters/conditions | Facts | Comments |
|---|---|---|
| Species | Rats (250–400 g) | All species disease-free |
| | Guinea pigs (400–500 g) | |
| | Dogs (15–25 kg) | |
| Anesthesia and drugs | Pentobarbital | |
| | Succinylcholine | |
| | Lidocaine | For posterior intercostal nerve block |
| | Post-operative antibiotics and analgesia | Trimethoprim-sulfadiazine Buprenorphine |
| Ventilator | Harvard apparatus | |
| Special surgical instruments for rat/guinea pigs | Microsurgery tweezers (45 ° and 90 °), mosquito clamps, scissors; small self-contained retractor; spatula as retractor during surgery | |
| Duration surgery and setup | Guinea pigs, rats: 2 h Dogs: 4 h | |
| Procedures/day/unit | Rodents: 2–3 Dogs: 1–2 | |

See *text for further details*

## *In situ* perfused LLL preparation

The perfusion circuit is diagrammed in Figure 6.1, with the equipment and materials in Table 6.3. The pumps and tubing are commercially available, whereas a plexiglass reservoir with two outlets at the bottom and one inlet at the top, and the cannulas are constructed locally; the reservoir measures about 3 cm diameter by 30 cm high, and is attached to a stand whose height can be varied. About 100–200 cm of tubing goes into a heated water bath to maintain perfusate blood at 37 °C. Priming the circuit requires about 300 ml of autologous blood, and care must be taken to

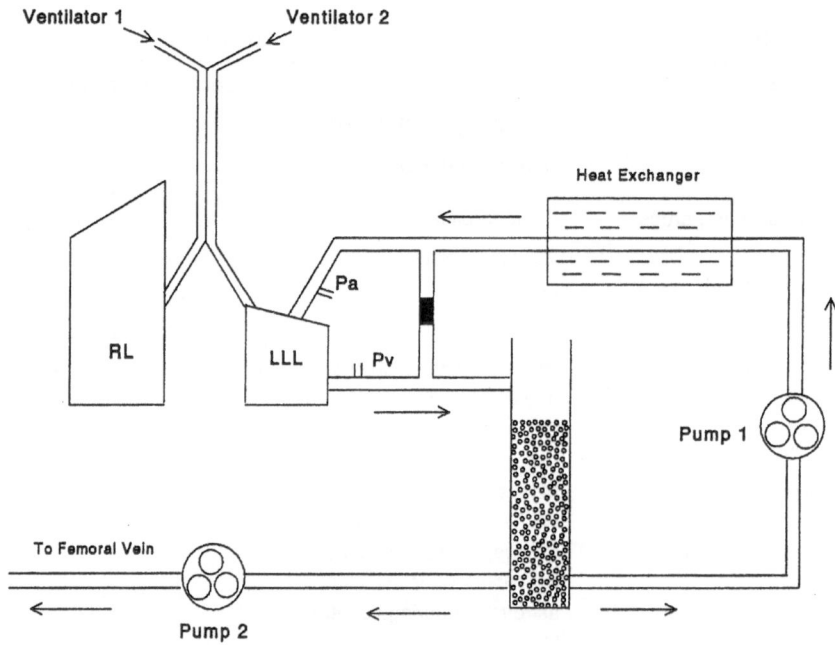

**Figure 6.1. Experimental setup for the in situ perfused left lower lobar preparation with high bronchial blood flow ($\dot{Q}_{br}$)**

The dog is kept alive by ventilation of its right lung (RL). Pump 2 measures $\dot{Q}_{br}$ entering the pulmonary circulation, draining into the reservoir and is returned to a femoral vein. Pump 1 is used to set the pulmonary arterial flow ($\dot{Q}_{pa}$) to the perfused left lower lobe (LLL). $P_a$ and $P_v$ are the pressures measured at the cannulas in the pulmonary artery and vein respectively, by transducers (not shown). See Section on Methods, for further details.

eliminate air bubbles. Foaming at the top of the reservoir is avoided by adding a tiny amount of antifoaming silicone emulsion (Instrumentation Lab., Watertown, MA) at the point of entry of the venous tubing.

To measure pressure in the bronchial collateral vessels on the pleura, additional equipment is required (Tab. 6.3 and below), with significant cost and time commitments. Most of the equipment is available commercially; the micropipettes are made before the experiment, but not necessarily in the same locale, and the equipment to make them can be borrowed from a nephrology laboratory or one doing microinjections.

*Table 6.3. Material and equipment for the* in situ *perfused canine left lower lobe preparation*

| Category | Equipment/material |
|---|---|
| 1. General equipment | |
| Perfusion circuit | 2 Harvard apparatus ventilators |
| | 2 Masterflex pumps with 7015-21 or 7016-21 heads and 6409-15 or 6409-16 tubing; |
| | Plastic reservoir on stand |
| | Water bath and heater |
| Occlusion and pressure measurements | 3–4 transducers (Sorenson, Trans-pac, Abbott, North Chicago, IL) |
| | Pressure recording system with link to computer |
| | Clamps or solenoid valves for occlusion |
| Approximate cost of equipment | $25 000–$30 000. |
| 2. Special equipment for micropuncture measurements | Servo-null pressure device |
| | Micropipettes and micropipette maker |
| | Micromanipulator |
| | Stereoscopic dissecting microscope |
| | Plexiglass ring and stand |
| Approximate cost | $50 000. |

## Morphological assessment of the bronchial and pulmonary vasculature using light microscopy and morphometry

The materials and equipment are in Table 6.4 and in the *Methods* section. The procedural details that follow the immediate excision of the tissues, their fixation and sampling, eg. embedding in paraffin for light microscopy, are not provided since they are routine and best done by a specialized laboratory. The morphometry and analyses are done on the prepared slides.

Table 6.4. Methods and equipment for light microscopic morphometry

| Parameter/conditions | Equipment | Source/comment |
|---|---|---|
| 1) Equipment for pigmented gelatin-barium mixture | Plastic bottles, tubing and cannulae | |
| | Pressure manometer | |
| | Household blender | |
| | Monastral blue and chrome yellow dyes | Dupont Canada, Pointe Claire, QC |
| | Gelatin (Bloom, granular) | Fisher Scientific, Fairlawn, NJ |
| | Barium sulphate | Mallinckrodt Canada, Pointe Claire, QC |
| | Vacuum pump | For degassing mixture |
| Approximate cost | $1 000–$2 000 | |
| 2) Equipment for morphometry and light microscopy | 10% buffered formalin | Fixation |
| | Optical microscope with calibrated ocular micrometer | |
| | Image analysis system useful | |
| Approximate cost | Varies: $10 000–$30 000 | |

See *also text for details, and Table 6.5.*

# Methods

## Surgical ligation of the left main pulmonary artery in dogs, rats and guinea pigs

### Canine model

Mongrel dogs free of respiratory or other diseases ("conditioned") are fasted overnight, anaesthetized with xylazine (1 – 1.5 mg/kg s.c.), atropine (0.04 mg/kg s.c.) and pentobarbital sodium (15 – 25 mg/kg i.v.), intubated and ventilated (Model 607 A Harvard Apparatus (Dover, MA) with 100 % $O_2$, and paralyzed with 20 mg succinylcholine. In the left lateral decubitus position and with the use of sterile surgical technique, a right thoracotomy through the fourth or fifth intercostal space is performed. The right lung is gently retracted and the pericardium incised to access the left main pulmonary artery; this requires gentle periodic manual retraction of the heart and adequate hydration to prevent hypotension. The left main pulmonary artery just beyond its bifurcation from the main artery is gently dissected and doubly ligated with #1 silk. Careful hemostasis is secured and a posterior intercostal nerve block with lidocaine at the appropriate level carried out to minimize postoperative pain. The pericardium and chest are closed in layers and the lung reinflated with temporary insertion of a chest tube. Postoperative care, and analgesics (Buprenorphine) and antibiotics (trimethoprim-sulfadiazine) are provided by an appropriate animal resources center.

*Rat and guinea pig model*

Hartley guinea pigs (Charles River, St. Constant, QC, Canada) weighing 400–500 g or rats of 200–300 g are anesthetized with pentobarbital sodium (35 mg/kg i.p.) and intubated in the prone position using the method of Thet [80]: under fiberoptic illumination, a 14 g polyethylene tubing with a stylet angled at about 15 ° is passed through the vocal cords into the trachea; it is connected to a Harvard Apparatus rodent ventilator model 680 (Dover, MA) and the animals ventilated with 30 % $O_2$ at 60 breaths/min with a tidal volume of 5–7 ml. For the ligation, they are placed in the supine position and using sterile technique, a left thoracotomy performed in the third or fourth intercostal space. The left pulmonary artery is ligated with 4 O silk approximately 2 mm beyond the bifurcation of the main pulmonary artery. The chest is closed in layers with 4 O Dexon sutures, the lung reexpanded with negative suction and positive pressure ventilation. Postoperatively and daily for 3 days, 5 mg/kg trimethoprim and 25 mg/kg sodium sulfadiazine are injected subcutaneously.

Survival in both the canine and rodent models of POPV is excellent (>90%) and the animals can be kept for months; they grow and develop normally. The other advantage of the technique described herein is that the contralateral right lung is a built-in paired control, although in one study, we found subtle alterations of impedance [46].

## *In situ* perfused LLL preparation to measure pulmonary and bronchial vascular flows, pressures and resistances using modified AO and VO and bronchial vascular micropuncture

### Procedure for the in situ *perfused LLL preparation*

The animals are anaesthetized with pentobarbital sodium, intubated, ventilated with 100 % $O_2$ and paralysed with 20 mg succinylcholine. Catheters are inserted into a femoral artery to measure systemic arterial pressure and into both femoral veins to inject drugs and to return bronchial blood to the dog. To expose the LLL, the animal is placed in the right lateral decubitus position and a left thoracotomy is performed at the fifth intercostal space. The left upper and middle lobes are excised and can be kept for morphological studies. The left main pulmonary artery and vein are carefully dissected free of surrounding tissue, avoiding the new bronchial vessels that bleed easily. The diagram in Figure 6.1 illustrates the preparation; both the animal and the perfusion circuit are heparinized. Rigid plastic or metal cannulae 7.5 and 6 mm outer and inner diameter, respectively are inserted into the LLL artery distal to the site of prior ligation and, through the left atrial appendage, into the LLL vein. The LLL is perfused with warm (37 °C) heparinized autologous blood using a Masterflex pump Model 6-600 RPM (Cole-Palmer Instrument Co., Chicago, IL) with precalibrated settings to measure precisely the flow to the pulmonary artery ($\dot{Q}_{pa}$). The venous effluent drains passively via the venous cannula into an open reservoir, the height of which can be varied to set venous pressure. In addition, bypass tubing is inserted between the arterial cannula and the occlusion site to directly drain anastomotic bronchial blood flow ($\dot{Q}_{br}$) from the pulmonary artery to the reservoir. The anastomotic $\dot{Q}_{br}$ to the *in situ* perfused LLL is measured by adjusting the flow rate of a second Masterflex pump which drains the venous reservoir in such a way that its volume of blood is kept constant. The excess blood is returned to the systemic circulation through a femoral vein access.

The LLL arterial ($P_a$) and venous pressures ($P_v$) are measured from side ports in the arterial and venous cannulae with transducers referenced to the top of the lobe. The dogs are kept alive and the right lung and LLL ventilated separately through a double-lumen tracheal tube (Willy Rusch AG, Waiblingen, Germany); the right lung receives 100% $O_2$ and the LLL a mixture of 95% $O_2$–5% $CO_2$; PEEP is set at 4–5 cmH$_2$O for both sides. The PO$_2$, PCO$_2$, and pH of the arterial blood perfusing the LLL are checked regularly and maintained at physiological levels, on occasion requiring small amounts of bicarbonate to maintain pH.

### AO and VO measurements

The elevated $\dot{Q}_{br}$ adds a new dimension to these and the possibility of examining several conditions. Those that we studied previously [59] are as follows (Fig. 6.2), and the rationale is presented below.

First, AO with retrograde $\dot{Q}_{br}$ only (Fig. 6.2, top panel). For this, the outflow from the venous cannula is clamped (beyond the sideport so that $P_v$ can still be measured) and $\dot{Q}_{pa}$ stopped ($\dot{Q}_{pa} = 0$); under these conditions, the $\dot{Q}_{br}$ that drains into the pulmonary vasculature exits in a retrograde direction via the arterial cannula and, with the bypass tube open, into the reservoir. An outflow AO is performed by rapidly occluding the arterial cannula tubing for about 2 s. The rapid rise in arterial pressure ($\Delta P_a$) is measured as the difference between $P_a$ before occlusion and $P_a$ at the breakpoint between its rapid and slow rise (corresponding to $P_{ao}$ in Fig. 6.2). Total resistance (Rt) of the system is calculated as $(P_v - P_a)/\dot{Q}_{br}$ and arterial resistance (Ra) as $\Delta P_a/\dot{Q}_{br}$.

Second, VO with antegrade $\dot{Q}_{br}$ only (Fig. 6.2, center panel). With $\dot{Q}_{pa}$ also zero, the bypass tubing is clamped so that $\dot{Q}_{br}$ entering the pulmonary circulation flows antegrade, exiting via the venous cannula into the reservoir. VO is performed by rapid occlusion of the venous cannula and the measured rapid rise of $P_v$ ($\Delta P_v$) is the difference between the $P_v$ before occlusion and the $P_v$ at the breakpoint between its rapid and slow rise (corresponding to $P_{vo}$ in Fig. 6.2). Rt is calculated as $(P_a - P_v)/\dot{Q}_{br}$ and venous resistance (Rv) as $\Delta P_v/\dot{Q}_{br}$.

Retrograde $\dot{Q}$br only

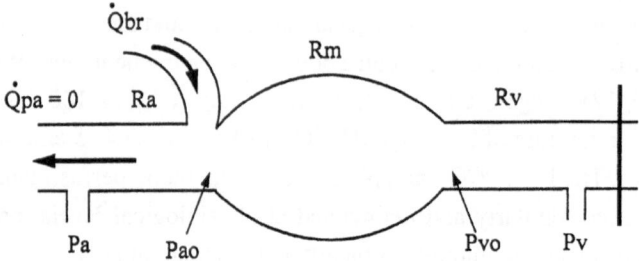

Antegrade $\dot{Q}$br only

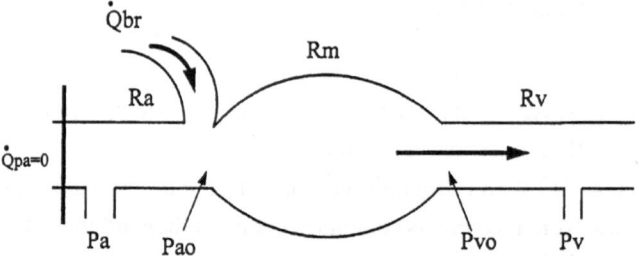

$\dot{Q}$pa plus antegrade $\dot{Q}$br

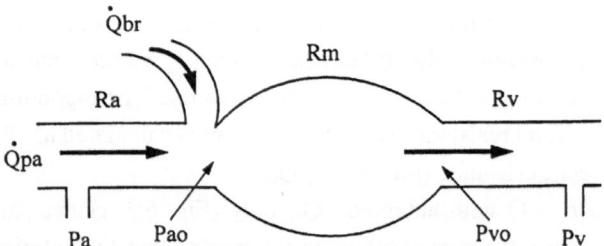

**Figure 6.2. Diagram of the model of the pulmonary and bronchial circulations in POPV as obtained with AO and VO, under three different conditions**

$\dot{Q}_{pa}$ and $\dot{Q}_{br}$ are the pulmonary and bronchial blood flows, Pa and Pv the arterial and venous pressures measured at the entry and exit of the lobe respectively. Pao and Pvo are the pressures at the downstream end of the arterial segment, and at the upstream end of the venous segment obtained by AO and VO respectively. Ra, Rm and Rv are the respective segmental arterial, middle and venous resistances calculated as detailed in the text. Arrows in the circulations show the direction of flow in each condition. (see Section on Methods for details)

Third, AO and VO with both $\dot{Q}_{br}$ and $\dot{Q}_{pa}$ (Fig. 6.2, bottom panel). For this, $\dot{Q}_{pa}$ is set at a physiological level and $\dot{Q}_{br}$ measured as above. AO and VO are performed in the classical manner (Chapter 7, [34]) except that $\dot{Q}_{br}$ is present. Total pressure drop ($\Delta Pt$) is $P_a - P_v$. For AO, the arterial inflow is occluded, with the rapid fall in $P_a$ before the slower exponential fall being the arterial pressure drop ($\Delta P_a$). For VO, the venous outflow is occluded, and the rapid linear rise before the slower linear rise of $P_v$ is the venous pressure drop ($\Delta P_v$). The middle segment pressure drop ($\Delta Pm$) is $\Delta Pt - (\Delta P_a + \Delta P_v)$. The Rt, Ra, Rv and middle (Rm) segmental resistances are calculated using formulas similar to those previously reported (Chapter 7, [34]) with the proviso that the arterial segment is perfused only with $\dot{Q}_{pa}$ not $\dot{Q}_{br} + \dot{Q}_{pa}$, since we had determined that the bronchial collateral flow entered the pulmonary circulation at the end of the arterial segment [47, 58, 60] (Fig. 6.2): thus Ra is computed as $\Delta P_a / \dot{Q}_{pa}$, Rv as $\Delta P_v / (\dot{Q}_{pa} + \dot{Q}_{br})$, Rm as $\Delta Pm / (\dot{Q}_{pa} + \dot{Q}_{br})$ and Rt as the sum of the three.

In addition, this preparation is amenable to examination of the effects of drugs such as serotonin and histamine, to the measurement of pressure-flow relationships, of vascular compliance using double occlusion [60], as well as calculation of bronchial vascular resistance. The results in the experimental lung or lobe with POPV can be compared with controls, either contralateral lobes or other, studied *in vitro* or *in situ* with conventional AO and VO.

The rationale for these different study conditions (retrograde and antegrade $\dot{Q}_{br}$) was previously discussed [60], and is briefly outlined here. At the outset of the experiments, we did not know exactly where the bronchopulmonary anastomoses occurred in POPV, pre or postcapillary. To address this question, we reasoned based on previous studies [24, 48, 86] that if their site was principally precapillary (Fig. 6.2), in the first condition with retrograde $\dot{Q}_{br}$ only between the point of entry of the bronchial circulation and the pulmonary arterial outflow, $\Delta P_a$ should nearly equal $\Delta Pt$; in the second condition, with antegrade $\dot{Q}_{br}$, $\Delta Pt$ should be significantly greater than $\Delta P_v$. Indeed, both hypothetical observations were confirmed. If in contrast, the anastomosis had been postcapillary, then in the first condition $\Delta Pt$ would be greater than $\Delta P_a$ and in the second, $\Delta Pt$ would be very close to $\Delta P_v$, which did not occur. With this information, we could compare the total and segmental resistances in the POPV lungs with the controls.

### Modified in situ perfused LLL preparation for bronchial collateral vascular pressure measurements by micropuncture

For micropuncture, wider exposure of the LLL is required: after a left thoracotomy, the fourth to seventh ribs are resected from mid-sternum to about 3 cm anterior to the vertebral column; careful hemostasis is important. Also, movement of the LLL due to vibrations transmitted from the beating heart and the ventilated contralateral lung must be minimized. Accordingly, the dogs are placed in the right lateral decubitus position and the LLL stabilized on a rigidly supported L-shaped plexiglass platform. The lobe rests on the horizontal plate and the upright plate separates it from the heart and right lung, with a hole to accommodate the hilum at the angle of the platform. Further stabilization is provided by maintaining the lung inflated at a distending pressure of 5 mm Hg. Bronchial collateral microvascular pressures (Pbr) are measured as previously [26, 33], by a servo-null pressure device (Model 900, World Precision Instruments, Sarasota, FL) with a micropipette as the pressure probe. The micropipettes (external diam 2–5 µm) are filled with 2 M KCl containing lissamine green dye for optical contrast and mounted on a micromanipulator (Narashige model MO-102, Japan) to control the precise location of the tip. A plexiglass ring is placed on the surface of the lobe over the area chosen for micropuncture and filled with saline. Vessels are viewed through the saline with a stereoscopic dissecting microscope (Model DV4 Zeiss, Oberkochen, Germany) at magnifications between ×40–80; their appearance is illustrated in [47]. The bronchial vessels of interest are brought into focus, their diameter determined by a calibrated eyepiece micrometer and then micropunctured. Measurements are considered valid if Pbr is stable for 30 s or longer, is greater than $P_v$, and responds to changes in $P_v$.

## Morphological assessment of the bronchial and pulmonary vasculature, using light microscopy and morphometry

*Measurement of pulmonary vascular medial thickness and muscularization in lungs injected with pigmented gelatin-barium mixtures [56–58]*

### Fixation and preparation

Lung lobes are excised after systemic heparinization and plastic cannulae of appropriate size tied into their artery, vein and bronchus. They are inflated with air to a pressure of 20 mmHg using an overflow system; the pulmonary artery and vein are cannulated, washed with saline or Ringer's lactate solution until clear of blood and injected with pigmented (chrome yellow and Monastral Blue respectively) gelatin barium mixtures (Tab. 6.5) prepared after a modification of the original method of Hales et al. [36]; the mixtures are poured into sealable plastic bottles with an inlet at the top for pressurization by a manometer and an outlet at the bottom for tubing to the lobar cannulae. After degassing, injection is done at pressures of 40–60 mmHg until the subpleural vessels are filled. The vessels are then tied off, and the lobe fixed by instillation of 10% buffered formalin at 20 mmHg, until it is distended. Following fixation overnight or for 24–72 h (on a constant pressure system if desired), the lobes are cut into 1-cm slices, and blocks selected (eg. from the midsagittal slice) for embedding in paraffin using standard histological technique, or in plastic, and 5 μm-thick sections cut and stained for descriptive assessment or for morphometry (see below). The adequacy of the injection can be verified by taking a radiograph [57]. After staining the sections, for example with hematoxylin and eosin, arteries and veins are readily distinguished from each other by the different color of the dyes within their lumina. The second purpose of the injection is to distend the vessels for morphometric measurements.

### Morphometry

The sections are examined through an optical microscope equipped with an ocular micrometer. Arteries and veins are identified by the color of the pigment, by location in the lobule (arteries with airways in most species,

*Table 6.5. Preparation of pigmented gelatin-barium mixture for vascular injection*

| | |
|---|---|
| Materials | 200 ml distilled water |
| | 26 g gelatin |
| | 26 g potassium iodide (KI) |
| | 2.5 ml 1 M NaH$_2$ PO$_4$, 2.0 ml 1 M Na$_2$H PO$_4$ 0.6 ml octanol-phenol (40:60% by volume) |
| | 240 g barium sulfate |
| | 4 g chrome yellow, 10 g monastral blue |
| Methods | Gently heat water and dissolve gelatin gradually until clear (stirring bar). Do not boil |
| | Slowly add KI, phosphates and octanol-phenol |
| | Slowly add barium sulfate |
| | Separate mixture into 2, put in blender and add dyes |
| | Pour into injection bottles and gently degas in vacuum |
| N.B. | Prepare fresh just before injection |
| | No formalin is added to the mixture |
| | Wash bottles and blender with plenty of water immediately after use |
| | Mixture is solidified by airways instillation of formalin (see text) |

*Modified from Hales and Carrington [36]. Recipe makes 100 ml each color, for one canine or ovine lung.*

veins in interlobular septa) and by structure [56]. The outer diameter (OD) at the external edge of the media, the inner diameter (ID) at the luminal edge, the medial thickness (MT) and if seen intimal thickness (IT) on both sides of the lumen, are measured (Fig. 6.3). Measurements are made on vessels selected systematically or randomly, that are circular or cut eccentrically with a maximal long/short axis of ~3:1. In the latter instance, OD, ID, MT, and IT are measured perpendicular to the long axis. From these values, the percentage of MT and IT (%MT and %IT respectively) are calculated as $(MT/OD) \times 100$ or $(IT/OD) \times 100$, taking the sum of the MT or IT from both sides of the vessel (Fig. 6.3). Arteries and

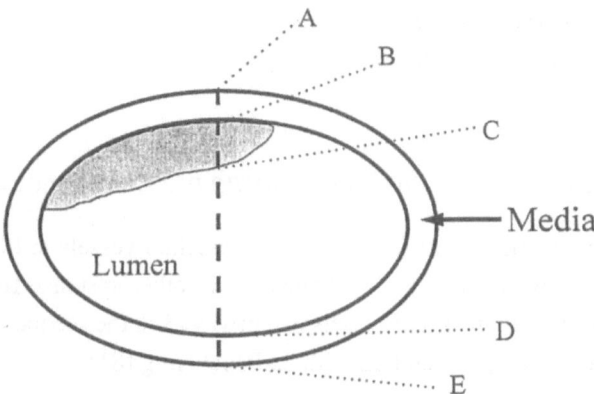

**Figure 6.3. Diagrammatic representation of an artery in eccentric cross-section**
**showing its lumen, media, and a patch of irregular intimal thickening (shaded area)**
Dashed line indicates the site of measurement of the structures. Medial thickness (MT) is AB
+ DE, intimal thickness (IT) BC, outer diameter (OD) AE, inner diameter (ID) CD. See text for
details of calculations from the data obtained.

veins can be divided into size categories eg. of < 50, 50–100, 101–200, 201–400, 401–600, 601–800, 801–1000, and > 1000 μm. The measurement of ID serves if one wants to study alterations of this parameter under experimental manipulation [58].

To assess extent of muscularization, a number of arteries and veins, e.g. 10–15, [56–58] in each size category are classified as elastic, transitional, muscular, partially muscular or nonmuscular; for the veins, only the last three categories are used. In addition, the arteries can be grouped with respect to adjacent airways (bronchi, bronchioles, respiratory bronchioles, alveolar ducts and alveoli). The advantage of this grouping is that it is independent of vessel size that can change with the experimental manipulation under study (e.g. in pulmonary fibrosis or in POPV) [58, 59]. Muscularization is expressed by grouping each type of artery by size and by accompanying airway, and veins by size only, since they do not run with the airways. Comparisons can then be made between control and experimental conditions in the %MT and %IT, and in the % of each type of artery or veins within a given size category, or for the arteries, of the % of each type of artery traveling with a given airway type.

For statistical analyses of the %MT or %IT, Student's *t*-test or analysis of variance are used, whereas for the data on the extent of muscularization, the chi-square test is appropriate.

## Assessment of proliferation in the bronchial vasculature

To quantitate proliferation of the bronchial vessels in POPV in rats, we recently adapted two methods used in other systems, first counting the number of bronchial vessels per airway [39], the second looking at endothelial cell proliferation with BrdU labeling [81].

### Bronchial vessel number per airway
Lungs are fixed by intrabronchial instillation of 10 % formalin at 20 mmHg for 18 h and embedded in paraffin as previously. Slides from control and experimental lungs are randomized and morphometry performed without knowledge of treatment groups: large and medium airways are typed as bronchi or bronchioles, their diameters measured at the luminal edge of the basement membrane and the mean number of bronchial arteries associated with each counted. In our data, we chose to examine the number of arteries per airway for bronchioles ≥ 220 μm diameter [39].

### Assessment of bronchial vascular endothelial proliferation using bromodeoxyuridine (BrdU) labeling
An important finding in the POPV model is bronchial vascular proliferation [24, 47, 48, 58, 73, 86]. To determine the time of maximal proliferation of the endothelial (and other) cells in POPV, we utilized the technique of *in vivo* BrdU labeling with immunohistochemical detection on rodent lungs at different times after ligation of the pulmonary artery. BrdU is a thymidine analog with minimal systemic toxicity that is incorporated into cellular DNA during synthesis. The method is as follows.

Using rats, the left pulmonary artery is ligated as previously and 24, 16 and 2 h prior to scheduled sacrifice, each rat receives BrdU (Sigma, St Louis, MO), 100 mg/kg in 0.9% saline i.p., to ensure labeling of the endothelial cells, since under normal circumstances their labeling index is very low. The rats are sacrificed by exsanguination after pentobarbital (40 mg/kg i.p.) and systemic heparinization. Through a midline abdominal incision, the inferior vena cava is cannulated and the circulation flushed with 30 ml 0.9% saline; the pulmonary circulation distal to the ligation is also flushed with saline solution through the left ventricle. The lungs are removed and fixed through the airways with 10% buffered formalin at 20 mmHg. The lungs are sliced in the sagittal direction and about four blocks from each lung embedded in paraffin; in addition, sections from the small or large intestine are sampled, fixed by immersion

*Table 6.6. Factors affecting bronchial blood flow*

| Factors | References |
|---|---|
| A. Hemodynamic | |
| *1. Upstream pressure: systemic arterial pressure* | [5] |
| *2. Downstream pressure: left atrial or pulmonary vascular pressure* | [5, 17, 82, 83] |
| *3. Perfusate temperature* | [4, 11] |
| B. Lung volume and airway-related | |
| *1. Lung volume and PEEP* | [2, 8, 82, 84] |
| *2. Relative humidity of inspired gas* | [3, 9, 10, 78] |
| C. Neural and pharmacological | [17, 87] |
| *1. Parasympathetic stimulation: dilation, via cholinergic and non-cholinergic* | |
| *2. Cholinergic agonists: dilation* | |
| *3. Alpha adrenergic agonists and sympathetic stimulation: vasoconstriction* | |
| *4. Beta adrenergic agonists: vasodilation* | |
| *5. Neuropeptides: VIP, NKA, CGRP, SP dilate the tracheal or bronchial vasculature* | |
| *6. Nonneural mediators, histamine, serotonin, PGs, leukotrienes, PAF, bradykinin: variable effects, species dependent* | |

*PEEP: positive end expiratory pressure; VIP: vasoactive intestinal peptide; NKA: neurokinin A; CGRP: calcitonin-gene related peptide; SP: substance P; PG: prostaglandins; PAF: platelet-activating factor.*

in formalin and processed with the lung tissues as positive controls for BrdU incorporation.

For the immunohistochemical demonstration of nuclear BrdU incorporation, a standard avidin biotin peroxidase complex (ABC) technique (Vectastain kit, Vector Labs, Burlingame, CA) adapted from Zeymner et al. [89] is used. For this, briefly, 4 µm-thick sections are cut from the paraffin blocks, deparaffinized with xylene and rehydrated through sequential alcohols, then treated with a methanol-hydrogen peroxide solution to block endogenous peroxidase activity. The tissues are permeabilized using 0.3 % triton-X100 in phosphate buffered saline (PBS) at pH 7.4, then treated with trypsin-$CaCl_2$ solution (37 °C, pH 7.6, 10 min) and 1N HCl (37 °C, 40 min) to denature the DNA. After neutralization of the HCl with two changes of borate buffer at pH 9, and two PBS washes, the primary antibody, anti BrdU-single-stranded DNA antibody prepared as previously described [71] is applied to the slides for 2 h at 37 °C; they are then incubated with the secondary antibody, biotinylated rabbit anti-mouse (DAKO, Carpinteria, CA) 60 min at room temperature, followed by incubation with ABC for 45 min. Immunoreactive sites are developed by immersion of the sections in a solution containing 0.01 % hydrogen peroxide and 0.025 % 3, 3'-diaminobenzidine (DAB) for 4 min. After washing in water, the sections are faintly counterstained with Harris' hematoxylin (diluted 1:10 to ensure good visibility of nuclear staining with the BrdU), dehydrated, cleared in xylene and mounted. For positive controls, the intestinal sections are stained in an identical manner, to show labeling of the epithelial cells at the bottom of the crypts; for negative controls, the primary antibody is omitted on one or more slides per batch stained. To assess the slides, they are randomized and examined without knowledge of treatment group to avoid bias. Bronchial vessels in the control and POPV lungs are identified by their location in the submucosa of the airways or in the adventitia of arteries and veins. The brown positive BrdU staining is seen in the nuclei of the endothelial cells, in our case of the bronchial vessels and pulmonary arteries and veins. At least 100 cells of each class under investigation for each lung of each animal are counted, and the proliferation fraction calculated as the ratio of BrdU positive nuclei/total nuclei. With this method, we found that 4 days after ligation of the pulmonary artery in rats, the mean proliferation fraction of the bronchial vascular endothelial cells was about 30%, compared with a fraction of about 4–5% in the controls [81].

# Discussion and troubleshooting

## Production of POPV

In the dog, the rationale of ligating the *left* pulmonary artery through a *right* thoracotomy is to avoid the extensive adhesions with substantial systemic collateral circulation and bleeding that develop after an ipsilateral ligation. Although morphological studies could be performed following the latter, animals destined for physiological measurements, for example in *in situ* perfused lobes [46, 47, 60] that require extensive dissection, should undergo artery ligation through a contralateral thoracotomy to minimize subsequent obstacles to mobilize the POPV lungs. Another method of overcoming this problem was recently described by Remy et al. [72] in pigs, and consists of embolization of coils *via* the endovascular route.

For the ligation in the rats and guinea pigs, problems were encountered initially with intubation and with infections; the latter were solved by antibiotic administration.

## *In situ* perfused left lower lobar preparation

The general methods for the arterial and venous occlusion are discussed in Chapter 7. The additional measurement of collateral bronchial blood flow after ligation adds little to the procedure, although bleeding from the new bronchial vessels is a concern. The method outlined here measures the $\dot{Q}_{br}$ that enters the pulmonary venous circulation and thus the left atrium, and does not take into account the "bronchial venous" drainage to the right atrium; thus, an underestimate of total $\dot{Q}_{br}$ is likely, although this is probably not too important, since in POPV, the anastomoses are mostly with the pulmonary circulation, and thus measured with our preparation. How much we obstruct the bronchial arterial inflow at the hilum with the cannulations is not clear, but also presumably not overly significant, since we obtained high values of $\dot{Q}_{br}$ [60].

The complex topic of the measurement of $\dot{Q}_{br}$ has been reviewed comprehensively by Baile and Pare [11], including the microsphere technique that measures accurately total $\dot{Q}_{br}$ to a lung or lobe; in our preparation, however, it would not be feasible since repeated measurements are required. Table 6.6 lists some of the factors that influence the measurement of $\dot{Q}_{br}$ and that can significantly alter the results. In a recent publication, Pearse et al. [68] found that microspheres could alter their own measurement of $\dot{Q}_{br}$ by mechanisms involving the release of adenosine and a dilator prostaglandin. Ashley et al. [7] also emphasized the complexities of $\dot{Q}_{br}$ measurement and systemic blood supply to the lung in sheep.

The measurement of pressure in bronchial vessels on the pleural surface in POPV using micropuncture is not a trivial undertaking. First, substantial bleeding occurs because of the bronchial collaterals and of the extensive surgery required to ensure adequate exposure. The second difficulty is isolation of the preparation from the motion of the heart and contralateral lung, since the animal is kept alive; it may be necessary, on occasion, to interrupt ventilation to the right lung to permit micropuncture. To our knowledge, Shepard and colleagues [75] are the only other group to have attempted micropuncture of the lung, in their case the pulmonary vessels, in anesthetized dogs. Other studies, including the most recent ones [27, 28], have been performed on isolated perfused lobes. Ballard et al. [12] examined the microvascular pressure profile of pulmonary airways using micropuncture and found that the major drop occurred in arteries between 10 and 100 µm diam.

## Morphological assessment of the bronchial and pulmonary vasculature

For the injection of the lungs with pigmented gelatin-barium mixtures, the procedure is straight forward; care must be taken, however, to minimize bubble formation by degassing. Even if the pressure of injection is applied to the bottle, the final pressure at the pulmonary end is uncertain, due to the viscosity of the mixture. The main purpose is to distend the lung vessels and obtain a constant denominator, i.e. external vascular diameter. There may be occasional crossing over into the opposite side of the circulation via the capillaries, but this is usually not significant. Our procedure is similar to the one of Meyrick and Reid [54, 55] in their studies on the pulmonary vasculature of several species, with the addition of venous injection and the use of two contrasting colors.

After the injection, fixation, slicing and sampling of the lungs, it is recommended that the embedding in paraffin, cutting sections and staining with hematoxylin and eosin be done by a histology laboratory (either in an anatomy or pathology department). Then only a good optical microscope with a micrometer is required for the morphometric measurements. Measurements and analyses can be made on a system using commercial or public domain software. For example, we recently studied in human lungs the relationship of bronchial arteries to plexiform lesions in pulmonary arteries that characterize certain forms of severe pulmonary hypertension [40], by measuring plexiform lesion-to-airway distances using an image analysis system consisting of a light microscope, video camera and readily available image analysis software (Image 1.44, National Institutes of Health). Other examples of results of %MT and extent of muscularization are found in refs [57–59].

For the assessment of bronchial vascular proliferation, the advantage of counting the number of bronchial vessels per airway is that it corrects for slight differences in experimental conditions, and for disparities in the amounts of tissue sampled; a similar advantage accrues to counting the number of myoendothelial junctions per unit length of basal lamina by electron microscopy [61]. One potential concern with the measurements of number of bronchial vessels per airway is that the size of airways may change with experimental manipulation, as they do for rats and guinea pigs in the lung with the ligated pulmonary artery compared with the contralateral side. To circumvent this problem, we have used the 10, 20 or 30 *largest* airways in each animal for study, irrespective of their size.

The method using BrdU labeling is not new and has been reviewed extensively [21, 22, 88]. In our experiments, we adopted a method involving multiple injections of BrdU to approximate a continuous rather than pulsed-labeling technique. This was done to enhance uptake of BrdU in occasional cycling endothelial cells in vessels not undergoing active proliferation, such as the pulmonary veins, as well as to ensure a measurable signal in bronchial artery endothelial cells. At the doses used, BrdU is well tolerated by the animals.

# Acknowledgements

The author is particularly grateful to Drs. J. Gordon, T. Hakim, F. Hu, B. Jamison, S. Kelly, B. Meyrick and A. Taylor, for much appreciated past and present collaboration related to the studies quoted in this chapter, and to Dr. B. Jamison for reading and commenting on the manuscript. The author's research presented herein was largely supported by the Medical Research Council of Canada, with support also from the Québec and Canadian Lung Associations.

# References

1   Abdi S, Herndon DN, Traber LD, Ashley KD, Stothert JC Jr., Maguire J, Butler R and Traber DL (1991) *J. Appl. Physiol.* **71**: 727

2   Agostoni P, Arena V, Biglioli P, Doria E, Sala A, Susini G (1989) *Chest* **96**: 1081

3   Agostoni P, Arena V, Doria E, Susini G (1990) *Chest* **97**: 1377

4   Agostoni P, Deffebach ME, Kirk W and Brengelmann GL (1987) *Respir. Physiol.* **68**: 259

5   Agostoni PG, Deffebach ME, Kirk W, Lakshminarayan S and Butler J (1987) *J. Appl. Physiol.* **63**: 485

6   Agostoni PG, Doria E, Bortone F, Antona C and Moruzzi P (1995) *Chest* **107**: 1247

7   Ashley KD, Herndon DN, Traber LD, Traber DL, Deubel-Ashley K, Stothert JC Jr. and Kramer GC (1992) *J. Appl. Physiol.* **73**: 1996

8   Baile EM, Albert RK, Kirk W, Lakshminarayan S, Wiggs BJR and Pare P (1984) *J. Appl. Physiol.* **56**: 1289

9   Baile EM, Dahlby RW, Wiggs BR, Parsons GH and Pare PD (1987) *J. Appl. Physiol.* **63**: 2240

10  Baile EM, Godden DJ and Pare PD (1990) *J. Appl. Physiol.* **68**: 105

11  Baile EM and Pare PD (1992) Methods of Measuring Bronchial Blood Flow. In: *The Bronchial Circulation,* Butler J (ed.), p. 101, Marcel Dekker New York

12  Ballard ST, Nations RH and Taylor AE (1992) *Am. J. Physiol.* **262**: H1303

13  Butler J (1992) *The Bronchial Circulation,* Marcel Dekker New York

14  Charan NB, Baile EM and Pare PD (1997) Bronchial vascular congestion and angiogenesis. *Eur. Respir. J.* **10**: 1173

15  Charan NB and Carvalho PG (1992) The Bronchial Circulation in Chronic Lung Infections. In: *The Bronchial Circulation,* Butler J (ed.), p. 535, Marcel Dekker New York

16  Charan NB, Carvalho P and Agostoni PG (1994) *J. Appl. Physiol.* **76**: 1836

17  Charan NB, Turk GM, Ripley R (1985) *J. Appl. Physiol.* **59**: 305

18  Cudkowicz L (1992) The Bronchial Circulation in the Human. A Historical Perspective. In: *The Bronchial Circulation,* Butler J (ed.), p. 3, Marcel Dekker New York

19  Daly RC and McGregor CG (1994) *Ann. Thorac. Surg.* **57**: 1446

20  Deffebach ME, Charan NB, Lakshmina-

rayan S and Butler J (1987) *Am. Rev. Respir. Dis.* **135**: 463

21  Dolbeare F (1995) *Histochem. J.* **27**: 339

22  Dolbeare F and Selden JR (1994) *Meth. Cell. Biol.* **41**: 297

23  Egan T (1995) Single Lung Transplantation. In: *Thoracic Transplantation.* Shumway SJ, Shumway NE (eds), p. 395, Blackwell Science Cambridge MA

24  Ellis FH Jr., Grindlay JH and Edwards JE (1952) *Am. J. Pathol.* **28**: 89

25  Ellis K (1992) The Bronchial Arteries and Anomalous Systemic Arteries to the Lungs in Congenital Heart and Lung Disease. In: *The Bronchial Circulation,* Butler J (ed.), p. 599, Marcel Dekker New York

26  Fein N (1972) *J. Appl. Physiol.* **32**: 560

27  Fike CD, Gordon JB and Kaplowitz MR (1993) *J. Appl. Physiol.* **75**: 1854

28  Fike CD and Kaplowitz MR (1994) *J. Appl. Physiol.* **77**: 2853

29  Folkman J (1995) *Molec. Med.* **1**: 120

30  Folkman J (1995) *N. Engl. J. Med.* **333**: 1757

31  Giaid A, Stewart DJ and Michel RP (1993) *J. Vasc. Res.* **30**: 333

32  Hakim TS, Dawson CA and Linehan JH (1979) *J. Appl. Physiol.* **47**: 145

33  Hakim TS and Kelly S (1989) *J. Appl. Physiol.* **67**: 1277

34  Hakim TS, Michel RP and Chang HK (1982) *J. Appl. Physiol.* **52**: 710

35  Hakim TS, Michel RP and Chang HK (1982) *J. Appl. Physiol.* **53**: 1110

36  Hales CA and Carrington CB (1971) *Yale J. Biol. Med.* **43**: 257

37  Hyde RW (1992) Circulation of Pulmonary Neoplasms. In: *The Bronchial Circulation,* Butler J (ed.), p. 551, Marcel Dekker New York

38  Jaffe EA (1994) *Biology of Endothelial Cells,* Nijoff Boston

39  Jamison BM, Hu F and Michel RP (1995) *Clin. Invest. Med.* **18**: B116

40  Jamison BM and Michel RP (1995) *Hum. Pathol.* **26**: 987

41  Jandik J, Endrys J, Rehulova E, Mraz J, Sedlacek J and De Geest H (1993) *Cardiovasc. Res.* **27**: 1076

42  Jayr C and Matthay MA (1991) *J. Appl. Physiol.* **71**: 1679

43  Kauczor HU, Schwickert HC, Mayer E, Schweden F, Schild HH and Thelen M (1994) *J. Comput. Assist. Tomogr.* **18**: 855

44  Kay JM (1995) Vascular Disease. In: *Pathology of the lung,* Thurlbeck WM and Churg AM (eds), p. 931, Thieme New York

45  Kelly SM, Bates JH and Michel RP (1995) *Eur. Respir. J.* **8**: 202

46  Kelly SM, Bates JH and Michel RP (1994) *J. Appl. Physiol.* **77**: 2543

47  Kelly SM, Taylor AE and Michel RP (1992) *J. Appl. Physiol.* **73**: 1914

48  Liebow AA, Hales MR, Harrison W, Bloomer W and Lindskog GE (1950) *Yale. J. Biol. Med.* **22**: 637

49  Liebow AA, Hales MR and Lindskog GE (1949) *Am. J. Pathol.* **25**: 211

50  Lockhart A, Dinh-Xuan AT, Regnard J, Cabanes L and Matran R (1992) *Am. Rev. Respir. Dis.* **146**: S19

51  Maddeus M (1995) The History of Lung Transplantation. In: *Thoracic Transplantation.* Shumway SJ and Shumway NE (eds), p. 15, Blackwell Science Cambridge MA

52  Malik AB and Tracy SE (1980) *J. Appl. Physiol.* **49**: 476

53  McGregor CG, Daly RC, Peters SG, Midthun DE, Scott JP, Allen MS, Tazelaar HD, Keating MR, Walker RC and McDougall JC (1994) *Ann. Thorac. Surg.* **57**: 1513

54  Meyrick B, Gamble W and Reid L (1980) *Am. J. Physiol.* **239**: H692

55  Meyrick B and Reid L (1982) *Am. Rev. Respir. Dis.* **125**: 468

56  Michel, RP (1982) *Am. J. Anat.* **164**: 227

57  Michel RP, Gordon JB and Chu K (1991) *J. Appl. Physiol.* **70**: 1255

58  Michel RP and Hakim TS (1991) *J. Appl. Physiol.* **71**: 601
59  Michel RP, Hakim TS and Freeman CR (1988) *J. Appl. Physiol.* **65**: 1180
60  Michel RP, Hakim TS and Petsikas D (1990) *J. Appl. Physiol.* **69**: 1022
61  Michel RP, Hu F and Meyrick BO (1995) *Exp. Lung Res.* **21**: 437
62  Mitzner W and Wagner E (1992) *J. Appl. Physiol.* **73**: 1196
63  Mitzner W and Wagner E (1994) *J. Appl. Physiol.* **76**: 1837
64  Moser KM, Auger WR and Fedullo PF (1990) *Circulation* **81**: 1735
65  O'Callaghan MW, Pascoe JR, Tyler WS and Mason DK (1987) *Equine Vet. J.* **19**: 411
66  O'Callaghan MW, Pascoe JR, Tyler WS and Mason DK (1987) *Equine Vet. J.* **19**: 428
67  Obermiller T, Lakshminarayan S, Willoughby S, Mendenhall J and Butler J (1992) *J. Appl. Physiol.* **73**: 195
68  Pearse DB, Fessler HE and Wagner EM (1995) *Am. J. Physiol.* **269**: H1037
69  Pearse DB and Wagner EM (1994) *J. Appl. Physiol.* **76**: 259
70  Perloff JK (1994) *The Clinical Recognition of Congenital Heart Disease*, WB Saunders, Philadelphia
71  Ratcliffe MJ (1994) *Eur. J. Immunol.* **24**: 458
72  Remy J, Deschildre F, Artaud D, Remy-Jardin M, Copin MC, Bordet R and Gosselin B (1997) *Invest. Radiol.* **12**: 218
73  Schlaepfer K (1924) *Arch. Surg.* **9**: 25
74  Schreinemakers H and Cooper JD (1992) The Human Bronchial Circulation. Anatomy and Lung Transplantation. In: *The Bronchial Circulation*, Butler J (ed.), p. 725, Marcel Dekker New York
75  Shepard JM, Gropper MA, Nicolaysen G, Staub NC and Bhattacharya J (1988) *J. Appl. Physiol.* **64**: 874
76  Shi W, Hu F, Eidelman DH and Michel RP (1995) *Clin. Invest. Med.* **18**: B112
77  Shi W, Hu F, Kassouf W and Michel RP (1996) *FASEB J.* **10**: A97
78  Soloway J (1992) Respiratory Air Conditioning and the Bronchial Circulation. In: *The Bronchial Circulation*, Butler J (ed.), p. 291, Marcel Dekker New York
79  Stocker JT and Dehner LP (1994) Acquired Neonatal and Pediatric Diseases. In: *Pulmonary Pathology*, Dail DH and Hammer SP (eds), p. 223, Springer-Verlag New York
80  Thet LA (1983) *Lab. Anim. Sci.* **33**: 368
81  Tiong I, Park S, Hu F, Jamison B and Michel RP (1996) *FASEB J.* **10**: A112
82  Wagner EM (1992) Mechanical Aspects of Physiological Regulation of the Bronchial Circulation. In: *The Bronchial Circulation*, Butler J (ed.), p. 219, Marcel Dekker New York
83  Wagner EM and Mitzner WA (1990) *J. Appl. Physiol.* **69**: 837
84  Wagner EM, Mitzner WA and Bleecker ER (1987) *J. Appl. Physiol.* **62**: 561
85  Wanner A and Long WM (1992) Airways. Asthma, Bronchitis and Emphysema. In: *The Bronchial Circulation*, Butler J (ed.), p. 493, Marcel Dekker New York
86  Weibel ER (1960) *Circ. Res.* **8**: 353
87  Widdicombe J and Webber SE (1992) Neuroregulation and Pharmacology of the Tracheobronchial Circulation. In: *The Bronchial Circulation*, Butler J (ed.), p. 249, Marcel Dekker New York
88  Yu CC, Woods AL and Levison DA (1992) *Histochem. J.* **24**: 121
89  Zeymner U, Fishbein MC, Forrester JS and Carcek B (1991) *Am. J. Pathol.* **141**: 685

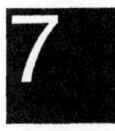

# 7

# Segmental vascular resistance and compliance from vascular occlusion

*C.A. Dawson*
*S.H. Audi and*
*J.H. Linehan*

When the pulmonary arterial inflow, venous outflow, or both arterial inflow and venous outflow, are rapidly occluded, the subsequent time varying arterial, $P_a(t)$ and venous, $P_v(t)$ pressures contain information regarding the longitudinal (arterial to venous) distribution of pulmonary vascular resistance, R, with respect to vascular compliance, C. The longitudinal distributions of geometric and mechanical properties of the pulmonary vascular bed are such that the longitudinal R and C distribution can be correlated with anatomical divisions (e.g., arteries, capillaries, and veins) to the extent that anatomical sites of changes in R and C can be inferred from the occlusion data. This concept was originally introduced by Hakim et al. [16] who observed that when the venous outflow from a pump-perfused, dog lung lobe was suddenly occluded, while the flow into the lobar artery continued at a constant rate, $P_a(t)$ and $P_v(t)$ followed a characteristic pattern (Fig. 7.1). The venous pressure jumped rapidly to a pressure near midway between the preocclusion arterial and venous pressures and then $P_a(t)$ and $P_v(t)$ increased more slowly with time almost linearly. They interpreted the data using the simple "two R, one C, T-section" electrical analog depicted in Figure 7.2. In this simple model interpretation, the rapid rise in the venous pressure was the result of the elimination of the pressure drop across a resistance, $R_2$, downstream from a region of high compliance, $C_T$. Then the difference between $P_a(t)$ and $P_v(t)$ after the rapid jump in $P_v(t)$ would be the preocclusion pressure drop across a resistance, $R_1$, upstream from the high compliance region, and the slopes of the slowly rising arterial and venous pressures would be the flow rate divided by $C_T$. A key observation linking the model elements to the anatomy of the vascular bed was that when the pulmonary venoconstrictor histamine was infused, the increase in the preocclusion arterial-venous pressure difference was about equal to the increase in the rapid jump in venous pressure following occlusion, i.e., an increase in $R_2$. Whereas, when the pulmonary arterial constrictor serotonin was in-

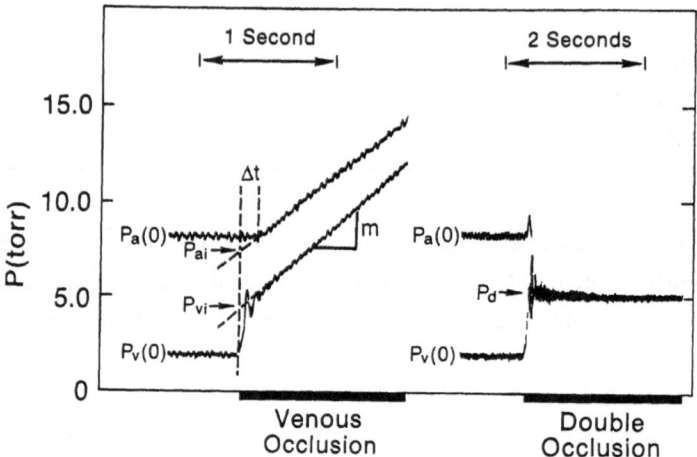

**Figure 7.1. Arterial, $P_a(t)$, and venous, $P_v(t)$, pressure tracings obtained during venous occlusion and double occlusion experiments on a dog lung lobe**

$P_{ai}$ and $P_{vi}$ are obtained by extrapolation of $P_a(t)$ and $P_v(t)$ back to the instant of occlusion. $P_d$ is the equilibrium pressure following double occlusion. The m is the slope of $P_v(t)$ (or as indicated in the text it could be the average of the slopes of $P_v(t)$ and $P_a(t)$) is inversely proportional to lobar vascular compliance. $\Delta t$ is the time delay before $P_a(t)$ begins to rise following venous occlusion. Adapted from [24] with permission from the American Physiological Society.

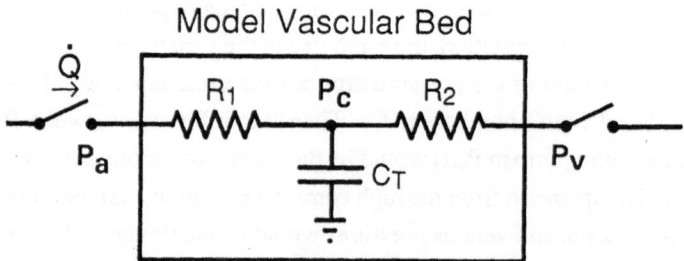

**Figure 7.2. An electrical analog T-section model used to explain the features of the arterial and venous pressure responses to occlusion of the venous outflow, arterial inflow, or both the arterial inflow and venous outflow**

Occlusion is analogized by opening the switches. Adapted from [13] with permission. For further explanation see text.

fused the increase in arterial-venous pressure difference was mainly in that part of the arterial-venous pressure difference remaining after the rapid jump, i.e., an increase in $R_1$ (Fig. 7.3). These results implied that a major fraction of the lobar vascular compliance was located between the muscular arteries and veins, i.e., in the capillaries, and that venous occlusion, VO, divided the lobar arterial-venous pressure difference into an arterial pressure drop upstream from the vessels responsible for most of the volume storage whose pressure is $P_c$ and a venous pressure drop downstream from $P_c$.

The model in Figure 7.2 also provides for an interpretation of the equilibrium pressure, $P_d$, that is obtained when both arterial inflow and venous outflow are simultaneously occluded in the double occlusion maneuver, DO, as in Figure 7.1 [13]. In addition, Hakim et al. [20] showed that, following arterial occlusion, AO, the $P_a(t)$ fell very rapidly followed by a slower exponential decay (Fig. 7.4), which is also predicted by the simple model in Figure 7.2. Thus, by accounting

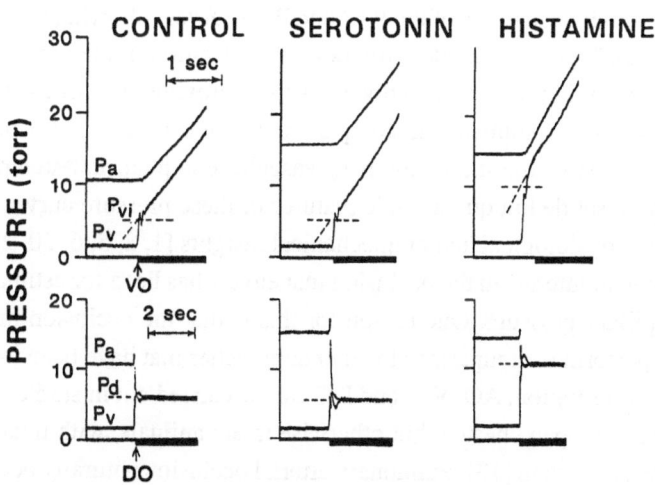

*Figure 7.3. The arterial and venous pressure curves obtained when the venous outflow, VO, or both the venous outflow and arterial inflow, DO, were occluded in an isolated dog lung lobe under normal conditions (control) or when serotonin or histamine were infused*
*Adapted from [13] with permission.*

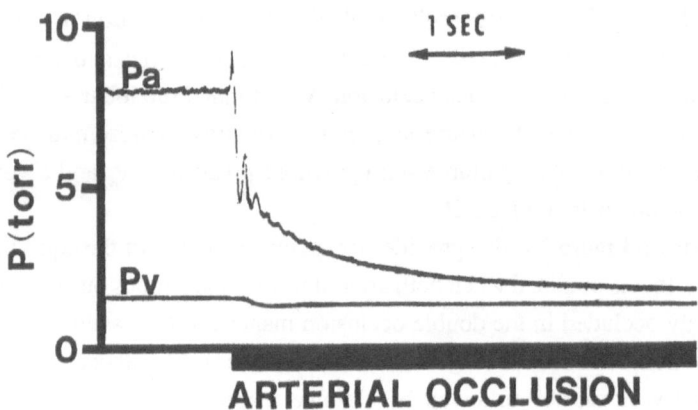

**Figure 7.4. The arterial and venous pressure curves obtained when the arterial inflow, AO, was occluded in an isolated dog lung lobe**
*Reprinted from [11] with permission from the American Physiological Society.*

for the most obvious features of the $P_a(t)$ and $P_v(t)$ curves following the occlusion maneuvers, the Figure 7.2 model provides a visualization of the intrapulmonary vasculature wherein the arterial and venous trees provide most of the resistance and relatively little compliance in comparison to the capillary bed which is responsible for most of the intrapulmonary vascular compliance. Attempts to explain the more subtle but quantifiable features of these pressure curves have led to additional physiological and biomechanical insights [1, 2, 5, 6, 20, 25]. However, a dominant interest in the occlusion maneuvers has been for estimating pulmonary capillary pressure. One reason for this is that the occlusion maneuvers are easy to perform in comparison to other approaches that have been used to obtain related information. AO, VO, and DO can be carried out in studies of isolated lungs [13], in open chested, but otherwise intact animals, with ligatures on a lobar artery and/or vein [13]. Pulmonary arterial occlusion naturally occurs at the end of each systole as the result of closure of the pulmonic valve [27], and whenever the balloon on the tip of a Swan-Ganz catheter located in a pulmonary artery is inflated [22]. The use of the balloon catheter in essence artificially extends the period between heart beats which is an advantage for data analysis.

The concept that the $P_c$'s estimated using the pressure data from the occlusion maneuvers and data analyses described below are useful estimates of capillary pressure comes in large part from the responses of the $P_c$'s when the pulmonary vasculature is exposed to various vasoconstrictor stimuli that have different sites of action [16, 13, 20] as indicated above. Other approaches used to address the anatomical location include comparison of $P_c$ with pressure obtained using isogravimetric [13, 29, 31] or isofiltration [7] methods or micropuncture of subpleural arterioles and venules [17]. These results appear to be generally confirmatory, although each carries its own caveats. Thus, there is not a clear gold standard for comparison.

The objective of what follows is to attempt to provide a perspective on the use of model interpretations of the occlusion data. In general, it is assumed that the data to be analyzed are obtained from systems wherein the forms of the recorded $P_a(t)$ and $P_v(t)$ are dominated by the geometric and biomechanical properties of the pulmonary vascular bed rather than by connecting tubing, catheters, or other components of the perfusion or data aquisition system.

# Methods

## The lumped parameter RCR model

The model in Figure 7.2 provides a basis for a fairly robust (relatively insensitive to real organ deviations from model assumptions and to correlations between model parameters) means for estimating the arterial and venous pressure drops, $C_T$, and $P_c$ in pump-perfused lungs. When the inflow is constant, linear extrapolation of the slowly rising portion of the venous pressure curve following VO back to the time of occlusion gives $P_{vi}$ (Fig. 7.1) which is one method used to estimate $P_c$ [13, 16]. The dynamic vascular compliance, $C_T$, can be estimated by dividing the flow rate, $\dot{Q}$ by the average of the slopes, m, of the slowly rising portions of $P_a(t)$ and $P_v(t)$ [13, 16]. $P_d$, commonly referred to as the double occlusion pressure, is probably the most robust estimate of $P_c$ obtainable from the occlusion maneuvers. $P_d$ can also be measured without changing capillary pressure. This is an advantage in studies wherein the transient changes in capillary pressure that occur when only the arterial inflow or venous outflow are occluded might interfere with other objectives of the study. According to the simple T-section model, if the slower exponential decay following AO were logarithmatically extrapolated back to the instant of occlusion, the resulting pressure intercept would provide the $P_c$ estimate. This approach would be advantageous when only the arterial inlet is accessible for occlusion, such as with the balloon-tipped catheter in the intact animal or patient, but, as will be discussed below, it apparently provides the least robust estimate of $P_c$, because it is the most sensitive to the inevitable real organ deviations from the simple model hypotheses. The combination of AO, VO, and DO has also been used along with more distributed models in an attempt to provide a more detailed evaluation of the RC distribution as discussed below. These various interpretations of the occlusion data are for the zone 3 condition (i.e. $P_c(0) >$ alveolar pressure), and, although zone 2 occlusion data are available [14, 15], a clear means of analysis, analogous to those described herein for the zone 3 conditions, has not been established.

## The continuous RC distribution

The model in Figure 7.2 provides a concise explanation for the post-occlusion pressure responses, and a method for estimating $P_c$. However, it is only an approximation to the complex pulmonary vascular bed. The additional complexity of the vascular bed can be appreciated by noting some of the details of the pressure curves that are not predicted by the simple model. An effort has been made to explain the deviations between the simple model and the data for two primary reasons. One is that the data may provide more detailed interpretable information about pulmonary vascular function than is exploited using the single T-section model. The other is the question of how deviations between the actual organ and any particular set of model assumptions affect the reliability of the model parameters as descriptors of organ function.

Deviations between the Figure 7.2 model predictions and the actual occlusion data include the fact that 1) the pressure intercept, $P_{vi}$, obtained by extrapolating the slowly increasing portion of $P_v(t)$ curve back to the time of VO, is consistently lower than $P_d$ [13]; 2) the sum of the rapid rise in $P_v(t)$ following VO and the rapid fall in $P_a(t)$ following AO do not quite equal the preocclusion arterial-venous pressure difference $(P_a(0) - P_v(0))$ [20]; 3) there is a time delay, $\Delta t$, before $P_a(t)$ begins to rise after VO (Fig. 7.1) [24], and 4) the rapid phases in $P_a(t)$ and $P_v(t)$ after AO and VO, respectively are not actually instantaneous. These observations reflect the fact that the R and C are more longitudinally distributed within the intrapulmonary vasculature than implied by the model in Figure 7.2. Therefore, attempts have been made to use more distributed models to determine whether the additional information not accounted for by the model in Figure 7.2 can be used to advantage and/or how it compromises the simple model interpretations.

Bronikowski et al. [5, 6] examined the implications of the additional information expressed by the above mentioned time delay, $\Delta t$, in $P_a(t)$ following VO and by the difference between $P_d$, and $P_{vi}$. The $\Delta t$ can be converted into the arterial intercept pressure, $P_{ai}$, by extrapolating the $P_a(t)$ back to the instant of VO as indicated in Figure 7.1. The approach was to assume that the resistance and compliance are actually continuously distributed from arterial inlet to venous outlet rather than compartmentalized as in the model in Figure 7.2, and then to determine the bounds on the actual distribution that can be identified by the occlusion data without a preconceived compartmental arrangement of R and C. To this end, one can visualize the longitudinal distributions of local vascular resistance, $R(x)$, and compliance, $C(x)$ as functions of a normalized spatial variable, x, that increases from $x = 0$ at the inlet artery to $x = 1$ at the outlet vein. The x variable might be, for example, the fraction of the distance from the arterial inlet to the venous outlet or the fractional cumulative vascular volume beginning from the arterial inlet and ending with the total vascular volume at the venous outlet. The structure of the occlusion data that led to the Figure 7.2 compartmental model interpretation indicates that the local vascular resistance and compliance are distributed differently with respect to x. One way to view the relationship between $R(x)$ and $C(x)$ is as cumulative functions, Rcum(x) and Ccum(x), respectively, where, between the arterial inlet and any x, Rcum(x) and Ccum(x) represent the total R and C normalized to the total resistance, $R_T$, and compliance, $C_T$, respectively. It can be shown that

Rcum, plotted as a function of Ccum, is a continuously increasing function within the region W (*see* Fig. 7.5) whose boundaries are defined by the preocclusion pressures, $P_a(0)$ and $P_v(0)$, and $P_{ai}$ and $P_{vi}$. Thus, the measurable pressure data put secure bounds on the vascular pressure at the mid point of the cumulative vascular compliance as shown in Figure 7.6. An estimate of $P_c$ is the pressure midway between these bounds on the pressure at the midpoint of the cumulative compliance, i.e.,

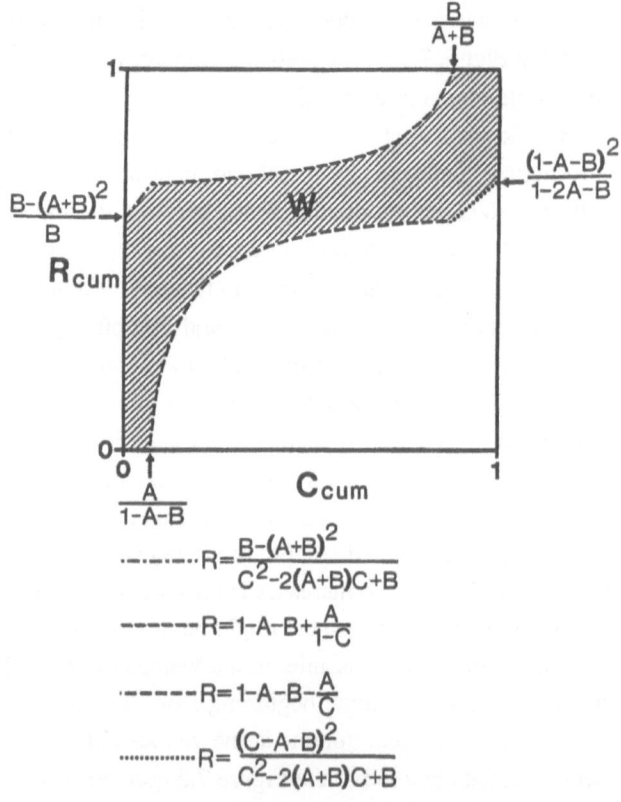

$$R = \frac{B-(A+B)^2}{C^2-2(A+B)C+B}$$

$$R = 1-A-B+\frac{A}{1-C}$$

$$R = 1-A-B-\frac{A}{C}$$

$$R = \frac{(C-A-B)^2}{C^2-2(A+B)C+B}$$

**Figure 7.5.** *The region W in the cumulative RC plane containing all the cumulative resistance, $R_{cum}$, versus cumulative compliance, $C_{cum}$, distributions compatible with $P_{ai}$ and $P_{vi}$*
*The boundaries of W are in terms of A and B where $A = (P_a(0) - P_{ai})/(P_a(0) - P_v(0))$ and $B = (P_{vi} - P_v(0))/(P_a(0) - P_v(0))$. In the equations for the boundaries of W, $R_{cum}$ and $C_{cum}$ are abbreviated by R and C, respectively. Adapted from [6] with permission.*

$P_c(0) - P_v(0) = (P_a(0) - P_{ai}) + (P_{vi} - P_v(0))$ as indicated on Figure 7.6. Also from Figure 7.6, it can be appreciated that when $(P_a(0) - P_{ai})$ is a small fraction of $(P_a(0) - P_v(0))$ the bounds on $P_c$ are narrow. In other words, the greater the difference in the shapes of Rcum(x) and Ccum(x), i.e., the more asymmetrical the graph of Rcum(Ccum) with respect to the diagonal connecting (0, 0) with (1, 1), the narrower the bounds on $P_c$. The utility of the model in Figure 7.2 for interpreting the venous occlusion data results from the fact that normally most of the compliance is located in the capillary bed while the intrapulmonary arterial and venous trees contribute most of the resistance and relatively little compliance. The same analysis can be carried out using $P_d$ in place of $P_{ai}$, in which case, A, defined in the Figure 7.5 legend, would be $(P_d - P_{vi})/(P_a(0) - P_v(0))$. From a practical point of view, the use of $P_d$ may be more reliable than $P_{ai}$ because $(P_a(0) - P_{ai})$ is a small fraction of small $(P_a(0) - P_v(0))$, and its

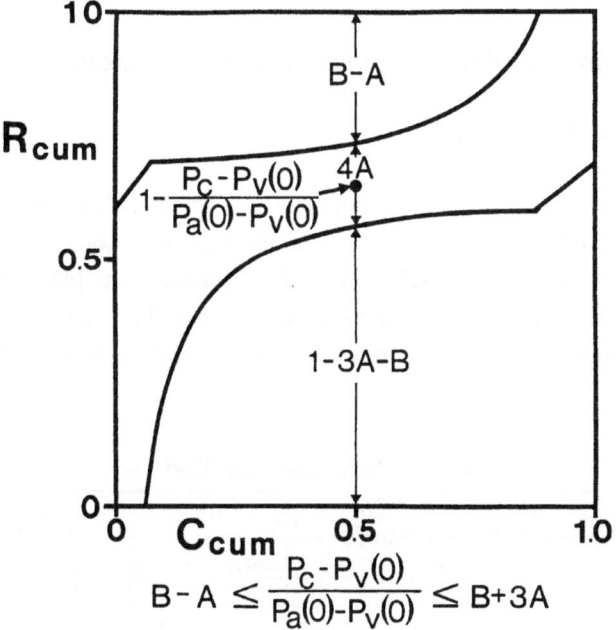

**Figure 7.6. The region W defined according to Figure 7.5**
$P_c$ *is located at* $C_{cum} = 0.5$. $P_c$ *is bounded such that* $B - A \le (P_c - P_v(0))/(P_a(0) - P_v(0)) \le B + 3A$.
*Adapted from [5] with permission.*

143

estimation involves linear regression analysis wherein the slope and intercept are correlated parameters.

To this point, we have focused on the information contained in the quasi steady-state portions of the pressure curves shortly after VO and/or the steady state following DO. The transient portions of the curves linking the preocclusion pressures to the post occlusion steady states also contain information about the distribution of R *versus* C. However, in this region, the data are confounded by the superposition of rarefaction and compression waves that travel from the sites of arterial and venous occlusion, respectively, revealing the impact of the inertance of the blood that is not anticipated by the usual RC models used to interpret the occlusion data. Small volume displacement resulting from the occlusion, and other mechanical effects external to the vascular bed make the transient portions of the venous and double occlusion pressure curves difficult to interpret in terms of RC distribution information [2, 26].

## More distributed lumped parameter models

### The 3C4R model

The useful information content of the occlusion data may be increased by incorporating data from arterial, as well as venous, and double occlusions in the analysis. Hakim [15] and Barman et al. [4] introduced the use of data from all three maneuvers to define the R *versus* C, distribution. Their data analysis is based on the 3C4R compartmental model of the

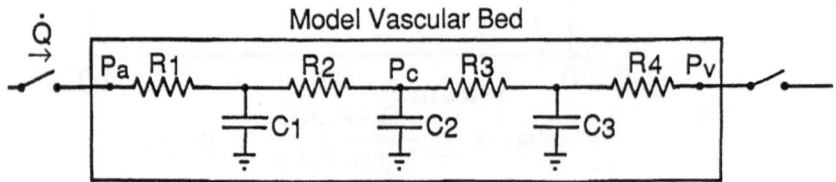

**Figure 7.7. A 3C4R compartmental model representation that has been used to interpret arterial, venous, and double occlusion data**
Reprinted from [2] with permission from the American Physiological Society.

vascular bed depicted in Figure 7.7. The three occlusion maneuvers provide the data used to identify each of the four R's. The magnitudes of the rapid decrease in $P_a$ after AO, and the rapid increase in $P_v$ after VO are interpreted as corresponding to the preocclusion steady state pressure drops across $R_1$ and $R_4$, respectively. Then, under the assumption that $C_1$ and $C_3$ are equal, the $P_d$ is used to specify the preocclusion steady state pressure drops across $R_2$ and $R_3$. This approach is an extension of the use of the individual occlusion maneuvers or other combinations of occlusion maneuvers [20], and it gives more structure to the distribution of R with respect to C. The interpretation has been that changes in $R_1$ and $R_4$ correspond to changes in the hemodynamic resistances in large arteries and veins, respectively, whereas changes in $R_2$ and $R_3$ correspond to changes in the resistances in small arteries and veins, respectively. What qualifies as a large or small vessel is not anatomically defined by occlusion data, but changes in the patterns of the pressure curves, summarized by the four R vector, clearly reveal changes in the distribution of R *versus* C within the vascular bed.


## The 3C2R model

As a result of the ambiguity with respect to the anatomical definition of large and small vessels in the application of the 3C4R model, we have considered an alternative approach to the use of the data from the three occlusion maneuvers motivated by the following two points. 1) When the 3C4R model has been used to interpret experimental data from the normal lung in the way described above, the estimates of the proximal and distal resistances ($R_1$ and $R_4$, respectively) designated as representing large arteries and veins, respectively, have been large fractions of the total vascular resistance. However, the morphometry of the pulmonary vascular bed [21] suggests that, if arteries and veins are to be categorized as large or small, a more anatomically based view would be that large arteries and veins have small resistance and relatively large compliance, whereas small arteries and veins have relatively large resistance and small compliance. 2) Identification of the four R's in the 3C4R model requires quantification of rapid jumps in $P_a(t)$ and $P_v(t)$ immediately following AO and VO. In the short time interval immediately following an occlusion, the inertance (within the vessels and the tubing connecting the vessels to the occluder, and possibly within the pressure measuring system), in the form of the rarefaction or compression waves referred to above, has a dominant influence on the recorded pressures [2] which can confound interpretations based on quantification of rapid jumps. Also, since the actual vascular resistances and compliances are continuously distributed within the vascular bed, it is difficult to unambiguously quantify the magnitudes of rapid pressure jumps in a way consistent with the model, even if the effects of system inertance could be effectively filtered.

As an alternative, we assume that the five parameter 3C2R model in Figure 7.8 is a useful representation of the aspects of the vascular bed that have a dominant influence on the post-occlusion pressure data. We view the larger arteries and veins as capacitance vessels, $C_1$ and $C_3$, respectively, with relatively small resistance, such that any hemodynamic influence of vasomotion is primarily on the vascular compliance. The smaller arteries and veins are resistance vessels, $R_1$ and $R_2$, respectively, having little compliance such that vasomotion mainly alters their hemodynamic resistance. According to this visualization, the largest segmental compliance would be in the capillaries, represented by $C_2$, and any capillary resistance would be partitioned equally among $R_1$ and $R_2$. This model concept appears compatible with available morphometric and vessel distensibility data [21], and the analysis of the data with this mod-

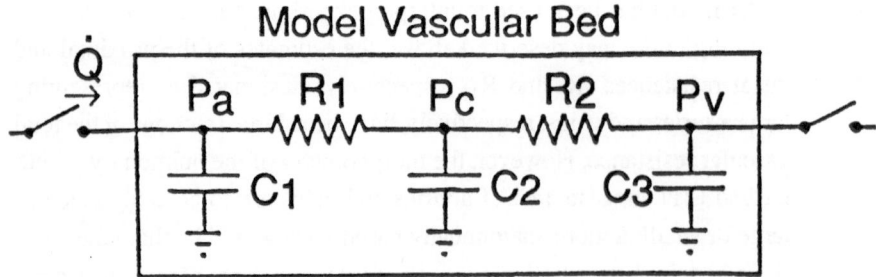

**Figure 7.8. A 3C2R compartmental model representation that has been used to interpret arterial, venous, and double occlusion data**
Reprinted from [2] with permission from the American Physiological Society.

el is less dependent on the details of the pressure changes at the instant of occlusion which are difficult to quantify consistently.

The five parameters of the 3C2R model are related by the following four equations derived in [6] in terms of the VO and DO data.

$$\tilde{R}_1 + \tilde{R}_2 = 1 \tag{1}$$

$$\tilde{R}_1 = \frac{B - (A + B)^2}{\tilde{C}_1^2 - 2(A + B)\tilde{C}_1 + B} \tag{2}$$

$$\tilde{C}_1 + \tilde{C}_2 + \tilde{C}_3 = 1 \tag{3}$$

$$\tilde{C}_3 = \frac{A - (1 - A - B)\tilde{C}_1}{A + B - \tilde{C}_1} \tag{4}$$

In Eqs (1–4), the $\tilde{R}$'s and $\tilde{C}$'s are the R's and C's indicated in Figure 7.8 each normalized by the total vascular resistance, $R_T$, and the total dynamic vascular compliance, $C_T$, respectively, (where $R_T = (P_a(0) - P_v(0))$ divided by the flow rate, $\dot{Q}$ and $C_T = \dot{Q}$ divided by the slope, m). The values of the dimensionless pressure ratios A and B obtainable from the VO and DO data are

$$A = (P_d - P_{vi})/(P_a(0) - P_v(0)) \tag{5}$$

and

$$B = (P_{vi} - P_v(0))/(P_a(0) - P_v(0)) \tag{6}$$

Equations (1–4) involve four pieces of readily quantifiable data from the VO and DO experiments. The AO data can be used to specify a fifth independent piece of information needed to identify each of the five R's and C's in Eqs (1–4) as follows. Eqs (7) and (8) describe the time variation in $P_a$ and $P_c$ following AO (assuming $P_v$ is constant):

$$C_1 \frac{dP_a}{dt} = -\frac{(P_a - P_c)}{R_1} \tag{7}$$

and

$$C_2 \frac{dP_c}{dt} = -\frac{(P_a - P_c)}{R_1} - \frac{(P_c - P_v(0))}{R2} \tag{8}$$

The solution of Eqs (7) and (8) has the form

$$P_a(t) = a_1 e^{-k_1 t} + a_2 e^{-k2t} + P_v(0) \tag{9}$$

where

$$k_1 = \frac{(\alpha + \beta + \gamma) + \left[(\alpha + \beta + \gamma)^2 - 4\alpha\gamma\right]^{1/2}}{2} \tag{10}$$

$$k_2 = \frac{(\alpha + \beta + \gamma) - \left[(\alpha + \beta + \gamma)^2 - 4\alpha\gamma\right]^{1/2}}{2} \tag{11}$$

$$a_1 = \frac{P_a(0)(\alpha - k_2) - \alpha P_c(0) + k_2 P_v(0)}{(k_1 - k_2)} \tag{12}$$

$$a_2 = P_a(0) - P_v(0) - a_1 \tag{13}$$

and $\alpha = (R_1 C_1)^{-1}$, $\beta = (R_1 C_2)^{-1}$, $\gamma = (R_2 C_2)^{-1}$, and $P_c(0) = \dot{Q} R_2 + P_v(0)$. Upon specification of the R's and C's, the $P_a(t)$ predicted by the model can be calculated for AO from Eqs (9–13).

In theory, $R_1$, $R_2$, $C_1$ and $C_2$ for the 3C2R model could be obtained from fitting Eq. (9) to the AO data alone. The total vascular compliance and $C_3$ could then be obtained from the VO data. However, there are at least two technical problems with this approach. First, correlations between the coefficients (a's and k's) of Eq. (9) and the presence of experimental noise in the pressure data significantly interfere with identification of an unequivocal set of coefficients for the purpose of R and C estimation. Second, the organ experimental data are being interpreted by a discrete compartmental model, but the organ R and C are coextensive. Thus, the experimental AO data are not consistent with the model in detail.

An alternative is to visualize the model as behaving as the AO data in only a general way and then to use a robust approach for identifying the model R's and C's that provide a useful representation of the vasculature when interpreted in terms of the compartmental model. We found [2] that

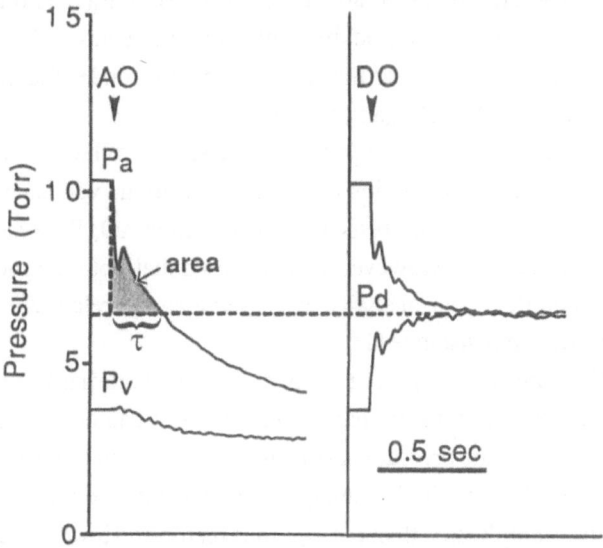

**Figure 7.9. An example arterial, AO, and double, DO, occlusion, showing the area on the arterial occlusion graph bounded by t=0, $P_a(t)$, and $P_d$. $\tau$ is the time following arterial occlusion when $P_a(t) = P_d$**
Adapted from [2] with permission from the American Physiological Society.

one could use the area bounded by t=0, $P_a(t)$, and $P_d$ shown in Figure 7.9 as the fifth independent piece of information consistent with this concept. Thus, the fifth model equation was introduced, namely,

$$\text{model area} = \frac{a_1}{k_1}\left(1 - e^{-k_1\tau}\right) + \frac{a_2}{k_2}\left(1 - e^{-k_2\tau}\right) - \tau(P_d - P_v(0)) \quad (14)$$

where $\tau$ is the time following arterial occlusion when $P_a(t) = P_d$.

To carry out the method, the venous occlusion data from 0.5 to 1 s following occlusion are used. This data epoch was chosen because the pressure curves will have generally approached the quasi-steady rate of increase necessary for extrapolation by 0.5 s. After about 1 s, at normal flow rates, the nonlinear pressure-volume relationship not included in the model becomes increasingly important [25]. The $R_T$, $C_T$, A, B and the experimentally obtained area bounded by $t=0$, $P_a(t)$, and $P_d$ are used in Eqs (1–4) and (14) to find, by nonlinear optimization [2], the best 3C2R model representation of the lung vasculature under the conditions that produced the AO, DO, and VO data.

In the derivation of Eq. (9), $P_v$ is assumed to be time invariant after AO. In practice, the tubing downstream from the venous pressure measuring site has a finite resistance. Thus, after AO, $P_v(t)$ is not precisely constant at $P_v(0)$. However, it was shown that both the model area, Eq. (14), and the experimentally measured area are relatively insensitive to downstream resistance [1].

One appealing aspect of the occlusion methods has been the ease with which apparently useful parameter estimates can be obtained by simple inspection of the pressure *versus* time data without requiring complex algorithms. The method of analysis described above for the 3C2R model is more complicated than the previous methods. However, under the simplifying assumption that following AO, and before $P_a(t)$ falls below $P_d$, $P_a(t)$ is determined almost exclusively by the $R_1C_1$ product, the following formulas can be used to directly estimate the 2R's and 3C's [1]:

$$R_1 + R_2 = R_T = (P_a(0) - P_v(0)) / \dot{Q} \tag{15}$$

$$R_1C_1 = \text{area} / (P_a(0) - P_d) \tag{16}$$

$$R_1 = (P_a(0) - P_d) / \dot{Q} \tag{17}$$

$$C_T = \dot{Q} / m \tag{18}$$

$$C_2 = C_T - (R_TC_1 / R_2) \tag{19}$$

When applied to simulated data obtained from the model itself, these estimates of the known model parameters are close but not exact. However, the method utilizes what appear to be the most reliably measured features of the experimental data, with the result that it can be more robust than the optimization method. The robustness is at least in part because it does not involve the zero time intercepts of the back extrapolated $P_a(t)$ and $P_v(t)$ curves following venous occlusion. These intercepts are sensitive to systematic time variations in the slopes of $P_a(t)$ and $P_v(t)$ following VO due to the viscoelasticity and volume-dependent compliance of the blood vessels and the influence of pressure dependence of vessel diameter on resistance [25] that are not contemplated in the constant parameter models depicted in Figures 7.2, 7.7, and 7.8.

One might question the notion of using a parameter estimation method that produces only approximate results when applied to simulations obtained from the compartmental model underlying the method. However, it should be appreciated that the compartmental model is itself only an approximation to the vascular bed. It serves as a guide for developing a systematic and objective way to estimate parameters that are physiologically interpretable. If the method of parameter estimation is entirely consistent with the model, i.e., recovers the exact input values when applied to model simulated data, it can sometimes be so sensitive to those differences between the model and lung that manifest themselves in the experimental data that the method can be unstable and unreliable. Thus, the objective is to find a method of data analysis sufficiently consistent with the model behavior that the model can be used as an aid in interpretation of the changes in parameter values, but also a method that is robust enough that the results are not so sensitive to small differences between model predictions and the experimental data that they are unreliable. In this regard, the single T-section (RCR) model (Fig. 7.2) and the $P_d$ following double occlusion probably provide the most robust combination of model and occlusion data available. The use of more independent features of the data allows for the calculation of more model parameters, but the price of the increased degrees of freedom can be increased sensitivity to the differences between compartmental model and the actual distributed vascular bed.

As in the methods described above, VO is commonly performed while the inflow remains constant, in which case after the rapid transients in $P_a(t)$ and $P_v(t)$ die out, a quasi steady-state is reached wherein the vascular volume expanding in the compliant vessels results in the constant rate of pressure increase throughout the vascular bed. Nonlinearities in the lung make the latter statement incorrect in detail, thus the use of the term "quasi" steady-state. Alternatively, in some studies the arterial pressure rather than the flow has been held constant following VO. In this case, the inflow rate falls continuously and the $P_v(t)$ rises until $P_v(t)$ and $P_a(t)$ are equal at $P_a(0)$. This maneuver is analogous to AO wherein the venous pressure is held constant and the venous outflow rate and $P_a(t)$ fall until the $P_a(t)$ and $P_v(t)$ are equal at $P_v(0)$. Baconnier et al. [3] provide the solution of the 3C2R model in terms of $P_v(t)$ after VO under conditions of constant arterial pressure and evaluate methods used for estimating $P_c$ from such data.

## Arterial occlusion *in vivo*

The use of the pressure decay at the tip of the Swan-Ganz catheter following balloon inflation to estimate $P_c$ was introduced by Holloway et al. [22]. Subsequently, several studies have utilized the approach in patients [8, 9] and in animals [18]. Figure 7.10 provides examples of the pressure curves obtained. The procedure is appealing because of the potential clinical importance of obtaining reliable estimates of pulmonary capillary pressure, and because it can be carried out so easily. The method is again based on the concept that the locus of most of the vascular compliance

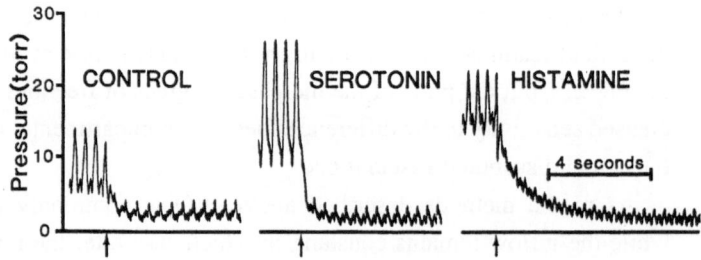

**Figure 7.10. Examples of the pulmonary artery pressure measured at the tip of a Swan-Ganz catheter before and after inflation of the balloon at the arrow**
Serotonin infusion was associated with an increase in pulse pressure and a rapid decrease in pressure after balloon inflation. Histamine infusion was associated with little change in pulse pressure and a slower decay after balloon inflation. Reprinted from [12] with permission.

between the catheter tip in a sublobar artery, and the outflow from the vein draining the portion of the vascular bed subtended by that artery is in the pulmonary capillaries. Accordingly, when the balloon is inflated, the pressure falls rapidly to $P_c$ and then decays more slowly as the capillary volume drains out through the veins. Because of the pulsatility of the preocclusion pressure and flow, the fact that vascular compliance is not confined only to the capillaries, and other factors, an unequivocal break in the pressure decay curve is not easy to identify. Thus, in an attempt to more objectively quantify the capillary pressure from the post occlusion pressure *versus* time data, alternative methods have been proposed. In general, exponential equations have been fit to the post occlusion $P_a(t)$. Then, using compartmental models of the vasculature, and the coefficients of the fitted exponential equation, an estimate of $P_c$ is obtained.

To characterize the AO data, the steady flow analysis leading to Eq. (9) has been used, where $P_v(0)$, the asymptotic value approached by $P_a(t)$, is the pulmonary arterial wedge pressure. The a's and k's can be determined by nonlinear regression analysis using the digitized pressure data starting with the time of occlusion and ending after the steady $P_v(0)$ is reached. The approaches to the data analysis then use the values of the coefficients, the a's and k's, to calculate $P_c$.

Based on the model represented by Eqs (7) and (8), Siegel and Pearl [30] derived the following formula for $P_c$ in terms of the coefficients in Eq. (9):

$$P_c = a_1 + a_2 - \frac{(a_1 k_1 + a_2 k_2)}{(k_1 + k_2) - \frac{(a_1 + a_2)k_1 k_2}{(a_1 k_1 + a_2 k_2)}} + P_v(0) \qquad (20)$$

Yamada et al. [32] also used Eqs (7) and (8), but included the assumption that $R_1 C_1 \ll R_2 C_2$, so that $P_c$ was defined as:

$$P_c = \left(1 - \frac{k_2}{k_1}\right) a_2 + P_v(0) \qquad (21)$$

Several studies [8, 10] have defined $P_c$ as:

$$P_c = a + P_v(0) \qquad (22)$$

where a is the coefficient of the exponential term in Eq. (9) with the smaller of the two k's.

Alternatively, the single T-section model predicts a sudden drop in $P_a(t)$ followed by a single-exponential decay. For this method the data epoch used in the regression analysis has generally started after the pressure oscillations immediately following arterial occlusion have died out (for example, 0.3 s after occlusion [12]).

We carried out an evaluation of the ability of Eqs (20) and (22) or the monoexponential extrapolation applied to the AO data to predict $P_d$ in anesthetized, open-chested dogs wherein both AO and DO could be performed [12]. The $P_d$, as a fraction of the total arterial venous pressure difference, $\tilde{P}_d$ (where $\tilde{P}_d = (P_d - P_v(0))/(P_a(0) - P_v(0))$, and $P_a(0)$ and $P_v(0)$ are the mean preocclusion pressures) was compared with $P_c$ as a fraction of the pulmonary arterial-venous pressure drop, $\tilde{P}_c$ where $\tilde{P}_c = (P_c - P_v(0))/(P_a(0) - P_v(0))$. We used vasoconstrictor stimuli that have different sites of action along the pulmonary vasculature to produced a wide range in $\tilde{P}_d$. When we compared the results obtained using the three methods of analysis, there were significant correlations between $\tilde{P}_c$ and $\tilde{P}_d$ for each, but the best predictor of $\tilde{P}_d$ from $\tilde{P}_c$ was, perhaps surprisingly, the single exponential extrapolation, the results of which are shown in Figure 7.11. The method based on the monoexponetial tends to predict $\tilde{P}_d$ at least as well as those based on the biexponential expression even though the biexponential tends to fit the pressure data better than the monoexponential fit and may be easier to accept theoretically. This result was obtained, at least in part, because high correlations exist between the coefficients (the a's and k's) in the biexponential fit to $P_a(t)$.

Siegel and Pearl [30] discussed why Eq. (20) is superior to Eq. (22) for the specific compartmental model shown in Figure 7.8. However, this model is only an approximation of the continuously distributed resistance and compliance of the vascular bed downstream from the occlusion site, and $P_c$ is designated as a pressure at a particular lumped vascular compliance in the model. Thus, it is not clear whether a value of $P_c$ based on such a model is a superior estimate of capillary pressure without empirical evidence. The significant correlations between each of the three definitions of $\tilde{P}_c$ and $\tilde{P}_d$ suggest that each of the $\tilde{P}_c$'s may be useful for detecting a change in the relative pressure drops upstream and down-stream from the microvascular bed if a sufficient number of observations is made. On the other hand, there is considerable variability in the relationship between $\tilde{P}_c$ and $\tilde{P}_d$. The motivation leading to attempts to interpret the AO data would appear to be to answer the question: under conditions wherein pulmonary diastolic pressure is abnormally elevated relative to pulmonary arterial wedge pressure, is pulmonary capillary pressure closer to the diastolic or to the wedge pressure? Based on the variability in the data in Figure 7.11, it is not clear that the methods used so

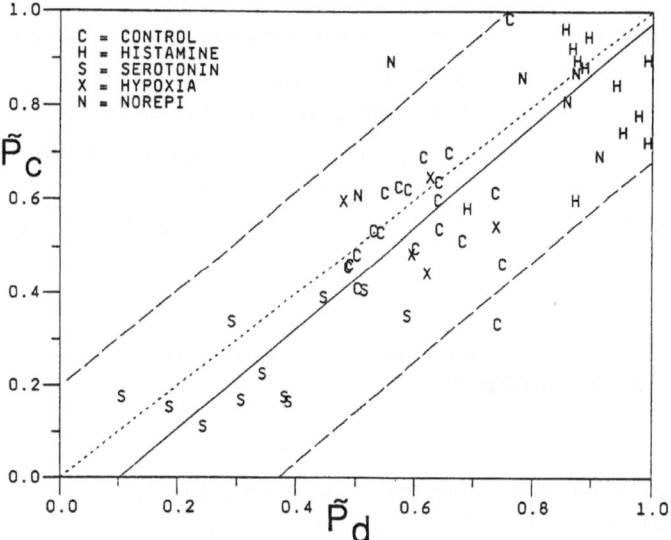

**Figure 7.11.** $\tilde{P}_c$ versus $\tilde{P}_d$ for the dog lungs
$\tilde{P}_c$ was calculated using the single exponential extrapolation method. The solid line is the regression line ($\tilde{P}_c = 1.09$; $\tilde{P}_d = 0.11$; $r = 0.82$). The dashed lines are 95% confidence interval for the individual values, and the dotted line is the line of identity. Each symbol represents a different condition used to obtain a wide range of $\tilde{P}_d$ values, i.e., infusion of histamine, serotonine, or norepinephrine, or ventilation with a hypoxic gas mixture. Adapted from [12] with permission.

far will reliably discriminate with a high degree of confidence using data from only an individual balloon inflation.

One factor that would appear to contribute to the variability of the results is the timing of the occlusion within the cardiac cycle [28, 32]. The methods described above are based on steady flow assumptions. Other considerations, such as the fact that the long, fluid-filled Swan Ganz catheter attached to a transducer does not necessarily provide optimal fidelity for recording rapid pressure changes may also be important. Attempts have been made to deal with some sources of variability [23].

Of course, any interpretation of the balloon catheter occlusion transient has the caveat that the pressure estimate is for the region subtended by the artery in which the catheter is located. Nonuniform parallel distribution of arterial to venous pressure gradients will not be detected in the observations made at one catheter tip location. Even within the subtended region other factors may need to be considered, such as the possibility that positive pressure inflation resulting in zone 2 conditions may distort the decay of the arterial occlusion pressure curve even though venous resistance is normal. In addition, it is conceivable that, under certain conditions associated with pulmonary hypertension, the pulmonary capillary compliance will be compromised. In which case, the anatomical compliance distribution which is the basis of the method, may not exist.

## Acknowledgements

The work by the authors included in this chapter was supported by NHLBI grant HL-19298 and the Department of Veterans' Affairs.

# References

1 Audi SH, Dawson CA and Linehan JH (1992) *J. Appl. Physiol.* **73**: 1190

2 Audi SH, Dawson CA, Rickaby DA and Linehan JH (1991) *J. Appl. Physiol.* **70**: 2126

3 Baconnier PF, Eberhard A and Grimbert FA (1992) *J. Appl. Physiol.* **73**(4): 1351

4 Barman SA, Senteno E, Smith S and Taylor AE (1989) *J. Appl. Physiol.* **67**: 1495

5 Bronikowski TA, Dawson CA and Linehan JH (1985) *Microvasc. Res.* **30**: 306

6 Bronikowski TA, Linehan JH and Dawson CA (1984) *Microvasc. Res.* **1984**: 289

7 Bshouty Z, Ali J and Younes M (1987) *J. Appl. Physiol.* **62**: 1174

8 Collee GG, Lynch KE, Hill RD and Zapol WM (1987) *Anesthesiology* **66**: 614

9 Cope DK, Grimbert F, Downey JM and Taylor AE (1992) *Crit. Care Med.* **20**: 1043

10 Corboz M, Sanou S and Grimbert FA (1995) *Eur. Respir. J.* **8**: 1122

11 Dawson CA (1984) *Physiol. Rev.* **64**: 544

12 Dawson CA, Bronikowski TA, Linehan JH, Haworth ST and Rickaby DA (1989) *Am. Rev. Resp.* **140**: 1228

13 Dawson CA, Linehan JH and Rickaby DA (1982) *Ann. NY Acad. Sci* **384**: 90

14 Dawson CA, Rickaby DA and Linehan JH (1986) *J. Appl. Physiol.* **60**: 402

15 Hakim TS (1988) *J. Respiration* **54**: 61

16 Hakim TS, Dawson CA and Linehan JH (1979) *J. Appl. Physiol.* **47**: 142

17 Hakim TS and Kelly S (1989) *J. Appl. Physiol.* **67**: 1277

18 Hakim TS, Maarek JM and Chang HK (1989) *Am. Rev. Respir.Dis* **140**: 217

19 Hakim TS, Michel RP and Chang HK (1982) *J. Appl. Physiol.* **53**: 1110

20 Hakim TS, Michel RP and Chang HK (1982) *J. Appl. Physiol.* **52**: 710

21 Haworth ST, Linehan JH, Bronikowski TA and Dawson CA (1991) *J. Appl. Physiol.* **70**: 15

22 Holloway H, Perry M, Downey J, Parker J and Taylor A (1983) *J. Appl. Physiol.* **54**: 846

23 Karrakchou M, Lambrecht CB and Kunt M (1995) *IEEE Eng. Med. Biol.* **1995**: 179

24 Linehan JH, Dawson CA and Rickaby DA (1982) *J. Appl. Physiol.* **53**: 158

25 Linehan JH, Dawson CA, Rickaby DA and Bronikowski TA (1986) *J. Appl. Physiol.* **61**: 1802

26 Linehan JH, deMora F, Bronikowski TA and Dawson CA (1988) *Advances in Bioengineering* **8**: 139

27 Liu Z, Brin KP and Yin FCP (1986) *Am. J. Physiol.* **251**: H588-H600

28 Maarek J-MI and Chang HK (1991) *J. Appl. Physiol.* **70**: 998

29 Parker JC, Kvietys PR, Ryan KP and Taylor AE (1983) *J. Appl. Physiol.* **55**: 964

30 Siegel LC and Pearl RG (1988) *Anesthesiology* **68**: 305

31 Townsley MI, Korthuis RJ, Rippe B, Parker JC and Taylor AE (1986) *J. Appl. Physiol.* **61**: 127

32 Yamada Y, Suzukawa M, Chinzei M, Chinzei T, Kawahara N, Suza K and Numata K (1989) *J. Appl. Physiol.* **67**: 2205

# Edema

# Experimental and clinical measurement of pulmonary edema

*S. Bayat and*
*F. Grimbert*

Pulmonary edema is defined as a pathological increase in extravascular lung water. Extravascular lung water lies within the interstitium as well as the alveoli, the lymphatics and the intracellular compartment. The lung interstitium and alveoli are the main sites of increase in extravascular lung water. Formation of edema reflects an imbalance between pulmonary microvascular filtration and lung liquid clearance, which are at equilibrium in the normal lung. An increase in microvascular filtration may result from an increase in the permeability of the microvascular-alveolar barrier or from the hydrostatic pressure gradient or both.

What do the investigator or the clinician expect from the measurement of edema, or extravascular lung water? Confirming the presence of edema induced in an experimental model and identifying factors that increase or decrease edema formation or its causal mechanism are important for the investigator. In the case of an increased permeability edema, quantifying extravascular lung water is currently used as an indirect measurement of the degree of inflammation in the experimental setting.

For the clinician the initial question is whether edema is present or not. In the early phase, identifying the mechanism of pulmonary edema and evaluating its severity is just as crucial as its diagnosis, although the immediate management of the patient is more based on gas exchange parameters and vital signs than on the precise quantification of edema. Moreover, injury to the microvascular-alveolar barrier, resulting in an increase in permeability and regional abnormalities in lung perfusion, often precedes edema *per se*. Measuring the effects of a particular therapy is another reason why the development of methods to quantitate edema, or its causal mechanism, is crucial in the clinical setting.

Measuring extravascular lung water, regardless of the method that is used, is rather insensitive for the early detection of injury to the microvascular-alveolar barrier [1]. Also, its variations in time are difficult to interpret for they may result from changes in filtration, clearance or both. If extravascular lung water is compared to the water level in a sink, filtration can be compared to water pouring into the sink out of a tap, and clearance to evacuation into a drain. If the water input is more than its output, the water level increases. Suppose that after a while both the water input and output return to their normal rate; the water level in the sink will remain elevated. In other words, extravascular lung water is a static parameter. Measuring pulmonary microvascular filtration rate may be a better indicator of edema formation. As we will see, the investigator is able to measure microvascular filtration experimentally, but quantifying filtration in the clinical setting presents practical difficulties. Dynamic methods have been developed to estimate the permeability of the microvascular barrier by measuring the passage of solute from the blood into the interstitium and alveoli. Theoretically, such methods should also allow indirect estimation of microvascular filtration, at a given permeability. However, such techniques are not practical in the clinical setting and their use has not become routine.

Measuring pulmonary microvascular filtration rate alone does not indicate the mechanism of pulmonary edema. Moreover there may be more than one mechanism involved. It seems that instead of considering a single parameter (such as lung water), combining the information from two or more parameters (such as extravascular lung water, transvascular permeability, anatomic distribution, capillary pressure, etc.) is much more helpful in identifying the mechanism(s) of edema.

In the following, we will review current techniques that allow the measurement of parameters that determine the formation and clearance of pulmonary edema in the experimental and clinical settings. The necessity for better quantitative techniques for early identification of lung injury, and for the evaluation of current and future therapy appears evident. In the meantime, interpretation of available data may be optimized, particularly in the clinical setting.

## Definitions

### Lung water filtration and clearance

Lung water can be separated into the intravascular and extravascular compartments. Intravascular lung water is contained in the blood vessels. Extravascular lung water is contained in the intracellular, interstitial, lymphatic, and alveolar compartments.

### Lung water filtration

The endothelial membrane can be compared to a semipermeable membrane. An ideal semipermeable membrane is impermeable to solutes, yet allows water to pass freely [2]. The concentration of solute on one side of the membrane exerts an osmotic pressure which pulls water to that side. Exchange of water across the membrane therefore depends on the osmotic and hydrostatic pressure differences across the membrane. Water exchange also depends on the capacity of the membrane to withhold solute, or reflection coefficient, and on its capacity to let water flow across, or hydraulic conductivity. The net amount of water that is exchanged also depends on the total surface of the membrane.

The forces commanding water filtration across the lung capillary endothelium are described by the Starling equation:

$$J_v = K_{f,\,c}[(P_{mv}-P_{pmv})-\sigma(\Pi_{mv}-\Pi_{pmv})]$$

where $J_v$ is the filtration rate or net transvascular fluid flow, $P_{mv}$ is the microvascular pressure or the hydrostatic pressure inside the capillary lumen, $P_{pmv}$ is the perimicrovascular pressure or the hydrostatic pressure in the interstitium, $\Pi_{mv}$ is the protein osmotic pressure in the capillary and $\Pi_{pmv}$ is the protein osmotic pressure in the interstitium. $K_f$ is the filtration coefficient, proportional to the permeability to water and to the exchange surface area, and $\sigma$ the reflection coefficient of the capillary wall to macromolecules such as proteins. An ideal semipermeable membrane would have a reflection coefficient of 1 (totally impermeable to protein macromolecules), real membranes have reflection coefficients to proteins of 0 to 1.

Several *safety factors* oppose pulmonary edema formation, namely the evacuation of interstitial fluid by the lymphatic system, the protein osmotic pressure gradient across the microvascular wall, the perimicrovascular liquid pressure, the low permeability of the alveolar epithelial, and capillary endothelial barriers to fluid and protein.

### Lung water clearance

*Alveolar epithelial fluid transport:* Active transport of sodium from the airway to the interstitium by the alveolar epithelium has been shown to be the principal mechanism of alveolar fluid clearance. The alveolar epithelium is composed of squamous type I cells and cuboidal type II cells. Active transport of sodium from the apical to the basolateral side has been essentially demonstrated in type II cells since they can be readily isolated and studied in vitro. It is not clear whether type I cells are involved in active sodium transport. Sodium enters the type II cell at the apical side through amiloride sensitive channels, and is then actively pumped into the interstitium by a Na, K-ATPase [3]. b-adrenergic agonists, through a cAMP-dependent mechanism, but also non-catecholamine-dependent mechanisms have been shown to increase sodium transport and alveolar fluid clearance. This active transport of salt and water seems to be preserved in the presence of mild to moderate lung injury [3]. Alveolar type II cells have also been shown to contain specialized water transporting proteins (aquaporins) [4]. The identification of these proteins has suggested channel mediated water movement, however their precise role in the exchange of water between the alveoli and the interstitium has not been defined. Water channels have been extensively reviewed recently by Matthay et al. [3].

Berthiaume et al. [5] found that fluid was removed at a rate of 8.3 %/h in the first 4 h after instillation of autologous serum in sheep lungs. Liquid removal progressively slowed to 3.3 and 1.4 %/h at 12 and 24 h, respectively, in relation to the rising protein osmotic pressure of the residual protein in the air spaces. By 24 h, approximately 80% of the instilled fluid had been removed. Similar *in vivo* studies have measured slower alveolar fluid clearance rates in dogs and faster clearance rates in rabbits and rats.

*Lymphatic clearance:* In normal conditions, a net transcapillary flow of fluid and solute occurs from the blood towards the interstitium. Maintenance of a normal hydration in the interstitium requires removal of fluid and solute through several escape pathways. The lymphatic system is one of these escape pathways.

Both passive mechanisms such as an increase in interstitial volume which pulls open the initial lymphatics by stretching their anchoring filaments, existence of lymphatic endothelial microvalves, and eventually external pressure changes during respiration, as well as active mechanisms such as collecting lymphatic contractility, and vesicular transport have been described. These mechanisms have been extensively reviewed by Aukland and Reed [6].

*Pleural clearance:* The pleural mesothelia are composed of cuboidal and of flat mesothelial cells with rather loose intercellular junctions. The surface of mesothelial cells is diffusely covered by microvilli. Blood vessels of the parietal pleura are of systemic origin in different animal species [7]. Visceral pleural vessels arise exclusively from the bronchial arteries in sheep [8], in humans however, the pulmonary circulation may contribute in part to the visceral pleural vessels [7]. The formation of pleural fluid is controversial. The balance of transpleural Starling forces would sustain fluid filtration from the parietal interstitium into the pleural space [9]. However, based on the observation that the presence of pleural effusions in patients with chronically elevated hydrostatic pressures correlates better with elevations in pulmonary wedge pressure than with systemic venous pressure, investigators have postulated that the excess pleural liquid arises from the interstitial space of the lung, or the visceral pleura [10], [11]. Pleural fluid is drained by the parietal pleura lymphatics, primarily in the lowermost areas of the pleural cavity [12]. Submesothelial lymphatics of the parietal pleura directly communicate with the pleural cavity through specialized openings in the mesothelial cells; the stomata, with diameters of 2 to 6 µm or larger [7], distributed over the lower parts of the pleural cavity. Pleural lymphatic flow has been shown to depend on respiratory movements (extrinsic mechanism) and on active contractions of lymphatic vessel walls (intrinsic mechanism) [13]. In normal conditions, very little fluid seems to filter, or drain through the visceral pleura [14]. Clearance of lung edema into the pleural space has been demonstrated in increased permeability pulmonary edema [15] as well as in increased hydrostatic pressure edema [16] in sheep.

*Edema formation = filtration − clearance*
Edema formation results from an imbalance between fluid transvascular filtration and clearance. The excess of fluid results first in an overhydration of the interstitium associated with accumulation of edema fluid in the loose connective

165

tissue (peribronchovascular liquid cuffs) [17]. Above a critical capillary pressure, the safety factors against edema formation are overcome and edema formation increases as alveolar flooding occurs. This situation coincides with an increase in extravascular lung water 50% above normal [57].

## Lung protein filtration and clearance

### Protein filtration

The transvascular transport of proteins occurs by two mechanisms which are convection and diffusion. Kedem and Katchalsky [18], described the transvascular transport of proteins by the following equation:

$$J_s = J_v(1-\sigma)Cp + Ps(Cp-Ci) \qquad (1)$$
$$\text{convection} \quad \text{diffusion}$$

where $J_s$ and $J_v$ are solute flux and water flux, respectively. Cp and Ci are protein concentrations in plasma and interstitial fluid, respectively, PS is the permeability-surface area product (which describes the diffusive capacity of the microvascular barrier), and $\sigma$ the reflection coefficient ($\sigma = 1$ when the barrier is impermeable to protein and $\sigma = 0$ when there is no resistance to protein flux). This equation separates convective (first term) and diffusive (second term) fluxes across the microvascular barrier and describes them as independent processes. In contrast, the Patlak equation, as modified by Granger and Taylor [19], describes solute convection and diffusion as phenomena occurring through the same pathways:

$$J_s = J_v(1-\sigma)Cp + (Cp-Ci)PS \ x/(e^x-1) \qquad (2)$$
$$\text{convection} \qquad \text{diffusion}$$

where x is a modified Peclet number, that is the ratio of convective water flux relative to diffusive water flux through the same pore:

$$x = \frac{(1-\sigma)J_v}{PS} \qquad (3)$$

The Peclet number itself is the dimensionless ratio of the superimposed solute velocity $V_{s.imp}$ relative to the solute diffusion velocity $V_{s.diff}$:

$$x = \frac{V_{s.imp}}{V_{s.diff}}$$

with $V_{s.imp} = \chi \cdot V_w$ where $V_w$ is the water velocity and where $\chi$ is a slip coefficient [20]. A solute which is small compared to the dimensions of the pore moves at a velocity very close to the water and $\chi = 1$.

When $J_v$ increases $[x/(e^x-1)]$ decreases, and the diffusive flux becomes very small as compared to the convective flux. Eq. (2) will therefore approach a constant value:

$$J_s = J_v(1-\sigma)C_p \qquad (4)$$

If it is assumed that protein concentration in the lymph (Cl) is equal to that in the interstitium (Ci) and $J_s = J_v\, C_l$, then:

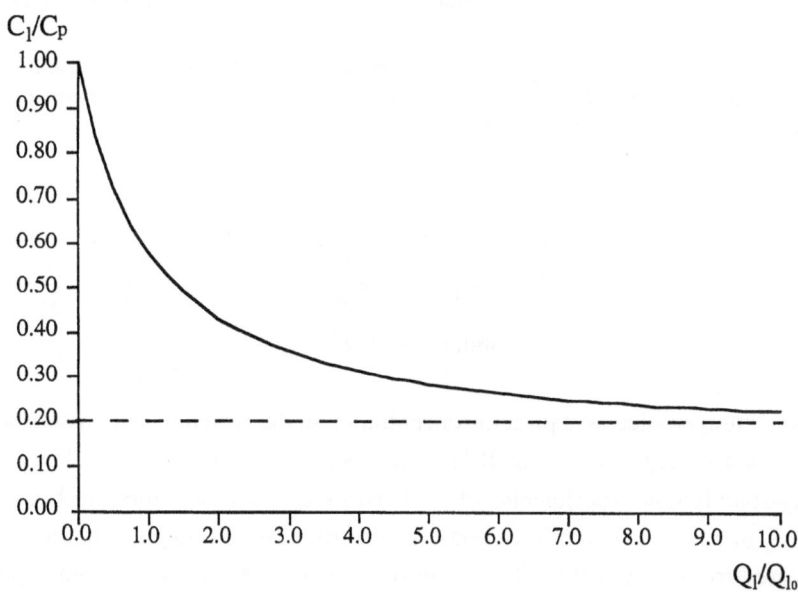

**Figure 8.1. Predicted relationship between $C_l/C_p$ and lymph flow $Q_l/Q_{l0}$ (relative to base line) with Patlak equation (Eq. 2)**
A reflection coefficient at 0.80 can be estimated by $\sigma = 1 - C_l/C_p$ at high lymph flows when $C_l/C_p$ is filtration rate independent. Adapted from [19] with permission.

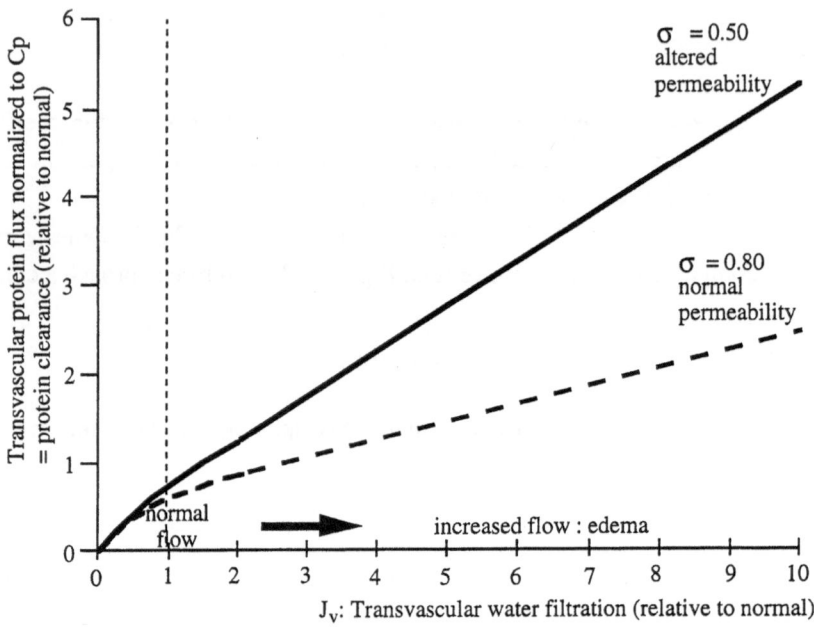

Figure 8.2. *Predicted relationship between transvascular protein clearance $C_l/C_p \times J_v$ and transvascular water flow $J_v$ (relative to normal) with the Patlak equation (Eq. 2) at normal ($\sigma = 0.80$) and altered transvascular protein permeability ($\sigma = 0.50$)*

$$J_v\, C_l = J_v(1-\sigma)C_p$$

$$C_l = (1-\sigma)C_p \tag{5}$$

$$\text{and: } \sigma = 1 - C_l/C_p \tag{6}$$

This equation predicts that protein concentration in the lymph reaches a constant value when $J_v$ is increased (Fig. 8.1). Taylor et al. used Eq. (6) to calculate $\sigma$ in steady-state lymph experiments, where $J_v$ was increased. According to Eq. (2), when $J_v$ increases (such as in edema), the diffusive flux becomes very small as compared to the convective flux, therefore macromolecule flux becomes proportional to filtration (Fig. 8.2). This suggests that measuring capillary–alveolar macromolecule flux can indirectly estimate fluid filtration when $J_v$ is large.

## Protein clearance

The mechanisms and pathways of protein clearance from the alveoli are not clearly defined. In the capillary-alveolar membrane, the alveolar epithelium is the major barrier to protein clearance [21–23]. Theodore et al. estimated that 90% of the total resistance of the capillary-alveolar barrier to the diffusion of large polar solutes such as dextrans (mol. wt. 60000–90000) resides in the alveolar epithelium.

Two of the identified mechanisms of protein passage across the alveolar epithelium are active transcytosis or vesicular transport and passive paracellular transport. Paracellular transport is the passage of protein macromolecules through openings or pores in between epithelial cells by diffusion. Berg et al. [24] estimated that the small pores (0.5 nm) occupy over 98%, and the large pores (3.4 nm) less than 2% of the total pore area, in isolated fluid filled rat lungs. Gee and Staub, however, suggested that when the airspace is fluid-filled, proteins cross the alveolar epithelium by bulk flow along a hydrostatic pressure gradient. They hypothesized that bulk flow of fluid and protein occurs through low resistance channels possibly at the level of terminal bronchioles [25]. However, filling the lung with large fluid volumes may have altered epithelial permeability to protein and induced bulk flow in their study.

Structure and permeability of the epithelial membrane at the tight junctions seems to be regulated by changes in cytoskeletal organization [26]. Data from alveolar to capillary clearance of tracer solutes of different size and labeled albumin has been used to calculate an alveolar to capillary PS [24, 27], and $\sigma$ [28]. Although vesicular uptake of tracer proteins such as horseradish peroxidase (mol. wt. = 40000) has been taken as evidence of vesicular transport of protein macromolecules by the alveolar epithelium [29] there is no sufficient data on the relative quantitative role of vesicular transport in the overall alveolar protein clearance [30, 27].

$^{125}$I-albumin instilled in the alveoli follows a slow monoexponential decline. A clearance rate of tracer albumin of 1 to 2% per hour has been measured in intact as well as isolated lungs, in different species over periods of up to 144 h [31, 32]. The rate of protein clearance from the alveoli seems to be size dependent in normal rabbit lungs and in patients recovering from pulmonary edema, confirming the sieving property of the alveolar epithelium [33]. Permeability of the alveolar epithelium to solutes has been described in terms of $\sigma$ and PS product. Data from alveolar to capillary clearance of tracer solutes of different size and labeled albumin has been used to calculate an alveolar to capillary PS [24, 27], and σ [28]. Once protein macromolecules have crossed the epithelium into the interstitium, they are removed through two major pathways: the pulmonary circulation and the lymphatic circulation. Berthiaume et al., in a long-term study of alveolar protein clearance in unanesthetized sheep found that over 50% of the [125]I-albumin instilled in the airway was cleared directly into the pulmonary circulation [34]. Only 25% of the instilled [125]I-albumin was cleared by the lymphatic circulation. Although macrophages can phagocytize protein, Berthiaume et al. found that their quantitative contribution to protein clearance may be minimal at least in the early phase after protein instillation into the airways of normal sheep lungs. The role of phagocytic cells may be more significant in the presence of inflammation and in the later stages of edema, or with hyaline membrane formation.

In summary, the precise routes and mechanisms of protein clearance from the alveoli have not been clearly identified. Both active and passive routes have been described, however restricted diffusion seems to be the predominant mechanism for removal of large amounts of protein [35]. Further correlation of ultrastructural and physiological data appears necessary to better define mechanisms of protein clearance from the alveoli.

### Protein accumulation = filtration − clearance

Alike the volume of extravascular lung water, the amount of protein macromolecules in the interstitium depends on the difference between the rates of filtration from blood to lung tissue on one hand, and clearance from lung tissue to blood on the other hand. It is important to consider this fact, particularly when labeled protein equilibration techniques are used (*see* Section on *Lung water clearance*, p. 173). In practice, tissue accumulation of radiolabeled proteins, whether counted in tissue specimens or externally detected, will underestimate transvascular protein mass transfer as most of the proteins will be cleared by lymphatic vessels. Ishibashi et al. documented this underestimation while increasing pulmonary capillary pressure for 2 h in anesthetized dogs. Tissue accumulation of labeled albumin increased only 20% whereas lymphatic removal accounted for 80% of the total transcapillary tracer flux [104]. If the rate constant of the clearance of labeled protein out of the lung is not taken into account, errors in the estimation of the permeability of the blood-tissue barrier may occur. In a comprehensive model of protein equilibration, the backward (tissue to blood) rate constant is estimated in order to account for clearance of tracer-protein.

## Mechanisms of pulmonary edema

Two general classes of pulmonary edema are usually described based on the Starling equation: (1) increased hydrostatic pressure edema, where the elevated hydrostatic pressure gradient across the microvascular barrier drives fluid into the interstitium and alveoli, such as in left ventricular failure, and (2) increased permeability edema.

The distinction of these two mechanisms of pulmonary edema must not lead to the erroneous interpretation that hydrostatic pressure is not an important determinant of edema formation in increased permeability edema. As illustrated in Figure 8.9, an identical increase in capillary pressure produces a larger increase in microvascular filtration when permeability is increased.

Decreased lymphatic clearance can contribute to the formation of edema. Impairment of lymphatic clearance is encountered in the post-operative period following lung transplantation, in lymphangitic carcinomatosis, and in fibrosing lymphangitis. An elevated central venous pressure impedes flow in lymphatic vessels which drain the lung into the venous circulation. that this may be a long-lasting hindrance remains uncertain [6]. This situation is encountered when positive end-expiratory pressure is applied to improve gas exchange [36].

---

# Material and methods

## Quantifying pulmonary edema formation and clearance in the experimental setting

### Lung microvascular filtration rate

Filtration rate can be determined by measuring the change in lung weight, assuming that weight change is not due to changes in blood volume, and that the density of the filtering fluid is approximately 1 g/ml. In isolated lung models, the lymphatic circulation is usually ligated, therefore weight gain is considered equal to filtration rate: $\Delta W/\Delta t = J_v$, where W is weight, t time, and $J_v$ transvascular flux.

## Isolated lung

Isolated lung preparations have been developed in different species (rats, rabbits, dogs, sheep; *see* Chapter 2). Generally, following anesthesia, blood is collected from a large artery, and the heart and lungs are removed and suspended from a strain-gauge force transducer that allows to monitor the weight of the preparation. The pulmonary vessels and the trachea are canulated and the preparation is ventilated and perfused. Venous and arterial reservoirs in the perfusion circuit allow changes in hydrostatic pressure simply by elevating and lowering the reservoirs.

Isolated lung preparations have several disadvantages. Some isolated lung preparations develop an increased resistance in the pulmonary circulation leading to lower perfusion rates and less homogenous perfusion than intact lungs. Isolated lungs tend to be leakier than intact lungs, and are suitable only for short-term experiments (up to a few hours). This may be due to microvascular damage caused by ischemia and reperfusion of the lung during the surgery.

## Intact lung

In intact lung preparations the thorax is opened and a single lung lobe is suspended from a force transducer in a manner such that it touches the animal only at the lobar hilus. A balloon catheter placed in the lobar vein allows to increase venous pressure by inflating the balloon. Measuring microvascular filtration rate in intact lung preparations assumes that lymph flow is either measured by canulating a lobar hilar lymph duct, or tied off. Intact lung preparations do not have the disadvantages of the isolated lung preparations mentioned above, probably since the pulmonary circulation is never interrupted.

Techniques have been developed [37] where the lungs are left in place but perfused through an extracorporeal circuit. The circuit includes a perfusate reservoir which is suspended from a force transducer. Changes in lung weight can be measured as the opposite in the reservoir weight changes. It is not clear whether this technique presents any advantage compared to the isolated lung preparation.

## Lung water clearance

### Lymph flow

In intact lung models, weight gain is equal to the difference between filtration rate and lymphatic clearance: $\Delta W/\Delta t = J_v - J_l$. In steady state conditions where there is no weight gain $J_v = J_l$, therefore filtration can also be estimated by measuring lymph flow, assuming that the total lung lymph flow is collected (*see* Chapter 11). This motivated investigators to develop techniques allowing measurement of lymph flow (and solute concentration) by cannulation of lymphatic vessels. Lymphatic cannulation techniques have been developed in sheep and in dogs, both in acute and chronic preparations [38], in intact and isolated lung models [39].

The assumption that lymph flow approximates microvascular filtration is reasonable in steady state conditions, however when edema develops, as lung lymph flow plateaus, other escape pathways drain interstitial fluid in parallel with the lymphatic system. The peribronchovascular spaces extending to the mediastinum, the pleural and alveolar spaces are among these pathways. This leads to progressive underestimation of microvascular filtration by lymph flow as filtration increases. Moreover, Drake et al. [39] observed that as lymph flow increases in hydrostatic edema, the resistance of the lymphatic cannula becomes significantly greater than that of the upstream lymphatic vessel, impeding lymph flow and leading to an underestimation of the increase in microvascular filtration. Flow from a cannulated lymphatic approaches flow in the intact lymphatic only when the cannula resistance and outflow height are adjusted to the resistance of the downstream lymphatic plus central venous pressure.

According to the assumption that $Jl = Jf$ in steady state conditions, in order to measure filtration, the total lymph drained from the lung should be collected. However, there is no single efferent lymphatic that drains the entire lung. Erdmann et al. report that approximately 70% of lung lymph was collected in sheep [40].

Another important point is that the collected lung lymph should not be contaminated by systemic lymph. In a sheep model developed by Staub et al. [38], the caudal mediastinal lymph node was canulated and the tail of the node was resected in order to avoid contamination by abdominal lymph. In a dog preparation, Martin et al. [41] found that lymph afferent to the left tracheobronchial node was not contaminated by extrapulmonary sources as opposed to the lymph collected at the right lymph duct [41]. The advantage of the model developed by Staub et al. is that it allows long-term lymph sampling in intact unanesthetized animals until the resected lymphatic vessels regenerate.

There is evidence that significant fluid exchange may take place when lymph traverses lymph nodes [42]. Postnodal lymph protein concentrations in the sheep model may not represent filtrate protein concentrations unless filtration and lymph flow are large. A solution to this problem is to collect prenodal lymph as in the above dog preparation [41]. Lung lymph flow rate approximates 30 [103] to 65 µl/min/100 g lung weight [43].

In summary, lymphatic cannulation techniques measure lymphatic clearance of fluid and solute from a given lung territory. Only if sufficient precaution is taken, microvascular filtration and protein flux can be estimated from lymph flow and protein concentration. Despite the problems mentioned above, measurement of lymph flow and protein content remains a valuable method for the monitoring of microvascular filtration in intact animals.

### Airway fluid clearance

*Isolated lung:* Isolated perfused lung preparations have been used to determine the rate of fluid clearance from the alveoli [3], with the difference that the lungs are usually not ventilated as absence of ventilation does not seem to affect alveolar fluid clearance [44]. A solution containing a labeled macromolecule is instilled in the air spaces. Changes in the concentration of this macromolecular indicator allow calculation of the net fluid movement between the alveoli and the interstitium. Measuring changes in lung weight allows estimation of the net fluid exchange between the lung and the perfusate, assuming that these changes are not due to variations in lung blood volume (*see* Section on *Isolated lung*, p. 184). Eventual loss of the labeled macromolecule out of the alveoli can be corrected for by measuring its concentration in the perfusate. The rate of fluid removal from the lung is proportional both to hydraulic conductance (or permeability to water) and surface area, neither of which can be separately estimated in these preparations.

Isolated non-perfused lung models have also been developed to study the rate of alveolar fluid clearance, based on observations that the absence of blood flow did not alter the rate of fluid removal from the alveoli for a few hours [5, 44–46]. This technique has been applied to surgically resected carcinomatous human lung lobes [47].

*Intact lung:* Alveolar fluid clearance has been studied in intact lungs of anesthetized and mechanically ventilated sheep [48], dogs [49] rabbits [50], and rats [51]. Berthiaume et al. [162] found that fluid was removed at a rate of 8.3%/h in the first 4 h after instillation of autologous serum in sheep lungs. Liquid removal progressively slowed to 3.3 and 1.4%/h at 12 and 24 h, respectively, in relation to the rising protein osmotic pressure of the residual protein in the air spaces. By 24 h, approximately 80% of the instilled fluid had been removed. Similar *in vivo* studies have measured slower alveolar fluid clearance rates in dogs and faster clearance rates in rabbits and rats. Measurement of lung lymph flow may also be performed in *in vivo* models, either to determine the fraction of alveolar fluid removed from the lung by the lymphatic circulation [33], or to estimate microvascular filtration of fluid and protein [3].

*Pleural fluid clearance*

A thorough review of experimental techniques used to measure the clearance of fluid and solute out of the pleural cavity can be found in [7]. In intact sheep lung, Wiener-Kronish et al. measured the rate of equilibration of intravenously injected radiolabeled albumin [52]. A pleural fluid turnover rate of 11%/h was calculated from the half time of equilibration between plasma and pleural liquid. In another study, the clearance of an experimentally induced hydrothorax was estimated by dilution of [111]In-labeled transferrin at various time intervals [53]. Pleural removal of radiolabeled albumin was measured simultaneously. The rate of lymphatic clearance of the instilled pleural fluid was estimated from the rate of removal of [51]Cr-labeled erythrocytes, which were assumed to leave the pleural cavity only through the lymphatic stomata due to their size. Pleural liquid was cleared at a rate of 0.28 ml/kg/h, 89% of which was cleared by the lymphatics. Negrini et al. studied the pleural distribution and clearance of small pleural boluses of $^{99m}$Tc-labeled albumin using external gamma detection in dogs [54]. The authors calculated an albumin egress rate of 0.24 mg/kg/h and a pleural liquid clearance rate of 0.024 ml/kg/h.

Clearance of lung edema into the pleural space was demonstrated in sheep, in increased permeability pulmonary edema by Wiener-Kronish et al. [15], and in increased hydrostatic pressure edema by Broaddus et al. [16]. Pleural clearance represented 21% and 23% of the total excess in lung water in the two studies respectively. The pleural space, and the parietal pleural lymphatics, therefore seem to play a significant role in the clearance of edema fluid from the lungs in early pulmonary edema.

In humans the rate of clearance of pleural effusions of various etiologies have been measured by dilution of T-1824 and radiolabeled human serum albumin [7] however, no data is available on the physiological rate of pleural fluid and protein clearance in humans

## *Lung water = filtration − clearance*

### *Lung weight (isolated lung)*
Changes in lung weight cannot monitor variations in extravascular lung water unless extravascular lung water and blood volume are measured independently or unless an elevation in microvascular pressure is imposed to separate these two variables (*see* Section on *Isolated lung*, p. 184)

### *Indicator dilution*
The methods for determining extravascular lung water using dilution of two indicators have been reviewed by Giuntini et al. [55]. This technique has received a wide application in the monitoring of pulmonary edema in intensive care patients. It will be described in the chapter on *Indicator dilution technique (extravascular thermal lung volume*, p. 197).

### Gravimetry

Considered as the gold standard for the measurement of extravascular lung water, this technique consists in the *post mortem* measurement of the wet to dry lung weight ratio. By definition this technique cannot be applied to intact lungs. In order to measure the dry weight, the lung is homogenized and samples of homogenate are weighed. Early methods used an oven or compressed air to dry lung specimens [2], however this procedure took up to 2 weeks. More recently a technique using a microwave oven was described [56]. Lung specimens were dried in approximately 1 h using this method.

The accuracy of the wet/dry weight ratio is affected by two technical problems: the water content of residual blood, and changes in dry lung weight [57] in high permeability pulmonary edema. Correction for the water content of residual blood can be made by measuring the hemoglobin concentration in blood and in the supernatant of homogenized lung after ultracentrifugation to determine residual blood. Drying blood specimens then allows to calculate the water content of the residual blood. The dog lung weighs approximately 0.8% of body weight. Its extravascular water normalized for dry blood-free lung weight is 3.6 or 4 ml/kg body weight [57]. The human lung weighs approximately 1% of body weight. Its wet/dry weight ratio is 5.2 and its extravascular water normalized for dry blood-free lung weight is 4.0 [57]. Increase in the dry weight of the lung may occur due to filtration of protein from plasma to the lung interstitium and alveoli in edema. Measurement of the dry weight of a sample of edema fluid with the measured increase in lung water, allows to correct for excess dry weight [57].

### Pathology

Investigators have developed and used scoring criteria to assess the degree of alveolar flooding based on the examination of lung tissue by light microscopy [2, 58]. Such methods can provide valuable information on the anatomic distribution of edema and lung injury, and may be used as an adjunct to physiological studies [2].

## Starling equation components

### Microvascular pressure

Pulmonary capillary pressure depends on pulmonary arterial and venous pressures. Pulmonary arterial pressure itself depends on venous pressure, blood flow, and pulmonary vascular resistances. Pulmonary venous pressure, in the absence of valvular disease reflects left ventricular end diastolic pressure. Pulmonary capillary pressure is influenced by the distribution of resistances along the pulmonary vascular bed; if most of the resistance is on the venous side, then capillary pressure will be closer to arterial rather than venous pressure and vice versa. This may explain why pulmonary arterial wedge pressure underestimates the effective pressure that commands filtration at the capillary level, under pathological conditions where venous resistance may represent over 50% of the total resistance of the pulmonary circulation, particularly in ARDS [59]. In such conditions, capillary pressure may be better approximated by pulmonary arterial pressure than by $P_{wp}$.

Finally, capillary pressure is a dynamic parameter. Vascular resistance is determined not only by transmural pressure and mechanical properties of the vessel walls, but also by changes in vascular smooth muscle tone in response to cellular mediators and pharmacological agents.

*Direct measurement by micropuncture:* Techniques to measure microvascular pressure by micropuncture in the lungs were initially developed by Bhattacharya et al. [60]. These methods have been used in intact [60, 61] as well as isolated [62] lungs. Subpleural arterioles and venules of approximately 20 μm in diameter can be punctured by means of a glass micropipette (tip diameter 3 μm). Micropuncture requires lung ventilation to be stopped for a few minutes to avoid interference with lung movements.

An important advantage of these techniques is that they allow determination of pressure in a microvessel whose diameter is precisely known. However, since morphological differences between superficial and deep lung microvessels have been shown [63], the microvascular pressures measured by this technique may not represent vascular pressures in the lung interior.

## Indirect measurements

*Isogravimetric filtration pressure:* This technique was developed by Gaar et al. in 1967 [64]. In an isogravimetric (not losing or gaining weight) isolated perfused lung, pulmonary arterial and venous pressures, and pulmonary blood flow are measured. For a given venous pressure, as pulmonary blood flow is decreased, pulmonary arterial and capillary pressures decrease, and the lung tends to lose weight. Gaar et al. decreased pulmonary blood flow in a stepwise fashion and at each step, increased the pulmonary venous pressure to keep the lung isogravimetric. When pulmonary arterial pressure at each step is plotted against blood flow, its pressure axis intercept is the isogravimetric filtration pressure. Isogravimetric filtration pressure is equal to capillary pressure if it is assumed that filtration occurs essentially in capillary vessels, however up to 25% of microvascular filtration may occur at extracapillary sites [65]. Isogravimetric filtration pressure is approximately half-way between pulmonary arterial and venous pressures. The technique assumes reaching a reliable isogravimetric condition which in practice requires 10 to 15 min for each pulmonary blood flow state. In injured lung, isogravimetric condition is obtained at low levels of vascular pressures, when derecruitment of injured capillaries may occur. Isogravimetric filtration pressure is then more representative of the less damaged capillaries.

*Retrograde catheterization:* Initially applied to the lung by Takahashi and Butler in 1967, this technique consists in introducing a fine (outside diameter: approx. 1 mm) polyethylene catheter in a pulmonary vein. The distal end of the catheter is threaded up a small vein and pushed out through the lung tissue. The distal extremity is then pulled until the flanged proximal extremity of the catheter occludes a small tributary to the pulmonary vein where pressure is being measured. The same maneuver can be performed through a pulmonary artery [66]. Hakim and Kelly estimated that the proximal catheter tips are lodged in tributaries less than 0.9 mm in diameter. Comparison of capillary pressures estimated by this method and by micropuncture and venous and arterial occlusion has shown consistent results [67], however retrograde catheterization is not applicable in *in vivo* lung preparations and its overall experimental use has been limited.

*Arterial, venous, and double occlusion:* If the pulmonary artery and vein of the same vascular territory, perfused at constant blood flow are simultaneously occluded, arterial pressure downstream to the occlusion site, and venous pressure upstream from the occlusion site, converge rapidly towards a common intermediate pressure level or *double occlusion pressure*, at the site of maximal vascular compliance, that is at the capillary level. Linehan et al. initially used this method to estimate capillary pressure in isolated perfused dog lung lobes [68]. However, due to difficulty in obtaining simultaneously the occlusion of both an artery and vein with the same vascular territory, this technique cannot be reliably executed *in vivo* using the inflation of balloon-tipped catheters.

In isolated lung preparations rapid occlusion of arterial inflow results in a characteristic arterial pressure profile with an initial nearly instantaneous drop followed by a slower exponential-like declining component. A few oscillations due to the occlusion itself may be observed in the rapid phase. Rapid occlusion of venous outflow results in a quick initial increase followed by a slow, almost linear elevation of the venous pressure profile as long as the venous occlusion is maintained [69]. If a single pulmonary vein is occluded, the slow component of the post occlusion venous pressure profile will be exponential, and will equalize with the pulmonary artery pressure.

Different methods have been proposed to determine capillary pressure. These methods consist in fitting a single or double exponential relationship to the post occlusion pressure tracings, whether an R-C-R (R: resistance, C: capacitance) or a C-R-C-R-C model of the pulmonary circulation is used to interpret the post-occlusion profiles. Capillary pressure has been estimated using the R-C-R model from either visual determination of the breakpoint between the fast and slow exponential components [70], or by back-extrapolation of the slow exponential component towards the instant of occlusion [66]. Capillary pressure may also been corrected using a double exponential fit of the post-occlusion pressure profiles and a C-R-C-R-C model which allows to interpret the fast phase of the arterial post-occlusion curve as the emptying of an arterial compartment, and the fast phase of the venous post-occlusion curve as the filling of a venous compartment [71].

Estimations of capillary pressure using a monoexponential fit of arterial post-occlusion and venous post-occlusion pressure profiles and an R-C-R model for interpretation are not identical. Capillary pressures estimated from arterial post-occlusion pressure profiles are slightly higher than those estimated by venous post-occlusion pressure profiles. Capillary pressure estimated from double occlusion is intermediate. These differences have been attributed to the existence of capillary resistances or to the interpretation of post-occlusion pressure curves by a R-C-R model. Double occlusion pressure has been used as a reference for capillary pressure and compared to estimates of capillary pressure by arterial and venous occlusions [66].

## Interstitial liquid pressure

Interstitial liquid pressure is determined by several factors; transpulmonary pressure, the elastic recoil of the lung, the water content of the interstitium, and alveolar surface tension are among these factors [72–74]. Both indirect and direct techniques have been used to estimate interstitial pressure. Using an indirect approach, Meyer and Guyton initially reported negative pressures in chronically implanted fluid-filled polyethylene capsules in dog lungs [75]. Snashall et al. estimated interstitial pressure in isogravimetric isolated lung lobes from the Starling equation, assuming that $\sigma = 1$ for the capillary endothelium [76]. Parker et al. measured the pressure in a small occluded lung segment, after instillation of Tyrode solution or plasma [77]. They allowed the pressure in the occluded lung segment to equilibrate for 30 min. They calculated subatmospheric interstitial pressures using the Starling equation, with simultaneous estimation of the osmotic reflection coefficient of the alveolar epithelium. Lai-Fook et al. used glass micropipettes to measure alveolar epithelial lining fluid pressure. They assumed that the pressure in the sub-phase of the epithelial lining fluid, which is reduced below the alveolar gas pressure due to surface tension forces comes into equilibrium with the interstitial fluid pressure.

Among direct approaches, wick catheters [78] and micropuncture techniques [72] have been used to estimate pressures within the interstitial compartment at the hilum. Using the latter technique, the inflated lung lobe is held in place using a vacuum ring and viewed through a ste-

181

reoscopic microscope. A beveled glass micropipette (tip diameter 2 μm) is introduced through the visceral pleura into the interstitium. The pressure at the distal extremity of the micropipette is recorded by the servo-null technique. The servo-null technique uses variations in micropipette electrical resistance to measure pressure. In a micropipette with a small quantity of buffer fluid in its tip, null resistance is established. Variations in the pressure of the fluid surrounding the tip will move fluid in or out of the micropipette. The resulting changes in resistance are opposed by a counter pressure to return the micropipette resistance back to null [79]. The micropuncture method has been used to estimate interstitial pressure in isolated lung [80] and in intact lungs [81]. Interstitial pressure can be estimated at alveolar junctions as well as in the adventitia of microvessels of approximately 50 μm, at a depth of about 50 to 200 μm below the visceral pleural level.

Using this method in isolated dog lung, Bhattacharya et al. found alveolar junctional and adventitial pressures, respectively 0.5 and −0.4 cm $H_2O$ that were below alveolar pressure set at 7 cm $H_2O$. The authors showed that a pressure gradient existed from the lung periphery to the hilum, which was reduced in edema and at increased alveolar pressure [61]. This pressure gradient could participate in the removal of interstitial fluid directly from the interstitium into the mediastinum [80]. However, it is not established whether this route plays a significant role in the overall removal of lung fluid. Interstitial fluid pressure seems height independent in the isolated lung in which lung recoil is uniform. Height-dependent variations in interstitial pressure have been observed in intact lungs [82] and may be related to variations in lung recoil [80]. The important decrease of interstitial pressure recently measured in several experimental models of inflammation in the systemic circulation may renew the interest in the measurement of interstitial pressure [83].

## Plasma protein osmotic pressure

Plasma colloid osmotic pressure can be measured directly using commercially available membrane osmometers. The apparatus was described by Prather et al. [84] and comprises two chambers separated by a synthetic polymer semipermeable membrane. One chamber is connected to an electronic pressure transducer, and filled with an isotonic saline solution with no colloid osmotic pressure. The other chamber is filled with the solution in which the colloid osmotic pressure is to be measured. The semipermeable membrane allows passage of water and solutes freely but retains macromolecules. Plasma colloid osmotic pressure can also be calculated from the measurement of total proteins using either refractometry or chemical technique as the Biuret method. This calculation is improved using albumin and globulin measurement by electrophoresis [85]. Plasma colloid osmotic pressure is approximately 27.5 mm Hg in man and 17.5 mm Hg in dog [85].

## Interstitial colloid osmotic pressure

The pulmonary interstitium is located between the capillary endothelium and the alveolar epithelial cells. The ground substance surrounding tissue cells consists of a collagen network, containing a gel phase made of glycosaminoglycans and proteoglycans that have a high affinity for water and tend to hold fluid within the gel matrix. The dense meshwork of the interstitial gel-phase allows free diffusion of water molecules, but restricts the diffusion of macromolecules such as albumin and globulin [86]. As microvascular filtration increases, tissue colloid osmotic pressure decreases. This is not only due to dilution of plasma proteins filtered into the interstitium by a protein-poor fluid, but also related to a convective protein washdown of the interstitium by transvascular fluid flow [104] and to an increase in the protein available space with increased hydration of the interstitium [87]. The rise in plasma to interstitial colloid osmotic gradient tends to limit an increase in microvascular filtration, and is considered as one of the safety factors against edema formation.

Techniques for direct sampling of interstitial fluid using glass pipettes, small catheters and wick methods, have been used to estimate interstitial colloid osmotic pressure in other organs. Normandin et al. [88] introduced a wick catheter through a mediastinoscope into the interstitium surrounding pulmonary vessels in dogs. They were able to collect sufficient interstitial fluid for analysis only after infusion of lactated Ringer's. They did not find significant differences between colloid osmotic pressures estimated by the wick method as compared to those estimated from the lymph protein concentration collected at the right lymph duct.

The most widely used method to estimate interstitial colloid osmotic pressure has been from lymph protein concentration. Colloid osmotic pressure is estimated from protein concentration using equations initially derived for plasma [89]. It is generally assumed that prenodal lymph protein concentration is representative of that of the protein available space in the interstitium, at least in steady state conditions. The lymph to plasma protein osmotic pressure gradient is in the 5 to 6 mm Hg range in dog in control conditions [190]. However, as discussed in the Section on *Analysis of lymph protein flux data*, p. 193, cannulation of a lymph vessel may alter resistance to lymph flow and possibly the protein concentration [6]. There is no single lymph vessel that drains the entire lungs, therefore it is usually assumed that the collected lymph is representative of lung lymph as a whole, and that it is not contaminated by lymph from other organs (*see* Section on *Isolated lung*, p. 173).

Interstitial protein osmotic pressure may also be measured using the accumulation in the interstitium of a radiolabeled diffusible protein infused in blood. This technique requires a second radiolabeled tracer restricted to the vascular space to differentiate protein activity in interstitium from combined protein activity in blood and interstitium. The protein tagged with a gamma-emitting tracer may be detected non invasively by external scintillation probes for 150–180 min. The regional interstitial volume of distribution of the tracer protein under the external probe may be calculated from transport rate constants of the radiolabeled protein from blood into and out of the extravascular space, allowing the calculation of interstitial protein concentration and colloid osmotic pressure [90]. In sheep, the results correlate with those of direct measurements in lung lymph.

### Filtration coefficient ($K_{f,c}$)

*Isolated lung:* Filtration coefficient can be determined by measuring the increase in filtration rate that results from an imposed elevation in microvascular pressure. $K_{f,c}$ is expressed as milliliters per minute per pressure units per 100 g lung weight assuming 1 ml = 1 g. When $\Delta W/\Delta t$ is plotted as a function of time following the microvascular pressure increase, there is an initial rapid weight gain phase (approximately 3 min) that represents mostly the change in lung vascular volume, followed by a slow weight gain phase which represents mostly transcapillary fluid filtration if lymphatic drainage is ligated (Fig. 8.3). Increases in lung capillary recruitment and vascular stress relaxation are usually minimized by perfusing the lung preparation in zone 3 conditions (pulmonary arterial pressure > pulmonary venous pressure > airway pressure) where recruitment is assumed to approach its maximum. Some investigators have also used vasodilators such as papaverine to reduce changes in vasomotor tone in isolated lung experiments.

$K_{f,c}$ *at time zero:* Since transcapillary Starling forces will change with time as fluid leaves the capillary bed, i.e., interstitial pressure will increase and tissue protein osmotic pressure will decrease, Drake, Gaar and Taylor recommended the extrapolation of the slow component of the weight gain curve back to time 0 when no changes in transcapillary Starling forces have yet occurred [91]. $K_{f,c}$ is calculated from:

$$K_{f,c}(0) = (\Delta W/\Delta t)/\Delta P_c \qquad (t = 0 \text{ min})$$

Alternatively, the weight transient shown in Figure 8.3 may be analyzed by a bi-exponential equation [92]:

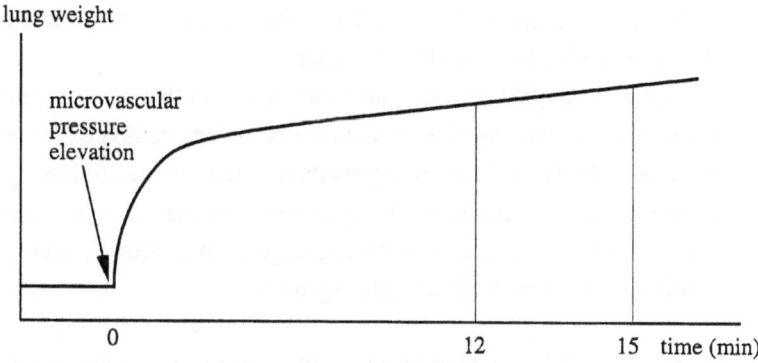

**Figure 8.3. Filtration coefficient measurement with lung weight**
See text.

$$W = a(1-e^{-bt}) + c(1-e^{-dt})$$
$$\text{vascular filling} \qquad \text{interstitial filling}$$

where the first and second term represent weight gain due to vascular and interstitial filling, respectively. a and c represent the maximum increase in weight associated with each term and may be used to calculate vascular and interstitial compliance. $K_{f,c}$ can be calculated as $c \cdot d/P_c$, as shown in [92].

$K_{f,c}$ *at time t:* A different approach in determining $K_{f,c}$ consists in measuring $\Delta W/\Delta t$ after a given time interval t (e.g. $\Delta t$ from $t = 12$ to $t = 15$ min) after $P_c$ elevation. $K_{f,c}$ is determined from the slope of the $\Delta W/\Delta t$ curve [93]:

$$K_{f,c(t)} = \frac{(\Delta W / \Delta t)}{\Delta P_c} \qquad t = 12 \text{ to } t = 15 \text{ min)}$$

*Hematocrit or protein densitometry:* A different approach to the measurement of transcapillary fluid filtration in isolated perfused lungs was proposed by Oppenheimer et al. [94] based on the hemoconcentration of the perfusing blood following an imposed elevation in microvascular pressure. Changes in the hematocrit of the perfusing blood were detected by changes in the absorbance of infrared laser light, provided flow remains constant. Transcapillary filtration is then calculated from the changes in hematocrit. Transcapillary filtration rate by this technique varies little during a constant $P_c$ elevation.

Parker et al. [95], in a dog lung model, found that $K_{f,c(0)}$ significantly overestimated transcapillary filtration coefficient compared to both the $K_{f,c(t)}$, and the laser densitometry method in the minutes following an increase in capillary pressure. However filtration rates by gravimetric and densitometric techniques tend to converge 20 min after $P_c$ elevation towards a value of 0.05 ml/min/mm Hg/100 g.

*Intact lung:* When the lung is not gaining or losing weight, it can be assumed that transcapillary fluid filtration is equal to lymph flow. In this case, the filtration coefficient can be estimated if lymph flow and the total Starling force imbalance are known:

$$J_l = J_v = K_{f,c} \left[ (P_{mv} - P_{pmv}) - \sigma(\Pi_{mv} - \Pi_{pmv}) \right]$$

or: $\quad K_{f,c} = J_l / \left[ (P_{mv} - P_{pmv}) - \sigma(\Pi_{mv} - \Pi_{pmv}) \right]$

Where $\left[ (P_{mv} - P_{pmv}) - \sigma(\Pi_{mv} - \Pi_{pmv}) \right]$ represents the Starling force imbalance. It can be assumed that the lymph protein osmotic pressure equals perimicrovascular protein osmotic pressure $\Pi_{pmv}$ and that perimicrovascular pressure ($P_{pmv}$) is constant and equal to the mean alveolar pressure i.e., zero. It can also be assumed that the microvascular wall is impermeable to protein macromolecules therefore $\sigma = 1$ [41]. Plasma and lymph protein osmotic pressures can be measured as well as microvascular pressure. Having made these assumptions, $K_{f,c}$ can be calculated by:

$$K_{f,c} = J_l / \left[ P_{mv} - \sigma(\Pi_{mv} - \Pi_{pmv}) \right]$$

The major disadvantage of this technique is that it requires multiple assumptions. The above calculated $K_{f,c}$ [41] underestimates by an order of magnitude $K_{f,c}$ measured by hemoconcentration [94]. This difference may be explained by a model including a high resistance pathway between the perimicrovascular space and the initial lymphatics [87].

## PS

While $\sigma$ is a measure of the selectivity of the microvascular barrier to a particular protein, the PS product contains both the selectivity and the total area available for exchange. The PS product measures the diffusive capacity of the membrane, and is expressed as $\mu l \cdot min^{-1}$.

*Small solute PS product:* This technique involves the simultaneous bolus injection of a vascular-restricted or reference indicator, and a diffusible indicator in the arterial circulation of the lung (Fig. 8.4). Repeated sampling of pulmonary venous blood leaving the lung or of systemic arterial blood allows to record a concentration-time curve for each indicator. The vascular or reference indicator reaches a higher peak concen-

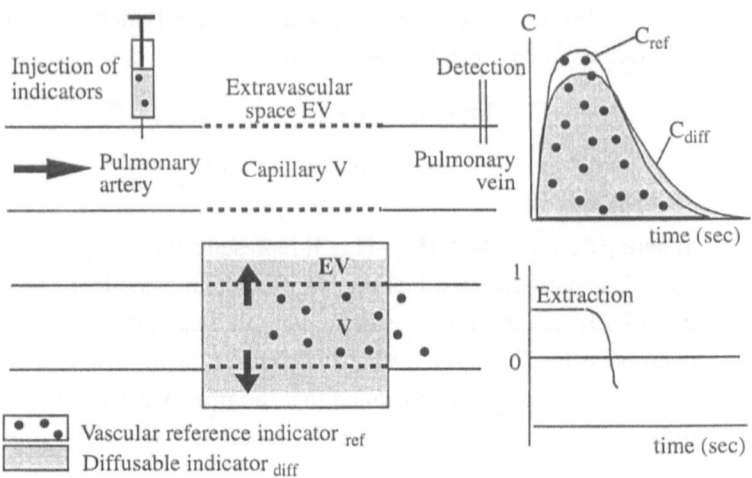

**Figure 8.4. Measurement of small solute PS product**
See text.

tration more rapidly than the diffusible indicator, and its concentration will fall more rapidly than the diffusible indicator. The proportion of the diffusible indicator that has left the circulation, or the *extraction* can be described by:

$$E = \frac{(C_{ref} - C_{diff})}{C_{ref}} \tag{1}$$

The total flux of the diffusible solute ($J_s$) across the microvascular barrier is described by:

$$J_s = \dot{Q}_p (C_{ref} - C_{diff}) \tag{2}$$

where $\dot{Q}_p$ is the plasma flow rate through the lung. For a few seconds following indicator bolus injection, diffusible solute flow is unidirectional from plasma to interstitium. $J_s$ can also be described as:

$$J_s = PS \, \overline{\Delta C} \tag{3}$$

where $\overline{\Delta C}$ is the average concentration gradient across the microvascular barrier. Combining Eqs (2) and (3) yields [96]:

$$PS = -\dot{Q}_p \ln(1 - E)$$

where $\dot{Q}_p$ is calculated from the integrated area for the reference indicator corrected for recirculation.

According to Crone [95], the indicator diffusion technique reaches maximal accuracy for extraction values of approximately 0.2 to 0.5. When the diffusibility of the tracer is high enough or the plasma flow rate low enough, the value of the PS product is determined more by blood flow rate than by permeability of the endothelial barrier and approaches 1. Such diffusible indicators are called "flow limited". When the diffusibility of the tracer is low, the measurement of extraction is affected by a low signal/noise ratio and PS product value approaches 0. Two corrections must also be achieved, a correction for the Taylor interlaminar effect related to the late appearance of diffusible indicator as compared to that of the reference indicator in the blood, and a correction for the red cell permeability of some diffusible indicators (e.g. urea) [96].

In order to minimize errors in the value of extraction due to flow inhomogeneity and interlaminar effect, extraction may be determined by calculating the difference in the areas of the reference and diffusible indicator curves. This is done by integrating the area difference over a given time interval. Usually this is the time interval between the appearance ($t_a$) of the reference indicator and its peak ($t_p$) to avoid backdiffusion of the diffusible indicator into the plasma.

$$E = \int_{t_a}^{t_p} \frac{(C_{ref} - C_{diff})}{C_{ref}} dt$$

Using this technique, PS products for various solutes such as sodium, urea, sucrose and inulin have been determined in different animal models as well as in humans.

*Macromolecule PS product:* The historical development of the methods for determining the protein PS product has been thoroughly reviewed by Taylor et al. [97]. Two problems must be considered. Since the solute flux equation used to determine $\sigma$ using the filtration-independent approach (*see* Section on *Small solute PS product*, p. 187), predicts that the diffusive component of solute exchange approaches zero at high filtration rate ($J_v$), PS cannot be measured in these experiments. Another difficulty in determining PS is that it is also contained in the non-linear term $[x/(e^x-1)]$ modifying PS$\Delta$C.

*Analysis of transcapillary labeled protein flux:* Analysis of the transcapillary flux of radiolabeled protein macromolecules such as albumin has been used to estimate the PS product. Kern et al. [98] described a single sample technique for determining PS in an isolated perfused rabbit lung model. Perfusate containing $^{125}$I labeled albumin is introduced in the arterial catheter. After 3 min, the perfusion is stopped and the lung vasculature is washed with perfusate not containing the indicator. The lung is weighed and homogenized and samples of the homogenate are counted for $^{125}$I activity. The flux of radiolabeled protein ($J_s$) can be described as:

$$J_s = \frac{A}{t}$$
(4)

Where A is the quantity of $^{125}$I-albumin measured in the tissue, and t is the exposure time in minutes. According to the Kedem and Katchalsky [18] equation (*see* Section on *Lung protein filtration and clearance*, p. 166), when the lung is not gaining or losing weight, i.e. there is no transvascular fluid filtration and the description of solute flux which simplifies to diffusive flux is

$$J_s = PS(C_p - C_i)$$
(5)

where Cp is the indicator concentration in the perfusate, and Ci is the indicator concentration in the interstitium. If it is assumed that the concentration of the indicator in the interstitium is negligible during the 3 min infusion of tracer, Ci can be deleted from the equation, therefore:

$$J_s = PSC_p$$
(6)

Combining Eqs (4) and (6) yields:

$$PS = \frac{A}{tC_p} \qquad (7)$$

This approach is based on the assumption that all of the tracer protein filtered across the microvascular barrier is retained in the interstitium. An advantage of this technique is that PS products are obtained per gram tissue weight. However, this technique will underestimate the PS product in an intact lung preparation, where the lymphatic circulation will remove a significant amount of tracer protein. Kern et al. [98] calculated a PS product of 2.28 $\mu l \cdot min^{-1} \cdot g^{-1}$ blood-free wet lung using this experimental approach in isolated rabbit lungs.

Using the same approach, $\sigma$ can be determined by cumulating data from several isolated lung experiments. When the lung is gaining weight, the Kedem and Katchalsky equation can be written for plasma protein clearance (or protein flux normalized to $C_p$) as:

$$J_s/C_p = PS + J_v(1-\sigma)$$

The weight gain ($J_v$) during the albumin infusion can be measured. Using the $J_s/C_p$ and $J_v$ from several experiments, a regression line of $J_s/C_p$ vs. $J_v$ can be determined. The slope of this regression line equals $(1-\sigma)$, and the y intercept equals PS [99] (Fig. 8.5).

The PS estimated by all of the methods discussed above is actually the product of PS and the modifying term $[x/(e^x-1)]$.

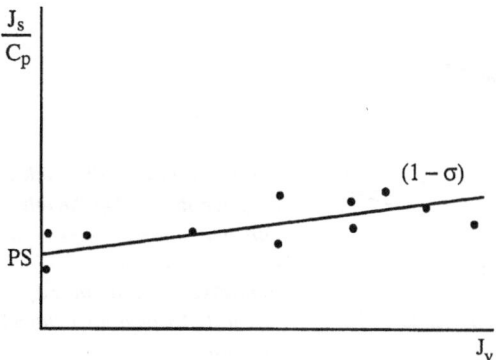

Figure 8.5. Analysis of transvascular labeled protein flux (normalized to Cp) $J_s/C_p$ using its relationship to transvascular water flow $J_v$ See text. Adapted from [99] with permission.

*Unique PS product:* Recently, Reed et al. [100] introduced a new approach to determine a unique PS product i.e. a PS product without the modifying term $[x/(e^x-1)]$, in other words independent of $J_v$, using lymphatic solute flux data. According to the solute flux equation (Patlak equation) as filtration increases, the diffusive component of solute flux first reaches a maximum, then slowly declines (Fig. 8.6). It is shown that at this maximum diffusion point, the peclet number ($x_{max, diff}$) is independent of $J_v$, and is determined by the reflection coefficient $\sigma$ only. When solute flux is measured as a function of lymph flow (filtration rate), the solute flux curve is initially curvilinear then becomes linear. The transition point can be determined graphically and represents the filtration rate at which maximal diffusion occurs or $J_{d, max}$. Thereafter $\sigma$ can be determined from the slope of the linear part of the solute flux curve. A unique peclet number can be calculated at $J_{d, max}$ by the following equation [100]:

$$\sigma = e^{x_{max,diff}} \left(1 - x_{max,diff}\right)$$

The derivation of this equation and the determination of x, once s is known is fully discussed by Reed et al. [101].

A unique PS product can be calculated using the filtration rate at the maximal diffusion point $J_{d, max}$, by modifying the equation defining the Peclet number (*see* Section on *Protein filtration*, p. 166):

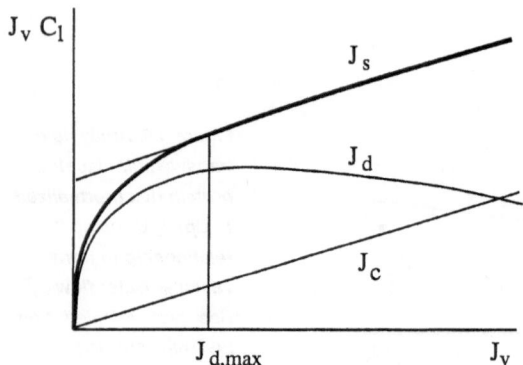

Figure 8.6. Unique PS Product determination using the relationship between transvascular labeled protein flux $J_s$ and transvascular water flow $J_v$ See text. Adapted from [10] with permission.

$$PS = \frac{(1-\sigma)J_{d,\max}}{x}$$

Ishibashi et al. [102] used this approach in an intact dog lung model to determine a PS product of 15 μl/min for total protein. This technique has the technical inconveniences associated with lymphatic cannulation. Its advantage is that it allows calculation of both a PS and a σ that are independent of microvascular filtration.

### Sigma (σ)

*Analysis of lymph protein flux data:* Different approaches have been used to estimate the reflection coefficient of the lung microvascular barrier to proteins by analysis of lymphatic protein flux. Granger and Taylor [19] used this equation to estimate σ in steady-state experiments where microvascular filtration $J_v$ (and consequently lymph flow) is elevated.

$$\sigma = 1 - \frac{C_l}{C_p}$$

As mentioned earlier (*see* Section on *Protein filtration*, p. 166), this estimation is theoretically possible because when $J_v$ is increased, the Peclet number x, (which describes the diffusive macromolecule flux capacity relative to convective flux capacity) increases, and the diffusive component of the Patlak equation approaches zero. This is exact only when $x = \infty$, however when the term $J_v/PS$ of the Peclet number exceeds 10 for a protein fraction, the lymph protein concentration decreases to a constant value, in other words becomes filtration independent.

$$x = (1-\sigma)\frac{J_v}{PS}$$

It is important to note that for a given filtration rate, plasma protein clearance will be higher for solutes with a larger effective hydrodynamic radius. Parker et al. found that $J_v/PS$ was sufficiently high for $C_l/C_p$ ratio to represent $(1-\sigma)$ only for protein fractions with a radius of 100 Å and above, and that σ was under-estimated for albumin (37 Å) by this method [103].

Reed et al. introduced a new approach to determine a unique PS (i.e. independent of $J_v$) and σ using lymphatic solute flux data [100]. This method is detailed in Section on *Unique PS product*, p. 192. When solute flux is measured as a function of lymph flow (filtration rate), the solute flux curve is initially curvilinear then becomes linear. σ is determined from the slope of the linear part of the solute flux curve. Ishibashi et al. calculated a σ of 0.67 for total protein in a dog lung model using this technique [103].

Methods using measurements of the lymphatic flux of macromolecules are limited by technical difficulties associated with lymphatic cannulation, the difficulty in obtaining lymph that is not contaminated by lymph from other organs, and the fact that they rely on the assumption that lymph macromolecule concentrations reflect that of the interstitium, therefore neglecting possible interstitial transport processes. Moreover, the effects of the height of the lymphatic cannula on lymph flow may be a source of error in the assumption that lymph flow equals filtration rate [39].

*Analysis of labeled macromolecule fluxes:* Labeled macromolecule fluxes from plasma to tissue have been used to estimate σ in isolated-perfused lung preparations (*see* Section on *Analysis of transcapillary labeled protein flux*, p. 190). An advantage of this technique is that it circumvents technical difficulties associated with lymphatic cannulation. Both σ and PS can be determined in isolated lung models using this approach, as long as lymphatic vessels have been ligated. Indeed, Ishibashi et al. demonstrated that in intact lung models (*see* above), σ may be overestimated by this technique due to the lymphatic removal of the tracer protein in the lung. They measured a σ of 0.99 for labeled albumin using plasma to tissue clearance, instead of a σ of 0.80 using combined plasma to tissue and lymph clearance [104].

*Osmotic transient studies:* This method uses the Starling equation to estimate σ in isolated lung preparations [105].

$$J_v = K_{f,c} (\Delta P - \sigma \Delta \Pi)$$

$\sigma$ is estimated by imposing a change in the concentration of a test solute in the perfusate of an isogravimetric lung, therefore non filtering lung. When the concentration of osmotically active substances is modified in the perfusate, this results in a change in $\Delta\Pi$, and the organ loses or gains weight accordingly. The weight-change curve obtained following the change in $\Delta\Pi$ is analyzed to obtain a time-zero weight-change slope or $(\Delta W/\Delta t)_0$. The following equation relates $(\Delta W/\Delta t)_0$ to the osmotic pressure change:

$$J_v = (\Delta W/\Delta t)_0 = K_{f,c}\, \sigma\Delta\Pi$$

Solving this equation for $\sigma$ yields:

$$\sigma = (\Delta W/\Delta t)_0 / K_{f,c}\, \Delta\Pi$$

$K_{f,c}$ is determined prior to the osmotic transient by elevating the capillary pressure and analyzing the weight transient as explained in Section on *Filtration coefficient*, p. 184. Changes in $\Delta\Pi$ can be induced by addition of osmotically active solutes [106, 22] or by dilution of the perfusate [106].

Technical problems with the use of osmotic transients are that a square wave of test solute concentration cannot be presented to the exchanging microvessels, and that fluid can be exchanged with both intracellular and extracellular compartments.

A second approach for measuring $\sigma$ requires measurement of capillary pressure in isogravimetric conditions $(P_{c,i})$ (*see* Section on *Isogravimetric filtration pressure*, p. 179). If $P_{c,i}$ is determined at different colloid osmotic pressures in isogravimetric conditions, the slope of the best-fit line relating $P_{c,i}$ to $\Pi$ is $\sigma$:

$$\Delta P_{c,i} = \sigma\, \Delta\Pi$$

## The filtered volume method

This approach is based on the determination of the masses of water and macromolecule which have left the circulation during a substantial microvascular pressure elevation over a given time. Weiser and Grande [107] initially demonstrated that in an isolated blood perfused organ, the volume of fluid that filters across the microvascular barrier during a given time interval (from $t = t_1$ to $t = t_2$) can be estimated from the rise in hematocrit:

$$V_{f,H} = V_1(1 - \frac{H_1}{H_2})$$

where $V_{f,H}$ is the filtered volume estimated from changes in hematocrit, $V_1$ is the initial perfusate volume, $H_1$ and $H_2$ are the initial and final hematocrits respectively.

Weiser and Grande also defined a volume of protein-free fluid ($V_{f,P}$) filtering across the microvascular barrier during the same time interval:

$$V_{f,P} = V_1(1 - H_1)(1 - \frac{C_1}{C_2})$$

Where C1 and C2 are initial and final perfusate protein macromolecule concentrations respectively. Pilati and Maron [108] first derived an equation to estimate $\sigma$ from calculated filtered volumes. Wolf et al. derived an alternative equation to estimate $\sigma$ in isolated perfused organs from measurements of hematocrit and protein concentrations [109]:

$$\sigma = 1 - \frac{C_2}{\overline{C}}(1 - \frac{V_{f,P}}{V_{f,H}})$$

Where $\overline{C}$ is the logarithmic mean of $C_1$ and $C_2$ [109]. The component

$$(1 - \frac{V_{f,P}}{V_{f,H}})$$

can be described as:

$$(1 - \frac{V_{f,P}}{V_{f,H}}) = \left[1 - \frac{(1 - H_1)(1 - C_1/C_2)}{(1 - H_1/H_2)}\right]$$

The derivation of the above equations relies on the assumption that during the time interval when $V_{f,H}$ and $V_{f,P}$ are measured, the product of filtration rate ($J_v$) and perfusate protein concentration C varies little [109]. It is also assumed that the diffusive protein flux is negligible.

Over-estimation of σ may result from hemolysis of the perfusate, and to a lesser extent, from evaporation of the perfusate. This technique requires a significant and sustained elevation of microvascular pressure and cannot be applied to intact lung models. It has the advantage of circumventing technical difficulties associated with lymphatic protein flux analysis techniques.

Using this experimental approach, White et al. found a mean albumin σ of 0.76 in isolated perfused ferret lungs [110].

## Quantifying pulmonary edema formation and clearance in the clinical setting

### Lung water and edema

### Indicator dilution technique: Extravascular thermal lung volume

When a nondiffusible or intravascular indicator and a freely diffusible indicator are injected together into the pulmonary circulation, the time required for the indicators to reach the outflow vessels or "mean transit time" is much longer for the diffusible indicator, because its volume of distribution is much larger. This difference in distribution volumes or the Extravascular Thermal Volume of the Lung (ETVL) is an estimate of extravascular lung water, assuming that during its transit the diffusible indicator equilibrates with all of the extravascular lung water volume. Extravascular lung water volume can therefore be calculated from mean transit time difference × proportion of water in the blood flow and is usually expressed as ml/kg. Gee at al. [111] initially reported the use of a thermal indicator as the diffusible indicator, and indocyanine green (cardiogreen) which binds to intravascular protein, as the intravascular indicator. The technique was then used at bedside in critically ill patients [112]. In humans, 5 mg indocyanine green and 10 ml cold normal saline are injected into the right atrium via a Swan-Ganz catheter. The indicator concentration curves are recorded in the distal aorta using a 5-F arterial catheter with a thermistor at the tip [113]. Fiberoptic catheters have been developed that allow spectrophotometric measurement of the indocyanine green concentration intravascularly, without sampling of arterial blood [114]. Temperature and concentration curves are recorded and integrated by a computer to calculate mean transit times.

Comparison between ETVL and gravimetric measurements of lung water in animals show good correlation [114]. The technique may not be sensitive to small changes in EVLW in humans [114]. One study reported better accuracy of this method in quantifying extravascular lung water in patients in comparison with portable chest radiogram [115]. ETVL values were found generally higher in permeability than in hydrostatic edema [116]. There is controversy concerning the dependence of ETVL on cardiac output. This dependency is refuted by some [117–119] and confirmed by others [120]. There is evidence however, that extravascular lung water is underestimated by this technique in the presence of regional abnormalities in perfusion [121–123], such as in ARDS or pulmonary embolism. This can be explained by the fact that the thermal indicator will diffuse in the extravascular space, only in areas that are perfused. In addition, there is conflicting experimental data on the effect of positive end expiratory pressure (PEEP) on ETVL [122–124]. ETVL values may vary with PEEP in humans but no objective data is available.

In summary, the thermal volume method is invasive, and subject to error due to perfusion inhomogeneity, which typically occurs in ARDS. However, it is the only quantitative method available in the clinical setting to measure extravascular lung water. In a recent study, Mitchell et al. successfully used ETVL measurement to monitor fluid restriction in patients with pulmonary edema [125]. They showed that the group managed with diuresis and fluid restriction required less mechanical ventilation and were in the intensive care unit for a shorter period of time. However, there is controversy concerning the usefulness of ETVL measurement apart from controlled studies. Although it is a quantitative means of estimating extravascular lung water at bedside, there is no evidence that the benefit/risk ratio of this method in routine is superior to portable chest radiography.

### Imaging techniques
*Chest radiography:* Chest radiography is the most commonly used technique to estimate lung water content in patients. The extravascular accu-

mulation of fluid increases the overall lung tissue density visualized on the chest roentgenogram. Quantitative measurements of extravascular lung water have been shown to correlate with radiographic findings [126]. While it is considered as a sensitive indicator of increased extravascular lung water, sometimes even prior to the onset of cardiorespiratory symptoms [126], the radiograph often lags behind gas exchange abnormalities in lung injury. In a study on patients with sepsis, Wheeler et al. found that over 20% of patients with a $Pa_{O_2}/FI_{O_2}$ ratio of $<300$ had normal radiographs or only mild abnormalities. The majority of patients at risk for ARDS however, will develop chest radiograph abnormalities within 24 h [127].

Milne et al. [128] have used a systematic approach to the interpretation of portable chest radiographs to distinguish increased permeability edema from increased hydrostatic pressure edema. In their study of 119 patients, the three most discriminating criteria were the distribution of pulmonary edema, the distribution of pulmonary blood flow, and the width of the vascular pedicle. They reported that increased permeability edema could be distinguished from hydrostatic edema in 91% of cases. Using a similar set of criteria, Aberle et al. [127] evaluated the distinction of increased permeability from hydrostatic edema by portable chest radiography. They used the ratio of edema fluid to plasma protein concentration as a reference method of distinction between the two mechanisms. These investigators found that a patchy, peripheral distribution of edema was the single most discriminating criterion, and relatively specific for increased permeability edema, however, this typical appearance occurred only in half of patients with permeability edema. In their study 87% of patients with hydrostatic edema, but only 61% of patients with permeability edema were correctly identified.

Although chest radiography is a practical and non invasive method to detect increased extravascular lung fluid and to evaluate its anatomic distribution, it is limited in the differentiation of the mechanism of edema. Estimations of the amount of edema by this method are semiquantitative, and the coexistence of more than one pathological process in the lung such as infection or atelectasis, further complicates interpretation. Also, therapeutic and diagnostic interventions such as positive end expiratory pressure or bronchoalveolar lavage may change the appearance of opacities, and should be considered in the interpretation of the chest radiograph.

*Computed tomography:* Computed tomographic studies have been performed in hydrostatic edema [129–131] as well as in permeability edema [132–134], both in experimental animal models and in patients. These studies have confirmed the patchy lung involvement interspersed with areas of normal appearing lung characteristic of lung injury [135], with predominant consolidation of dependent lung regions.

Gattinoni et al. described a densitometric analysis method that allows estimation of lung weight based on the mean CT number and its frequency distribution [136]. They measured lung gas volume using a helium dilution method, then derived lung tissue volume. Lung tissue mass was estimated by assuming that the specific weight of the lung = 1. Lung tissue mass computed by this method combines the intravascular and extravascular compartments.

Bombino et al. compared analysis of chest radiograms by a standardized scoring system with densitometric CT analysis (CT number, excess tissue mass), and found a significant correlation between the two methods in patients with ARDS [137]. They concluded that the sensitivity of standardized chest radiographic readings in detecting pulmonary edema is at least as good as computed tomography. Although computed tomography allows better assessment of the distribution of pulmonary edema compared to chest radiography [136], it is not clear whether it is more sensitive in detecting increased lung water. Also, the ability of computed tomography to distinguish the mechanism of pulmonary edema has not been objectively evaluated. Computed tomography is particularly useful in detecting the complications of permeability edema or its therapy such as superimposed infection or barotrauma [128]. However, the benefit of computed tomography *vs.* portable chest radiography in the evaluation of lung edema alone is limited according to current data. Also, the risk associated with the transport of critically ill patients limits the routine use of computed tomography.

*Nuclear magnetic resonance (NMR) and magnetic resonance imaging (MRI):* MRI is an imaging technique that detects hydrogen protons aligned using a strong magnetic field. The emission of a radiofrequency wave pulse displaces the protons which absorb some of the transmitted energy. When the radiofrequency pulse is stopped, part of the energy absorbed by the protons is emitted as a weak radiofrequency signal. This signal is detected and digitally processed into an image [138]. Also, the time taken by the hydrogen nuclei to return to their resting state can be measured as a "relaxation time". Although proton MRI has an excellent contrast resolution for soft tissue, it is limited in imaging lung tissue due to its low average signal intensity. Lung imaging is further complicated by artifacts due to cardiac and respiratory movements. Artifacts due to cardiovascular motion can be reduced by synchronizing (gating) data acquisition with cardiac motion.

Several experimental studies have shown correlation between gravimetric measurements of lung water and relaxation times measured by NMR, both in hydrostatic and permeability edema in different species [139–145]. Preliminary observations in humans have suggested that NMR estimations of lung water should be feasible [146]. MRI may detect increased lung water earlier than CT in increased permeability edema according to one experimental study [147]. However, it should be kept in mind that this technique cannot distinguish between hydrogen proton signals originating in the intracellular or extracellular compartments, or the intravascular or extravascular compartments. Recently an original technique using sodium – as opposed to proton – MRI has been developed, where macromolecule coated magnetite particles are used as an intravascular indicator. These particles suppress the signal from plasma sodium, allowing a better estimation of extravascular lung water [148].

Alike CT, MRI requires transport of a critically ill patient. Prospects of routine application of MRI in pulmonary edema in humans are as yet limited.

*Positron emission tomography (PET):* PET is an imaging technique that allows measurement of the regional concentration of compounds labeled with a positron emitting radioactive tracer. It is an interesting technique in that it allows quantitative estimation of both extravascular lung water and microvascular permeability to a macromolecular indicator [149].

Regional lung water measurements can be obtained by PET, after equilibration of intravenously infused $^{15}O$ water between the blood and lung tissue. Details of this technique are thoroughly reviewed by Schuster et al. [150]. The regional lung water estimated by this method includes intravascular and extravascular water. The intravascular component can be estimated from the regional activity of [11]C- or [15]O-labeled carbon monoxide, administered by inhalation. The labeled carbon monoxide avidly binds to hemoglobin, and is confined to the intravascular compartment. Extravascular water content of a region is then calculated by subtracting the intravascular water content from the regional lung water. Extravascular lung water estimated by PET has been shown to correlate well with gravimetric lung water determinations [150]. However, its spatial resolution is limited, and PET estimations of regional extravascular lung water will be underestimated when blood flow to an edematous area approaches zero, particularly in the injured lung. Also, like computed tomography, PET studies require transport of a critically ill patient, which is not without risk. Another limitation to this technique is that few institutions in the world are able to perform PET.

### Transthoracic bioimpedance

In this technique, an alternating electric current is applied to the subject's thorax through two electrodes, and the resistance to the current is measured using two other electrodes. The impedance (proportional to resistance) is inversely proportional to the amount of water contained in the tissue within the electric field. The technique is safe, non invasive and may be performed at bedside. Estimations of lung water by bioimpedance have been attempted in humans [150] and animals [151]. However, thoracic impedance depends on many factors such as; body weight, body position, respiratory variations in lung volume, and IV fluid infusion [150 151]. Impedance measurements cannot distinguish between increased lung water and reduced lung volume, differentiate increased intrathoracic blood volume from increased lung water, nor can they distinguish extravascular from intravascular, or extrapulmonary lung water [150]. Decreased impedance has been observed in pleural and pericardial effusions [150]. A period of 40 to 80 min seems necessary to obtain a steady state in control animal experiments [151, 152]. Finally, due to the wide scatter of normal impedance values and considerable overlap between values obtained in normal and edematous lungs, single impedance measurements are of limited use in detecting or quantifying edema [150].

## Solute filtration: Capillary-alveolar macro-molecule transport

### External radioflux detection

Gorin et al. measured transport of a diffusible indicator; [113m]Indium-labeled transferrin, from blood to the interstitium in sheep. They used technetium labeled red blood cells as an intravascular indicator. The activity of both indicators was measured simultaneously using an external scintillation probe over the lung and a well counter for serial blood samples (Fig. 8.7). The increase in extravascular activity of the diffusible tracer was normalized to blood activity and analyzed with a compartmental model. Three transport coefficients for tracer flux (ml/min) were identi-

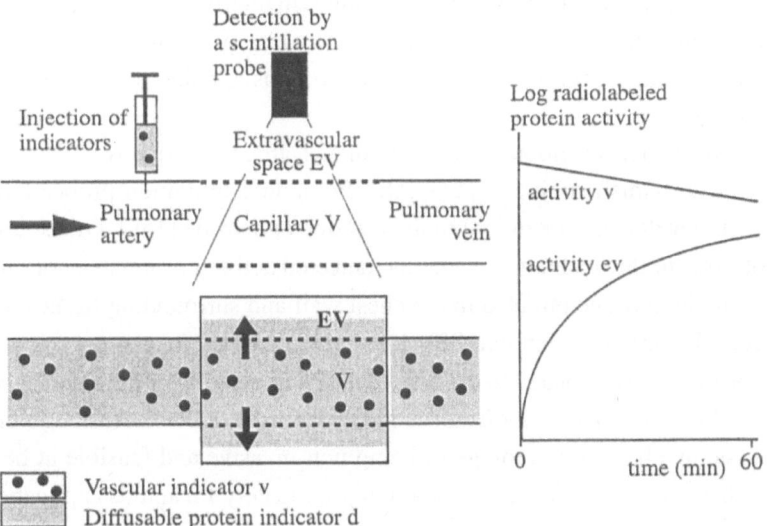

**Figure 8.7. External detection of extravascular radiolabeled protein accumulation**
See text.

fied, one from plasma to interstitium, a second from interstitium to plasma, and a third one from plasma into non-pulmonary spaces. Transport coefficients for tracer flux from plasma to interstitium obtained under control, increased microvascular pressure and high transvascular permeability conditions were similar whether using external detection or lymph data [153]. Gorin et al. later adapted this technique to man using external counting for 60 min [154]. This is a short period of time compared to the time of equilibration of protein tracer fluxes in and out of the interstitium. The accumulation of tracer protein in interstitium is therefore influenced mainly by the transport coefficient from plasma to interstitium. Since this transport coefficient depends both on permeability and on fluid filtration, that is on microvascular pressure and the available exchange surface area, the authors normalized it to the regional pulmonary plasma volume (assuming that the latter varies linearly with exchange surface area) to obtain a mean Pulmonary Trans Capillary Escape Rate or PTCER of 0.0038 $min^{-1}$. It was later demonstrated in sheep [90] that PTCER is increased by alteration in transvascular permeability and not by an increased microvascular pressure. Using a two-pore model, Roselli et al. [154] analyzed the factors influencing PTCER and concluded that PTCER is relatively insensitive to changes in microvascular pressure but is greatly affected by changes in microvascular permeability. It may be inferred that PTCER expresses mainly transvascular protein permeability.

Originally developed in a sheep model, this technique was later applied to human subjects [155–158]. Portable scintillation probes have been developed for external radiodetection at bedside [159]. One source of error in this technique is that the detected activity originates not only in the lung tissue but also in the chest wall and surrounding tissues, for both the intravascular and diffusible indicator. Data from one region of the lung is extrapolated to the entire lung. Dissociation of the radioactive label and the protein indicator is another source of error. Although this technique has the advantage of being non-invasive and feasible at bedside, it requires data acquisition for approximately 1 h and its application has not become routine in patients. Further discussion of this technique can be found in [1].

## Positron emission tomography (PET)

Transvascular protein transport can be estimated by measuring the rate constant of the transport of a radiolabeled protein such as [68]Ga-Transferrin across the pulmonary endothelial barrier [149]. Because PET cannot distinguish between the activity of labeled protein originating in the intravascular or extravascular compartments, the intravascular component is estimated separately, then subtracted from the total measured activity. Since it is assumed that all of the labeled protein activity is confined to the vascular compartment at the time of intravenous injection, intravascular activity as well as regional blood volume are estimated from activity measurements at the beginning of the scan.

PET is a non-invasive technique that not only allows to measure PTCER and to estimate microvascular permeability, it also allows to visualize the anatomic distribution of permeability to a protein indicator. Spatial resolution of PET is low (5 mm). The time required for data collection is from 20 to 60 min. Also, respiratory movements are a potential source of error. As already mentioned, a limitation to this technique is that few institutions in the world are able to perform PET.

## Magnetic resonance imaging (MRI)

Berthezene et al. introduced a paramagnetic macromolecular contrast agent (Polylysine-gadopentetate dimeglumine), MW = 40 000) into the bloodstream in a rat model of hydrostatic and increased permeability edema. They found that the MRI signal was enhanced 200% and 250% in hydrostatic and increased permeability edema respectively, due to passage of the macromolecular contrast agent across the microvascualr endothelium. Although the authors did not measure a transport rate constant, they showed a significant difference in MRI signal intensity with increased microvascular permeability as well as the ability to characterize the anatomic distribution of changes in permeability to a macromolecular indicator using MRI.

## Edema fluid protein and Bronchoalveolar Lavage fluid

Standard Bronchoalveolar Lavage (BAL) involves instillation of normal saline into the lower respiratory tract followed by aspiration and recovery of the fluid through a fiberoptic bronchoscope. The instillation—aspiration sequence is then repeated five to six times. Only 50% to 70% of the instilled fluid is recovered. BAL is widely used in the clinical setting, including in patients with ARDS [160], often to investigate an infectious etiology. As BAL fluid mixes with epithelial lining fluid (ELF), cells and solute in the ELF are greatly diluted by lavage fluid. The final concentration of ELF substances in lavage fluid depends on several factors. Significant exchange of fluid occurs between the blood and the alveoli during lavage [161]. Also, the distribution of lavage fluid within the lavaged segment must be complete, mixture with ELF or edema fluid must be homogeneous, and distribution of lavage fluid should be limited to the lavaged segment. Standard bronchoalveolar lavage does not account for most of these factors, therefore solute and cell concentrations in the lavage fluid are difficult to interpret, and to compare in between subjects. Although several studies have reported higher BAL fluid protein/plasma protein ratios in lung injury as compared to normal lung, there is considerable overlap between hydrostatic and increased permeability edema reducing the clinical utility of this ratio [1]. Moreover, because of different clearance rates of protein and fluid from edematous lungs [162] protein concentration in edema fluid will change with time, further complicating interpretation. Various inflammatory cells and proteins have been retrieved in lavage fluids of patients with increased permeability edema however there is no evidence for a mediator specific to ARDS.

We developed a new lavage protocol allowing to progressively saturate the lavaged lung segment in dogs [163, 164]. We used this lavage technique to measure capillary—alveolar transport of fluorescein labeled dextran (D-FITC, MW = 70 000) infused at constant plasma concentration 30 min prior to lavage. We used lavage fluid to plasma concentration ratio of D-FITC to compute a capillary-alveolar D-FITC clearance (ml/min$^{-1}$) and normalized this clearance to the lavaged alveolar volume to obtain a capillary-alveolar transport rate (min$^{-1}$). The mean capillary—alveolar transport rate for D-FITC was $4.1 \cdot 10^{-5}$ min$^{-1}$ at baseline and $61.4 \cdot 10^{-5}$ min$^{-1}$ in oleic acid-induced lung injury [164].

## Starling equation components

### Microvascular pressure

*Pulmonary capillary pressure:* In the clinical setting, capillary pressure may be estimated by analysis of the arterial pressure profile after rapid occlusion. This technique requires the insertion of a balloon flotation pulmonary artery (Swan-Ganz) catheter, through a subclavian vein. Occlusion of pulmonary arterial vessels may be performed by rapidly inflating the balloon of the catheter [165]. In patients, apnea is required to record the occlusion curves. The time required to inflate the balloon is significantly longer than with mechanical occluders used in isolated lung experiments, and the instant of occlusion cannot be determined as precisely. Also, artifacts generated by balloon occlusion may modify the initial fast phase of the post-occlusion curves, interfering with the double exponential fit which is required to correct the capillary pressure estimate using a C-R-C-R-C model [166]. Therefore, capillary pressure is most often estimated using the R-C-R model from either visual determination of the breakpoint between the fast and slow exponential components [70], or by back-extrapolation of the slow exponential component towards the instant of occlusion (Fig. 8.8) [65]. Pulsatility of capillary pressure is important to consider in clinical measurement. Maarek et al. [167] have shown that capillary pressure estimated from post occlusion arterial pressure profile varies with the instant of occlusion in the cardiac cycle. The capillary pressure estimate is higher if blood flow is stopped at peak systole and lower when occlusion is performed during diastole. Therefore, each capillary pressure estimate has to be normalized to an instant of occlusion corresponding to the mean arterial pressure level [168].

The constraints of $P_c$ measurement may be discouraging when time and equipment are not available. However, $P_{wp}$ should not be substituted for a measurement or estimation of $P_c$. $P_{wp}$ underestimates the effective pressure that drives microvascular filtration at the capillary level, particularly under pathological conditions where venous resistances are elevated, such as in ARDS (*see* Section on *Starling equation components (microvascular pressure)*, p. 178). It must therefore be emphasized that $P_c$ may always be approximated using the Gaar equation which states that

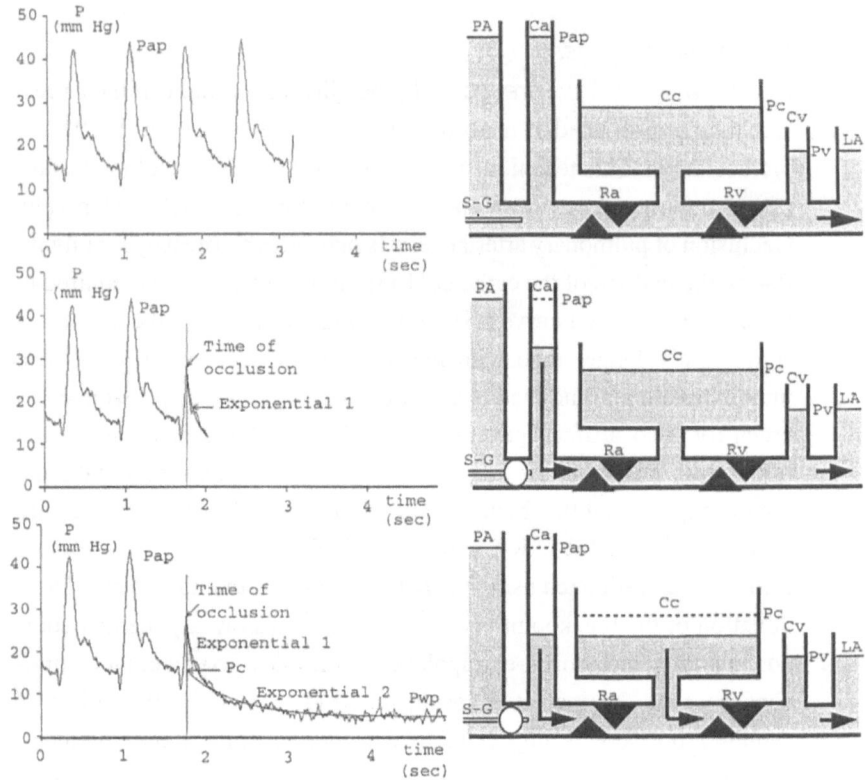

**Figure 8.8**

Left: Post-occlusion pressure transient from pulmonary arterial pressure (Pap) to wedge pressure (Pwp) using the balloon inflation and distal pressure recording of a balloon-tipped Swan-Ganz (S-G) catheter dwelling in a sublobar pulmonar artery

Right: Interpretation of the post-occlusion pressure transient using a C-R-C-R-C model of pulmonary circulation with poorly compliant arterial (Ca) and venous (Cv) compartments and a highly compliant capillary compartment (Cc) separated by an arterial (Ra) and a venous (Rv) resistance. AP: pulmonary artery; LA: left atrium.

Middle part of Figure 8.8: Following occlusion, the pressure transient presents a steeply decreasing exponential-like segment (exponential 1). This segment is interpreted in the model as the fast emptying of a low compliant arterial compartment through the downstream resistances.

Lower part of Figure 8.8: The pressure transient then presents a slow decreasing exponential-like segment (exponential 2) until reching the level of Pwp. This segment is interpreted in the model as the slow emptying of a highly compliant capillary compartment through the venous resistance. Pulmonary capillary pressure (Pc) has been estimated here by back-extrapolation of exponential 2 to the time of occlusion, according to a R-C-R model neglecting the Ca and Cv compliances. If a C-R-C-R-C model is used to estimate Pc, the mathematical formalization is more complex [166].

mean $P_c = P_{wp} + 0.4$ (mean $P_{ap} - P_{wp}$). $P_c$ calculated by the Gaar equation will be considerably less in error than is $P_{wp}$ to estimate the effective filtration pressure.

*Pulmonary arterial wedge pressure:* $P_{wp}$ can be measured by right heart catheterization with a Swan-Ganz catheter. In the absence of pulmonary venous occlusive disease or mitral stenosis, it reflects left atrial pressure, and thus the left ventricular filling pressure. Measuring $P_{wp}$ is therefore useful in identifying left ventricular failure ($P_{wp} > 18$ mm Hg).

The decision to use pulmonary artery catheterization must involve the assessment of risks compared to benefits. Several complications associated with the use of Swan-Ganz catheters have been reported. Pneumothorax, ventricular arrhythmias, pulmonary infarction, local vascular thrombosis, pulmonary artery rupture, and catheter related sepsis are among these complications [169].

*Estimation of pulmonary arterial and wedge pressures by echocardiography:* Several investigators have used echocardioghraphy to estimate pulmonary arterial ($P_{ap}$), and pulmonary arterial wedge pressures ($P_{wp}$). One approach consists in measuring the blood flow velocity (V) through a stenotic, regurgitant, or shunt lesion, between two cardiac or vascular compartments. Using the Bernouilli equation, the pressure gradient between the two compartments can be calculated as $\Delta P = 4 \, V^2$. The pressure in both compartments can be calculated if the pressure in one of them is estimated from clinical parameters, or assumed. Pulmonary arterial systolic pressure has been estimated from the peak tricuspid regurgitation velocity using this method [170–172], and pulmonary artery diastolic pressure has been estimated from the flow velocity profile of pulmonary regurgitation [172, 173] with strong correlations between echocardiographic estimations and catheterization in both cases. Regurgitant flows may be inexistant, or difficult to record in some patients, however this may be improved by contrast enhancement with injection of agitated dextrose or saline [171], or sonicated albumin [174].

Right ventricular isovolumic relaxation time (from the closure of the pulmonary valve to the opening of the tricuspid) has been shown to correlate with pulmonary arterial systolic pressure [172, 175]. However, this method is heart rate dependent, and limited by significant tricuspid stenosis or regurgitation or right-sided heart failure [175]. The ratio of acceleration time (AT: time from the onset to the peak of right ventricular ejection flow velocity) to right ventricular ejection time (ET: time from the onset of ejection to zero flow) has been used to estimate mean Pap. AT/ET has been shown to correlate with mean Pap values measured by catheterization [172, 176].

Mitral flow velocity recordings obtained by Doppler echocardiography have been used to estimate $P_{wp}$. In early diastole, blood flow across the mitral valve occurs down a pressure gradient generated during systole; in late diastole active contraction of the atrium empties blood into the left ventricle. The ratio of early to late transmitral diastolic filling velocity (E/A ratio) has been shown to directly correlate with $P_{wp}$ [177]. This may be explained by the fact that as left ventricular end-diastolic pressure rises, flow across the mitral valve following atrial contraction decreases. Several studies have demonstrated a close correlation between $P_{wp}$ measured by right-heart catheterization, and estimated by Doppler echocardiography [177–179]. This technique has the advantage of being simple, non-invasive, and feasible at bedside. However, mitral flow velocity variables are influenced by age, loading conditions, significant mitral or aortic regurgitation, and mitral stenosis [179, 180]. The E/A ratio will decrease as heart rate increases [180]. Also, arrhythmias, particularly atrial fibrillation, are a problem due to the loss of the mitral A wave [179].

Another approach uses simultaneous ECG and Doppler echocardiographic tracings to estimate $P_{wp}$. This technique is based on the direct correlation of $P_{wp}$ with the time interval from the onset of the QRS complex of the ECG to the point C of the systolic closure of the mitral valve (Q-MVC interval) on the echogram, and its inverse correlation with the interval from the onset of the aortic valve closure, or the $A_2$ sound on the phonocardiogram, to the maximal early diastolic opening point E of the echogram of the anterior mitral leaflet (AVC-E interval, or left ventricular isovolumetric relaxation time) [181]. The AVC-E interval can also be calculated from (Q-E)–(Q-AVC), where AVC is the aortic valve closure point on the echogram [182]. The (Q-MVC)/(AVC-E) ratio has been shown to closely correlate with $P_{wp}$ measured by catheterization [181,

182]. However, Q-MVC varies with the preceding R-R interval, and the AVC-E interval depends on factors other than the left atrial pressure [182].

In summary, echocardiographic techniques to estimate $P_{ap}$ and $P_{wp}$ are simple, non-invasive, and in selected patients, may help establish the indication for, or represent an alternative to catheterization when the latter is contraindicated.

## Small solute PS

Details of this technique were discussed above (*see* Section on *Small solute PS product*, p. 187). Several studies have measured the $^{14}$C-Urea PS product in patients with pulmonary edema [35, 183–185]. A non-diffusible indicator such as $^{51}$Cr-labeled red blood cells is used as an intravascular tracer. The advantage of this technique is that it is relatively easy to use in the intensive care unit, and may be a sensitive test in early lung injury [1]. Normal values for $^{14}$C-PS in humans are approximately 2 ml/s/l total lung capacity [183]. $^{14}$C-Urea PS product was found to correlate with the degree of hypoxemia and outcome, suggesting it may have some predictive value [183].

Disadvantages of this technique are that it is invasive, requiring pulmonary arterial and aortic catheters, use of isotopes, and a considerable delay in processing of the data [1]. $^{14}$C-Urea PS product depends on cardiac output. Its value increases with decreased cardiac output due to a prolonged capillary residence time allowing for $^{14}$C-Urea to equilibrate with a larger volume. On the other hand, zero PS products may be observed when flow through capillaries is so high that the capillary residence time is shorter than the transcapillary escape time, resulting in zero extraction of the diffusible tracer [183]. Also, in an experimental study, dramatic changes in surface area may result in a low PS product when permeability is actually increased, in the presence of regional defects in lung perfusion due to microemboli or oleic acid injury [186].

## Lung water clearance

Alveolar fluid clearance has been studied experimentally in patients with hydrostatic and increased permeability edema, by measuring protein concentration in sequential edema fluid samples obtained within 15 min of intubation through the following 12 h [187]. Edema fluid was samp-led using a 14-F suction catheter passed through the endotracheal tube and wedged in a distal airway [33]. Although clearance of protein and fluid occur simultaneously, protein clearance is much slower than fluid clearance. The validity of this method requires the assumption that mas-sive exchanges in protein across the epithelium do not occur during the sampling interval. Using this method, evidence for active removal of edema from the alveoli was demonstrated in humans [187]. The rate of fluid clearance can be estimated by this technique in pulmonary edema at its early phase. However, it is not clear which exchange surface area this clearance rate applies to, since with the same clearance rate the vol-ume of fluid cleared by the epithelium should vary in proportion to ex-change surface area. Also, the sequential samples may come from differ-ent lung territories whereas the distribution of fluid clearance from the alveoli may not be homogeneous particularly in the injured lung. Alto-gether, this is a simple technique to use at bedside and may provide valuable information about the epithelial capacity to remove edema fluid from the alveoli in early pulmonary edema.

## Epithelial permeability: DTPA clearance

This technique consists in the inhalation of an aerosol containing $^{99m}$Tc-DTPA ($^{99m}$Tc-diethylenetriaminepentaacetic acid) for approximately 1 to 3 min. The aerosol particles are deposited in the distal airways and al-veoli and their clearance rate may be determined externally using a port-able scintillation probe or a gamma camera. The chest is scanned for 7 to 30 min. Since the permeability of the capillary endothelium is much higher to $^{99m}$Tc-DTPA, it is rapidly cleared from the pulmonary intersti-tium by the circulation. $^{99m}$Tc-DTPA clearance rate is therefore considered to be an index of lung epithelial permeability. Normal $^{99m}$Tc-DTPA clearance rate is approximately 1%/min [1].

The technique is easy to perform and non invasive. It is sensitive, however increases in lung volume or minor injury to the epithelium such as that caused by cigarette smoking also increase the $^{99m}$Tc-DTPA clearance rate. Thus clearance of $^{99m}$Tc-DTPA is influenced by factors other than lung injury making its interpretation difficult. This high sensitivity may be due to the small size of the DTPA tracer (MW = 495, radius = 0.6 nm) [2]. Other potential problems with this method are the delivery of aerosol particles to the region of interest. This may be a significant problem in the presence of alveolar flooding, where tracer deposition may primarily occur in the better ventilated regions of the lung [2].

A similar method was developed experimentally using $^{99m}$Tc labeled serum albumin, and was found more specific for increased permeability. Loss of the $^{99m}$Tc label from the albumin tracer however, was a technical problem [32].

## Identifying pulmonary edema and its mechanism in the clinical setting

The choice among the methods of measurement of pulmonary edema is different according to whether it is necessary to diagnose pulmonary edema in a general practitioner's office or in the intensive care unit of a university hospital. This is also true for the identification of the mechanisms of pulmonary edema. Regardless of the medical environment, the history and physical examination remain important components of the diagnosis.

The mechanisms of pulmonary edema so far described are not exclusive. There does not seem to be a single parameter that can identify the mechanism(s) of pulmonary edema by itself but rather the combination of the information from at least two parameters that may or may not include lung water. Clinical scoring systems have been developed to define, grade the onset of lung injury, or evaluate its response to treatment, based on criteria such as chest radiographic findings, hypoxemia, compliance of the respiratory system, etc. [188]. The discussion of such clinical scores is beyond the scope of this chapter. Also, the discussed methods that may be used to identify the mechanism of edema, particularly lung injury at its early phase, do not predict its late evolution or allow to distinguish patients who will go on to develop organizing infiltrations and lung fibrosis along with other complications.

## Present

### Diagnosis and quantification of pulmonary edema

Suspicion of pulmonary edema is usually confirmed by chest radiography. The thermal volume indicator dilution technique has the advantage to measure extravascular lung water at bedside. Although it requires an invasive arterial access, it has received a wider application than protein and small solute detection. However, its sensitivity to evidence pulmonary edema does not seem to surpass that of bedside chest X-ray.

The measurement of lung water is more sensitive to an increase in pulmonary edema than to its reduction. The measurement of extravascular lung water is therefore poorly adapted to evaluate therapies aimed at lowering water and solute transvascular filtration. Altogether, capillary pressure better reflects filtration than lung water. $P_c$ commands transvascular filtration, whether transvascular permeability is low or high, and therefore varies in the same direction as transvascular filtration.

### Identification of mechanisms

It has long been recognized that two mechanisms are important to identify: (1) an imbalance in Starling forces which results in high pressure pulmonary edema, a paradigm of which is left ventricular failure; (2) an increased transvascular permeability which may be the consequence of an inflammatory process, either localized in the lung or reflecting a systemic inflammatory response.

## Identification of an imbalance in Starling forces

*Increased hydrostatic pressure gradient: $P_c - P_i$:* The range of variation of $P_c$ is usually considered larger than that of $P_i$. Also, the occurrence of an increase in $P_c$, such as resulting from a left ventricular failure, is considered more frequent than a decreased interstitial pressure. Moreover, $P_c$ may be monitored and modified by therapy. For the above reasons, $P_c$ is presently the most important variable to identify and to modify among the Starling forces. Its monitoring requires the presence of a balloon-tipped catheter in the pulmonary artery. If time or equipment for signal processing of the pulmonary arterial occlusion profile is not available, $P_c$ may be approximated using the Gaar equation which states that $P_c = P_{wp} + 0.4 \, (P_{ap} - P_{wp})$ where $P_{wp}$ is the pulmonary artery wedge pressure. This estimate of $P_c$ is considerably less in error than is $P_{wp}$ in estimating the effective pressure that commands filtration at the capillary level.

*Decreased protein osmotic pressure gradient: $\pi_c - \pi_i$:* The range of variation of $\pi_c$ is less than the range of variation of $\pi_i$. $\pi_i$ decreases with an increase in microvascular filtration induced by an elevation of $P_c$. The rise in plasma to interstitial protein osmotic gradient tends to limit such an increase in microvascular filtration, and is considered as one of the safety factors against high pressure edema formation. However, it must be emphasized that the efficiency of this safety factor is limited when the reflection coefficient is decreased as a consequence of an altered transvascular protein permeability. By comparison, a moderate hypoproteinemia and its consequence, the decrease of $\pi_c$, is less deleterious as it is associated with a concomitant decrease in $\pi_i$, with an even protein osmotic pressure gradient [189].

*The $P_c - \Pi_c$ pressure gradient:* This popular pressure gradient is actually more confusing than $P_c$ alone because it has a curtailed scientific foundation, $\pi_c$ being an oversimplified version of the effective protein osmotic pressure gradient $\sigma \, (P_c - \Pi_c)$. Using $\pi_c$ instead of $\sigma \, (P_c - \Pi_c)$ masks the very important decrease in $\sigma \, (P_c - \Pi_c)$ that occurs when transvascular protein permeability is altered and $\sigma$ is low. One may be easily tempted to restore a diminished plasma protein level and $\pi c$ by an albumin infusion. In such conditions, the restoration of $\Pi_c$ is short-lived as albumin crosses the leaky pulmonary capillaries resulting in an increase in transvascular protein transport [190]. Moreover, the albumin infusion may be very efficient to withdraw interstitial fluid through the walls of intact capillaries in the systemic circulation. This could result in an increased plasma volume, increased $P_c$ and more edema in the lung.

*Identifying high pressure pulmonary edema:* As long as transvascular permeability is not altered, $P_c$ measurement, not pulmonary wedge pressure measurement, is the best criterion for diagnosis and monitoring of high pressure pulmonary edema when a balloon-tipped pulmonary arterial catheter is inserted. Most patients with acute hydrostatic pulmonary edema present physical signs pointing to acute left ventricular failure [191]. Lung opacities on chest X-ray may be observed consistently following acute myocardial infarction when $P_{wp}$ increases beyond 18 mm Hg [192]. This is true for an acute elevation in microvascular pressure, however, tolerance to an elevated microvascular pressure increases with time. Anderson et al. observed in 116 patients with chronic left ventricular failure that no signs of pulmonary edema were present despite $P_{wp} > 25$ mm Hg [193].

Central distribution of lung opacities on chest X-ray is also a discriminating sign [126, 128]. If the pulmonary edema fluid is sampled within 1 h of the acute phase of pulmonary edema, a low edema fluid/plasma protein concentration ratio ($< 0.50$) is in favor of high pressure pulmonary edema [194].

Pulmonary PTCER is not sensitive enough to differentiate high pressure edema from normal because interstitial protein concentration decreases as transvascular fluid filtration increases [154, 158].

*Identification of an altered transvascular permeability*
Measurements of permeability in the experimental setting cannot be transposed in the clinical setting. Except for small solute PS product determination, all experimental measurements of transvascular permeability, either to water (filtration coefficient) or to proteins (reflection coefficient), require to elevate vascular pressure in order to increase filtration. Such an elevation in filtration worsens pulmonary edema and

therefore cannot ethically be attempted in patients. Other limitations will be mentioned below.

*Increased permeability to water:* Lung microvascular filtration cannot be measured in patients. Several techniques, either qualitative or quantitative, are available to measure extravascular lung water in patients. Therefore, the measurement of transvascular permeability to water relies on the relation between the level of extravascular lung water and the level of capillary pressure. In other words, the diagnosis of high permeability to water relies on the following observation: the level of capillary pressure is too low for the level of extravascular lung water (Fig. 8.9) [195].

*Increased permeability to proteins:* Transvascular protein permeability during pulmonary edema is associated with high transvascular filtra-

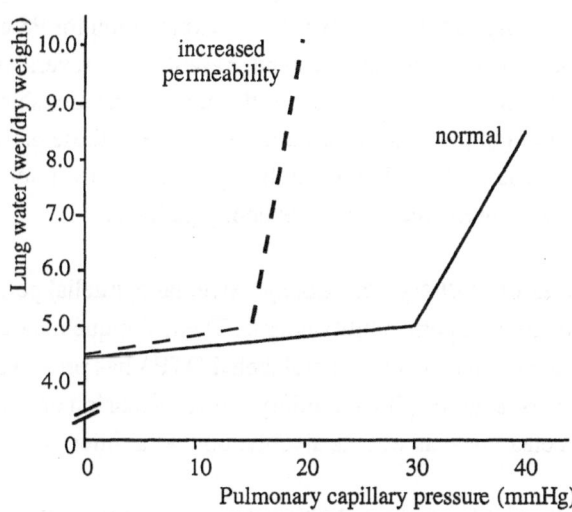

**Figure 8.9. Relationship between lung water and pulmonary capillary pressure (estimated by left atrial pressure + 5 mm Hg)**

The normal relationship has been estimated from wet/dry lung weight ratios following 30-min left atrial pressure elevation in dog [195] The increased permeability relationship is speculative. Adapted from [195] with permission.

tion (with predominance of convection) and more specifically quantified by the reflection coefficient than by PS product. The reflection coefficient in lymph studies is calculated when the lymph to protein ratio becomes independent of lymph flow, as the latter is increased (*see* Section on *Analysis of lymph protein flux date*, p. 193). Such a continuous measurement of transvascular fluid flow and protein transport is not available in patients. The measurement of transvascular protein permeability is usually approached in patients by the measurement of the pulmonary protein transcapillary escape rate (PTCER) with two radiolabeled indicators: an intravascular indicator and a diffusible protein indicator (*see* Section on *Solute filtration: Capillary–alveolar macromolecule transport (external radio flux detection)* p. 203).

*PS product for small solutes:* PS product for small solutes may be measured in patients using dilution curves of $^{14}$C-urea and of an intravascular radiolabeled indicator. $^{14}$C-urea PS product is higher in patients presenting nonreversing rather than reversing high permeability pulmonary edema [196]. An increased pulmonary transvascular permeability in nonreversing patients is only a partial explanation for PS elevation, as an increased surface area may also be present in nonreversing patients. The latter possibility is supported by the inverse relationship observed between PS and pulmonary vascular resistance in these patients. The most likely cause of this relationship being a lack of diversion of blood flow from the injured areas in non reversing patients.

*Alveolar epithelial permeability:* Alveolar epithelial permeability is increased in high permeability edema. The technique measuring the clearance rate of an aerosol of radiolabeled DTPA has proven simple but non specific of a large epithelial injury. Lung distension or smoking increase DTPA clearance, as well as alveolar epithelial injury [1].

*Identifying high permeability pulmonary edema:* The techniques *currently* used to measure transvascular transport of solutes all require radioactive tracers. Pulmonary protein transcapillary escape rate measurement requires a steady-state for 1 h to count external thoracic radioactivity, a demand which is difficult to satisfy in critically ill patients. PS product determination of small solutes requires extensive laboratory and counting procedures. These constraints may explain why these techniques are not used routinely even in university hospitals.

The measurement of extravascular lung water alone does not identify the mechanism of pulmonary edema. It must be coupled with the measurement of pulmonary capillary pressure to identify increased permeability edema (Fig. 8.9). If the level of capillary pressure cannot explain the level of extravascular lung water, an increase in transvascular permeability must be suspected. However, it must be emphasized that a high $P_c$ or $P_{wp}$ can coexist with high permeability edema [197]. In other words, a high $P_c$ or $P_{wp}$, does not exclude high permeability edema. It should be pointed out that the same elevation in $P_c$ increases edema formation far more in the presence of increased permeability than when permeability is normal (Fig. 8.9).

In the presence of risk factors such as aspiration, sepsis, or multiple transfusions, or physical signs in favor of pulmonary inflammation either from direct pulmonary injury or from a non-pulmonary origin (i.e. systemic inflammatory response) increased permeability should be suspected. Patchy distribution of lung opacities on chest radiography is a relatively specific sign of increased permeability pulmonary edema. If the edema fluid is sampled within 1 h of the acute phase of pulmonary edema, a high edema fluid/plasma protein concentration ratio (> 0.50) is in favor of permeability edema [194].

## Future

### Role of edema clearance

Previous studies have underlined the important role of the pulmonary and bronchial circulations, the lung lymphatic clearance, and the pleural clearance in the evacuation of pulmonary edema fluid. An important recent finding in this field is that reabsorption of fluid from distal airspaces of the lung is driven by active sodium transport. Catecholamine dependent and independent mechanisms have been identified. The capacity of the alveolar epithelium to reabsorb edema fluid seems to recover rapidly after injury. Also, a family of molecular water channels has been identified whose role in the epithelial permeability to water are yet to be explored. So far, investigators have estimated alveolar liquid clearance in humans by measuring the total protein concentration in sequential samples of edema fluid [3]. Further research should focus on improving and developing techniques to study the clearance of edema in man, and on methods to enhance this clearance.

### Role of exchange surface area

An increase in lung microvascular exchange surface area increases fluid filtration. This increase in exchange surface area is essentially due to recruitment of pulmonary capillaries when microvascular pressure or pulmonary blood flow increases. Alternatively, microvascular exchange surface area decreases with regional defects in lung perfusion [186]. There is evidence to suggest that the outcome of patients with lung injury may depend not only on the degree of increased permeability, but also on the ability to decrease exchange surface area through derecruitment of the injured areas of the lung microcirculation [196].

Experimentally, exchange surface area may be estimated while microvascular permeability and microvascular pressure are kept constant. Experimental techniques have been developed that allow indirect measurement of the pulmonary microvascular exchange surface area by measuring substrate metabolism by the pulmonary vascular endothelium [198]. In the clinical setting however, available techniques cannot measure exchange surface area independently of microvascular permeability. It would be of great interest to develop techniques that allow to advance our understanding of the role of the pulmonary microvascular exchange surface area and particularly its variations with microvascular pressure, pulmonary blood flow, and lung injury in humans.

### Macromolecule transport

An increased pulmonary microvascular permeability remains the hallmark of acute lung injury [197] and efforts should be made to develop techniques to measure pulmonary microvascular permeability at bedside, ideally without using radioactive tracers.

Several different techniques have been developed that measure the passage of macromolecules from the blood to the interstitium and the alveoli. As was mentioned earlier, when microvascular permeability is increased, convective transport of macromolecules across the endothelium becomes the predominant mechanism. This convective transport is proportional to microvascular filtration, which is in turn determined by capillary pressure. This suggests that changes in transcapillary transport flux of macromolecules may be not only due to changes in permeability, but also to changes in capillary pressure, particularly when permeability is elevated. Accounting for changes in microvascular pressure may therefore increase the specificity of these methods in recognizing increased permeability. Although pulmonary transcapillary escape rate for macromolecules is normalized for the underlying blood volume and is presumed to be less sensitive to changes in microvascular pressure [154], its relationship to $P_c$ may provide an additional discrimination factor between high permeability and high pressure edema (Fig. 8.10).

In summary, future methods to estimate lung microvascular permeability by measuring a macromolecule transcapillary transport should consider normalizing this transport to capillary pressure when possible. Accounting for changes in microvascular pressure may increase the specificity of these methods in recognizing increased permeability.

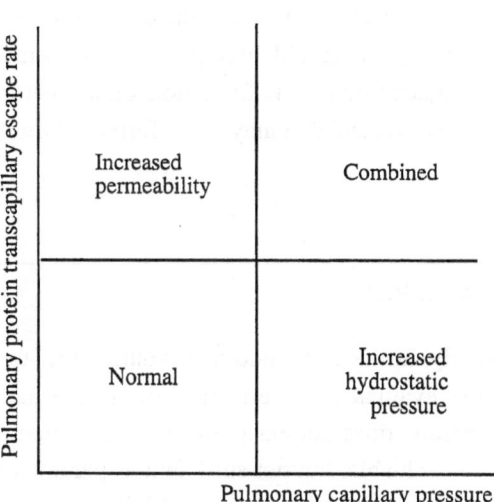

*Figure 8.10. Relationship between pulmonary protein transcapillary escape rate and pulmonary capillary pressure* This relationship allows to identify the main mechanisms of pulmonary edema in a given in vivo situation.

### Anatomic distribution

In distinguishing high pressure from permeability edema, the anatomic distribution of edema seems to be a relatively specific criterion. Indicator dilution methods that allow estimation of extravascular lung water cannot assess its distribution. Imaging techniques such as chest radiography or computed tomography provide static information on the distribution of the excess lung fluid, i.e. they do not distinguish regions where edema formation is active from those where edema is being removed. Several dynamic techniques were reviewed above that allow estimation of microvascular permeability by measuring transcapillary exchange of labeled macromolecules. It is interesting to note that an increase in the transcapillary transport of macromolecules, therefore in permeability, is not specific to lung injury but is generally the consequence of inflammation [199]. What characterizes ARDS seems to be the severity, but also the widespread distribution of increased permeability [135]. Therefore, techniques that measure increased permeability should ideally allow to evaluate its anatomic distribution also. Techniques such as positron emission tomography (PET) visualize the distribution of actively leaking microvessels and allow a quantitative measurement of transmicrovascular transport of macromolecules. Unfortunately, such techniques that have the advantage of being noninvasive, require sophisticated equipment, cannot be performed at bedside, and their lack of practicality has kept them from being used outside of the experimental setting. Future work in this field should attempt to design methods that provide dynamic information on edema formation, on its anatomic distribution, that are noninvasive, and that may be performed at the bedside of a critically ill patient.

## Conclusion

Currently, an ideal method that would allow to diagnose pulmonary edema at bedside, evaluate its severity, identify its mechanisms, and to measure the effect of a therapy does not exist. Sensitive detection of increased extravascular lung water is valuable, but not sufficient as parameters that determine the formation and clearance of edema are multiple. However, measuring the severity and identifying the mechanism of edema can now be improved by coupling the information from two or more parameters (such as extravascular lung water, transvascular permeability, anatomic distribution, capillary pressure, etc.). Capillary pressure, not wedge pressure, should be repeatedly estimated whenever a balloon-tipped pulmonary arterial pressure catheter is available. The risks and benefits of the above measurements for critically ill patients should be identified through clinical trials. Identifying the subjects who will go on to develop severe permeability edema remains challenging and complex. Regional changes in lung perfusion, and increased permeability may precede the development of detectable edema, therefore new methods should aim at early evaluation of these parameters.

# References

1  Staub NC, Hyde RW and Crandall E (1990) *Am. Rev. Respir. Dis.* Apr; **141**(4 Pt 1): 1071

2  Peterson BT (1992) *Am. J. Physiol.* **262**(3 Pt 1): L243

3  Matthay MA, Folkesson HG and Verkman AS (1996) *Am. J. Physiol.* **270**(4): L487

4  Folkesson HG, Matthay MA, Hasegawa H, Kheradmand F and Verkman AS (1994) *Proc. Natl. Acad. Sci. USA* **2491**(11): 4970

5  Berthiaume Y, Staub NC and Matthay MA (1987) *J. Clin. Invest.* **79**(2): 335

6  Aukland K and Reed RK. (1993) *Physiol. Rev.* **73**(1): 1

7  Pistolesi M, Miniati M and Giuntini C (1989) *Am. Rev. Respir. Dis.* **140**(3): 825

8  Albertine KH, Wiener-Kronish JP, Roos PJ and Staub NC (1982) *Am. J. Anat.* **165**(3): 277

9  Negrini D, Townsley MI and Taylor AE (1990) *J. Appl. Physiol.* **69**: 438

10  Wiener-Kronish JP, Matthay MA, Callen PW, Filly RA, Gamsu G and Staub NC (1985) *Am. Rev. Respir. Dis.* **132**(6): 1253

11  Wiener-Kronish JP, Goldstein R, Matthay RA, Biondi JW, Broaddus VC, Chatterjee K and Matthay MA (1987) *Chest* **92**(6): 967

12  Negrini D, del Fabbro M and Venturoli D (1993) *J. Appl. Physiol.* **74**(4): 1779

13  Negrini D, Ballard ST and Benoit JN (1994) *J. Appl. Physiol.* **76**(6): 2267

14  Miserocchi G, Venturoli D, Negrini D and Del Fabbro M (1993) *J. Appl. Physiol.* **75**(4): 1798

15  Wiener-Kronish JP, Broaddus VC, Albertine KH, Gropper MA, Matthay MA and Staub NC (1988) *J. Clin. Invest.* **82**(4): 1422

16  Broaddus VC, Wiener-Kronish JP and Staub NC (1990) *J. Appl. Physiol.* **68**(6): 2623

17  Staub NC, Nagano H and Pearce ML (1967) *J. Appl. Physiol.* **22**(2): 227

18  Kedem O and Katchalsky A (1989) *Biochim. Biophys. Acta* **1000**: 413

19  Granger DN and Taylor AE (1980) *Am. J. Physiol.* **238**(4): H457

20  Curry F-RE (1984) Mechanics and thermodynamiccs of transcapillary exchange. In: *Handbook of Physiology. The Cardiovascular System. Microcirculation*, Sect. 2, Vol. IV, Pt. 1, Chapt. 8, p. 309. *Am. Physiol. Soc.*, Bethesda, MD

21  Taylor AE and Gaar KA, Jr (1970) *Am. J. Physiol.* **218**(4): 1133

22  Theodore J, Robin ED, Gaudio R and Acevedo J (1975) *Am. J. Physiol.* **229**(4): 989

23  Gorin AB and Stewart PA (1979) *J. Appl. Physiol.* **47**(6): 1315

24  Berg MM, Kim KJ, Lubman RL and Crandall ED (1989) *J. Appl. Physiol.* **66**(5): 2320

25  Gee MH and Staub NC. (1977) *J. Appl. Physiol.* **42**(2): 144

26  Schneeberger EE and Lynch RD (1992) Structure, function, and regulation of cellular tight junctions. *Am. J. Physiol.* **262** (6 Pt 1): L647

27  Serikov VB, Grady M and Matthay MA (1993) *J. Appl. Physiol.* **75**(2): 940

28  Egan EA (1982) *J. Appl. Physiol.* **53**(1): 121

29  Schneeberger-Keeley EE and Karnovsky MJ (1968) *J. Cell Biol.* **37**: 781

30  Hostetter MW, Dawson CA and Moore VL (1981) *Proc. Soc. Exp. Biol. Med.* **167**: 412

31  Berthiaume Y, Albertine KH, Grady M, Fick G and Matthay MA (1989) *J. Appl. Physiol.* **67**(5): 1887

32  Peterson BT, Dickerson KD, James HL, Miller EJ, McLarty JW and Holiday DB (1989) *J. Appl. Physiol.* **66**(5): 2374

33  Hastings RH, Grady M, Sakuma T and Matthay MA (1992) *J. Appl. Physiol.* **73**(4): 1310

34  Berthiaume Y, Albertine KH, Grady M, Fick G and Matthay MA (1989) *J. Appl. Physiol.* **67**(5): 1887

35  Hastings RH, Wright JR, Albertine KH, Ciriales R and Matthay MA (1994) *Am. J. Physiol.* **266**(5 Pt 1): L544

36  Allen SJ, Drake RE, Laine GA and Gabel JC (1991) *J. Appl. Physiol.* **71**: 314

37  Patterson GA, Mitzner WA and Sylvester JT (1985) *J. Appl. Physiol.* **58**(3): 882

38  Staub NC, Bland RD, Brigham KL, Demling R, Erdmann AJ 3rd and

Woolverton WC (1975) *J. Surg. Res.* **19**(5): 315

39  Drake RE, Scott RL and Gabel JC (1983) *Am. J. Physiol.* **245**(1): H125

40  Erdmann AJ 3d, Vaughan TR, Jr, Brigham KL, Woolverton WC and Staub NC (1975) *Circ. Res.* **37**(3): 271

41  Martin DJ, Parker JC and Taylor AE (1983) *J. Appl. Physiol.* **54**(1): 199

42  Adair TH, Moffatt DS, Paulsen AW and Guyton AC (1982) *Am. J. Physiol.* **243**(3): H351

43  Parker JC, Crain M, Grimbert F, Rutili G and Taylor AE (1981) *J. Appl. Physiol.* **51**(5): 1268

44  Sakuma T, Pittet JF, Jayr C and Matthay MA (1993) *J. Appl. Physiol.* **74**(1): 176

45  Effros RM, Mason GR, Sietsema K, Silverman P and Hukkanen J (1987) *Circ. Res.* **60**(5): 708

46  Jayr C, Matthay MA (1991) *J. Appl. Physiol.* **71**(5): 1679

47  Sakuma T, Okaniwa G, Nakada T, Nishimura T, Fujimura S and Matthay MA (1994) *Am. J. Respir. Crit. Care Med.* **150**(2): 305

48  Matthay MA, Landolt CC and Staub NC (1982) *J. Appl. Physiol.* **53**(1): 96

49  Berthiaume Y, Broaddus VC, Gropper MA, Tanita T and Matthay MA (1988) *J. Appl. Physiol.* **65**(2): 585

50  Smedira N, Gates L, Hastings R, Jayr C, Sakuma T, Pittet JF and Matthay MA (1991) *J. Appl. Physiol.* **70**(4): 1827

51  Jayr C, Garat C, Meignan M, Pittet JF, Zelter M and Matthay MA (1994) *J. Appl. Physiol.* **76**(6): 2636

52  Wiener-Kronish JP, Albertine KH, Licko V and Staub NC (1984) *J. Appl. Physiol.* **56**: 459

53  Broaddus VC, Wiener-Kronish JP, Berthiaume Y and Staub NC (1988) *J. Appl. Physiol.* **64**: 384

54  Negrini D, Pistolesi M, Miniati M, Bellina CR, Giuntinni C and Miserocchi G (1985)

J. Appl. Physiol. **58**: 2062

55 Giuntini C Pistolesi M Miniati M and Fazio F (1988) *J. Thorac. Imaging* **3**(3): 36

56 Peterson BT, Brooks JA and Zack AG (1982) *J. Appl. Physiol.* **52**(6): 1661

57 Staub NC (1974) *Physiol. Rev.* **54**(3): 678

58 Michel RP, Hakim TS, Smith TT and Poulsen RS (1983) *Lab. Invest.* **149**: 412

59 Collee GG, Lynch KE, Hill RD and Zapol WM (1987) *Anesthesiology* **66**(5): 614

60 Bhattacharya J and Staub NC (1980) *Science* **210**(4467): 327

61 Bhattacharya S, Glucksberg MR and Bhattacharya (1989) *J. Circ. Res.* **64**(1): 167

62 Raj JU, Bland RD and Lai-Fook SJ (1986) *J. Appl. Physiol.* **60**(2): 539

63 Weibel ER (1983) *Morphometry of the Human Lung.* p. 78, Springer-Verlag, Berlin

64 Gaar KA Jr., Taylor AE, Owens LJ and Guyton AC (1967) *Am. J. Physiol.* **213**(4): 910

65 Gropper MA, Bhattacharya J and Staub NC (1988) *J. Appl. Physiol.* **65**(1): 343

66 Hakim TS, Maarek JM and Chang HK (1989) *Am. Rev. Respir. Dis.* **140**(1): 217

67 Hakim TS and Kelly S (1989) *J. Appl. Physiol.* **67**(3): 1277

68 Linehan JN, Pawson CA, Rickaby PA (1984) *J. Appl. Physiol.* **57**: 309

69 Hakim TS, Dawson CA and Linehan JH (1979) *J. Appl. Physiol.* **47**(1): 145

70 Cope DK, Grimbert F, Downey JM, Taylor AE (1992) *Crit. Care Med.* **20**(7): 1043

71 Baconnier PF, Eberhard A, Grimbert FA (1992) *J. Appl. Physiol.* **73**(4): 1351

72 Lai-Fook SJ (1982) *Lung* **160**(4): 175

73 Glucksberg MR, Bhattacharya J (1991) *J. Appl. Physiol.* **70**(2): 914

74 Hida W, Hildebrandt J (1984) *J. Appl. Physiol.* **57**(1): 262

75 Meyer BJ, Meyer A and Guyton AC (1968) *Circ. Res.* **22**(2): 263

76 Snashall PD, Nakahara K and Staub NC (1979) *J. Appl. Physiol.* **46**(5): 1003

77 Parker JC, Guyton AC and Taylor AE (1978) *J. Appl. Physiol.* **44**(2): 267

78 Goshy M, Lai-Fook SJ and Hyatt RE (1979) *J. Appl. Physiol.* **46**(5): 950

79 Kelly SM and Macklem PT (1991) *Am. J. Physiol.* **260**(3 Pt 1): C652

80 Bhattacharya J, Gropper MA and Staub NC (1984) *J. Appl. Physiol.* **56**(2): 271

81 Miserocchi G, Pistolesi M, Miniati M, Bellina CR, Negrini D and Giuntini C (1984) *J. Appl. Physiol.* **56**(2): 526

82 Miserocchi G, Negrini D, Pistolesi M, Bellina CR, Gilardi MC, Bettinardi V and Rossitto F (1988) *J. Appl. Physiol.* **64**(2): 577

83 Reed RK, Rubin K, Wiig H and Rodt SA (1992) *Circ. Res.* **71**: 978

84 Prather JW, Gaar KA, Jr and Guyton AC (1968) *J. Appl. Physiol.* **24**(4): 602

85 Navar PD and Navar LG (1977) *Am. J. Physiol.* **233**(2): H295

86 Parker JC, Falgout HJ, Parker RE, Granger DN and Taylor AE (1979) *Circ. Res.* **45**(4): 440

87 Taylor AE (1981) *Circ. Res.* **49**(3): 557

88 Normandin D, Tung H, Hargens AR and Peters RM (1990) *J. Surg. Res.* **48**(1): 91

89 Landis EM and Pappenheimer JR (1963) Exchange of substance through the capillary walls. In: *Handbook of Physiology*, Hamilton WF and Dow P (eds), Circulation, Vol. II., Section 2, p. 972. Washington DC

90 Gorin AB (1988) *J. Appl. Physiol.* **64**(4): 1561

91 Drake R, Gaar K and Taylor AE (1978) *Am. J. Physiol.* **234**(3): H266

92 Uhlig S and von Bethmann AN (1997) *J. Pharmacol. Toxicol. Meth.* 37 (3): 119

93 Parker JC, Townsley MI and Cartledge JT (1989) *J. Appl. Physiol.* 66(4): 1553

94 Oppenheimer L, Unruh HW and Skoog C, Goldberg HS (1983) *J. Appl. Physiol.* 54(1): 64

95 Parker JC, Prasad R, Allison RA, Wojchiechowski WV and Martin SL (1993)

*J. Appl. Physiol.* **74**(4): 1981

96 Crone F-RE and DG Levitt (1984) Capillary permeability to small solutes. In: *Handbook of Physiology. The Cardiovascular System. Microcirculation.* Sect. 2, Vol. IV, Pt. 1, Chapt. 10, p. 411. *Am. Physiol. Soc.*, Bethesda, MD

97 Taylor AE and Granger DN (1983) Exchange of macromolecules across the circulation. In: *Handbook of Physiology, Section 2, Vol. 4, Microcirculation,* EM Renkin and CC Michel (eds), *Am. Physiol. Soc.,* Bethesda, MD

98 Kern DF, Levitt D and Wangensteen D (1983) *Am. J. Physiol.* **245**(2): H229

99 Vincent PA Kreienberg PB, Minnear FL, Saba TM and Bell DR (1992) *J. Appl. Physiol.* **73**(6): 2440

100 Reed RK, Townsley MI and Taylor AE (1989) *Am. J. Physiol.* **257**(3 Pt 2): H1037

101 Reed RK, Townsley MI, Korthuis RJ and Taylor AE (1991) *Am. J. Physiol.* **261** (*Heart Circ. Physiol.* **30**): H728

102 Ishibashi M, Reed RK, Townsley MI, Parker JC and Taylor AE (1989) *Physiologist,* **32**(4): 201

103 Parker JC, Parker RE, Granger DN and Taylor AE (1981) *Circ. Res.* **48**(4): 549

104 Ishibashi M, Reed RK, Townsley MI, Parker JC and Taylor AE (1991) *J. Appl. Physiol.* **70**(5): 2104

105 Rippe B, Townsley MI and Taylor AE (1985) *J. Appl. Physiol.* **58**(5): 1521

106 Wangensteen OD, Lysaker E and Savaryn P (1977) *Microvasc. Res.* **14**(1): 81

107 Weiser PC and Grande F (1974) *Am. J. Physiol.* **226**(5): 1028

108 Pilati CF and Maron MB (1984) *Am. J. Physiol.* **247**(1 Pt 2): H1

109 Wolf MB, Watson PD and Scott DR 2d (1987) *Am. J. Physiol.* **253**(1 Pt 2): H194

110 White P Jr., Brower R, Sylvester JT, Permutt T and Permutt S (1993) *J. Appl. Physiol.* **74**(3): 1374

111 Gee MH, Muller PD, Stage AF and Blanchero N (1971) *Proc. Natl. Acad. Sci. USA* **30**: 379

112 Lewis FR, Jr and Elings VI (1978) *Surg. Forum* **29**: 182

113 Byrne K and Sugerman HJ (1988) *J. Surg. Res.* **44**(2): 185

114 Pfeiffer U, Birk M, Aschenbrenner G, Petrowicz O and Blümel G (1980) *Eur J. Surg. Res.* **12** (suppl):106

115 Sivak ED, Richmond BJ, O'Donavan PB and Borkowski GP (1983) *Crit. Care Med.* **11**(7): 498

116 Sibbald WJ, Warshawski FJ, Short AK, Harris J, Lefcoe MS and Holliday RL (1983) *Chest* **83**(5): 725

117 Lewis FR, Elings VB, Hill SL and Christensen JM (1982) *Ann. NY Acad. Sci.* **384**: 394

118 Wickerts CJ, Jakobsson J, Frostell C and Hedenstierna G (1990) *Intensive Care Med.* **16**(2): 115

119 Boldt J, King D, Scheld HH and Hempelmann G (1990) *J. Cardiothorac. Anesth.* **4**(1): 73

120 Fallon KD, Drake RE, Laine GA and Gabel JC (1985) *Anesthesiology* **62**(4): 505

121 Effros RM (1985) *J. Appl. Physiol.* **59**(3): 673

122 Noble WH and Kay JC (1988) *J. Appl. Physiol.* **65**(1): 156

123 Carlile PV and Gray BA (1984) *J. Appl. Physiol.* **57**(3): 680

124 Gray BA, Beckett RC, Allison RC, McCaffree DR, Smith RM, Sivak ED and Carlile PV, Jr (1984) *J. Appl. Physiol.* **56**(4): 878

125 Mitchell JP, Schuller D, Calandrino FS and Schuster DP (1992) *Am. Rev. Respir. Dis.* **145**(5): 990

126 Aberle DR, Wiener-Kronish JP, Webb WR and Matthay MA (1988) *Radiology* **168**(1): 73

127 Wheeler AP, Carroll FE and Bernard GR (1993) *New Horiz.* **1**(4): 471

128 Milne EN, Pistolesi M, Miniati M and

Giuntini C (1985) *Am. J. Roentgenol.* **144**(5): 879

129 Forster BB, Muller NL, Mayo JR, Okazawa M, Wiggs BJ and Pare PD (1992) *Chest* **101**(5): 1434

130 Kato S, Nakamoto T and Iizuka M (1996) *Chest* **109**(6): 1439

131 Morooka N, Watanabe S, Masuda Y and Inagaki Y (1982) *Jpn. Heart. J.* **23**(5): 697

132 Murata K, Herman PG, Khan A, Todo G, Pipman Y and Luber JM (1989) *Invest. Radiol.* **24**(9): 647

133 Hedlund LW, Effmann EL, Bates WM, Beck JW, Goulding PL and Putman CE (1982) *J. Comput. Assist. Tomogr.* **6**(5): 939

134 Hedlund LW, Vock P, Effmann EL and Putman CE (1985) *Invest. Radiol.* **20**(1): 2

135 Maunder RJ, Shuman WP, McHugh JW, Marglin SI and Butler J (1986) *JAMA* **9255**(18): 2463

136 Gattinoni L, Presenti A, Torresin A, Baglioni S, Rivolta M, Rossi F, Scarani F, Marcolin R and Cappelletti G (1986) *J. Thorac. Imaging* **1**(3): 25

137 Bombino M, Gattinoni L, Pesenti A, Pistolesi M and Miniati M (1991) *Chest* **100**(3): 762

138 Hansell DM (1995) Thoracic imaging. In: *Respiratory Medicine*, Brewis RAL, Corrin B, Geddes DM and Gibson GJ (eds) 2nd Edition, Vol. 1, Part B, Diagnostic Methods, Section 6.1, p. 278. WB Saunders, London

139 Cutillo AG, Morris AH, Ailion DC, Case TA, Durney CH, Ganesan K, Watanabe F and Akhtari M (1988) *Am. Rev. Respir. Dis.* **137**(6): 1371

140 Siefkin AD, Nichols BG (1986) *Am. Rev. Respir. Dis.* **134**(3): 509

141 Hayes CE, Case TA, Ailion DC, Morris AH, Cutillo A, Blackburn CW, Durney CH and Johnson SA (1982) *Science* **18216**(4552): 1313

142 Skalina S, Kundel HL, Wolf G and Marshall B (1984) *Invest. Radiol.* **19**(1): 7

143 Schmidt HC, McNamara MT, Brasch RC and Higgins CB (1985) *Invest. Radiol.* **20**(7): 687

144 Wexler HR, Nicholson RL, Prato FS, Carey LS, Vinitski S and Reese L (1985) *Invest. Radiol.* **20**(6): 583

145 Vinitski S, Pearson MG, Karlik SJ, Morgan WK, Carey LS, Perkins G, Goto T and Befus D (1986) *Magn. Reson. Med.* **3**(1): 120

146 Cutillo AG, Morris AH, Ailion DC, Durney CH and Ganesan K (1988) *J. Thorac. Imaging* **3**(3): 51

147 Awai K, Utsumi T, Kajima T, Fukuda H, Nakamura S, Fujikawa K, Azuma K and Ito K (1995) *Nippon Igaku Hoshasen Gakkai Zasshi* **55**(9): 633

148 Lancaster L, Bogdan AR, Kundel HL and McAffee B (1991) *Magn. Reson. Med.* **19**(1): 96

149 Schuster DP (1989) *Am. Rev. Respir. Dis.* **139**(3): 818

150 Fein A, Grossman RF, Jones JG, Goodman PC and Murray JF (1979) *Circulation* **60**(5): 1156

151 Nierman DM, Eisen DI, Fein ED, Hannon E, Mechanik JI and Benjamin E (1996) *J. Surg. Res.* **65**: 101

152 Newell JC, Edic PM, Ren X, Larson-Wiseman JL and Danyleiko MD (1996) *IEEE Trans. Biomed. Eng.* **43**(2): 133

153 Gorin AB, Weidner WJ, Demling RH and Staub NC (1978) *J. Appl. Physiol.* **45**: 225

154 Roselli RJ and Riddle WR (1989) *J. Appl. Physiol.* **67**(6): 2343

155 Gorin AB, Kohler J and DeNardo G (1980) *J. Clin. Invest.* **66**(5): 869

156 Basran GS and Hardy JG (1988) *J. Thorac. Imaging* **3**(3): 28

157 Campbell JH, McCurrach GM, McBeth F, Bessent RG, McKillop JH and Banham SW (1991) *Nucl. Med. Commun.* **12**(4): 288

158 Raijmakers PG, Groeneveld AB, Teule GJ and Thijs LG (1996) *J. Nucl. Med.* **37**(8):

1316

159 Basran GS, Byrne AJ and Hardy JG (1985) *Nucl. Med. Commun.* **6**(1): 3

160 Steinberg KP, Mitchell DR, Maunder RJ, Milberg JA, Whitcomb ME and Hudson LD (1993) *Am. Rev. Respir. Dis.* **148**(3): 556

161 Kelly CA, Fenwick JD, Corris PA, Fleetwood A, Hendrick DJ and Walters EH (1988) *Am. Rev. Respir. Dis.* **138**(1): 81

162 Matthay MA, Berthiaume Y and Staub NC (1985) *J. Appl. Physiol.* **59**(3): 928

163 Bayat S, Menaouar A, Anglade D, Perez N, Lafond JL, Ettinger H, François-joubert A and Grimbert FA (1995) *Eur. Respir. J.* **8**(S19): 398s

164 Bayat S, Menaouar A, Anglade D, Perez N., Lafond JL, Ettinger H and Grimbert FA (1996) *Am. J. Respir. Crit. Care Med.* **153** (4): A384

165 Swan HJ, Ganz W, Forrester J, Marcus H, Diamond G and Chonette D (1970) *N. Engl. J. Med.* **283**: 447

166 Baconnier PF, Eberhard A and Grimbert FA (1992) *J. Appl. Physiol.* **73**(4): 1351

167 Maarek JM, Hakim TS and Chang HK (1990) *J. Appl. Physiol.* **68**: 761

168 Grimbert F, Amardeil P, Ettinger H, Peyrin JC and Girardet P (1994) *Am. J. Respir. Crit. Care Med.* **149** (4, 2): A435

169 Matthay MA and Chatterjee K (1988) *Ann. Intern. Med.* **15109**(10): 826

170 Riedel M, Dennig K, Henneke KH and Rudolph W (1988) *Eur. Heart J.* **9**: 355

171 Himelman RB, Stulbarg M, Kircher B, Lee E, Kee L, Dean NC, Golden J, Wolfe CL and Schiller NB (1989) *Circulation* **79**(4): 863

172 Stevenson JG (1989) *J. Am. Soc. Echocardiogr.* **2**(3): 157

173 Lee RT, Lord CP, Plappert T and Sutton MS (1989) *Am. J. Cardiol.* **64**(19): 1366

174 Tanabe K, Asanuma T, Yoshitomi H, Kobayashi K, Nakamura K, Okada S, Shimizu H, Sano K and Shimada T (1996) *Am. J. Cardiol.* **78**(10): 1145

175 Burstin L (1967) *Brit. Heart J.* **29**: 396

176 Yagi H, Yamada H, Kobayashi T and Sekiguchi M (1990) *Am. Rev. Respir. Dis.* **142**: 796

177 Channer KS, Culling W, Wilde P and Jones JV (1986) *Lancet* **1**: 1005

178 Störk TV, Müller RM, Piske GJ, Ewert CO, Wienhold S and Hochrein H (1990) *Crit. Care Med.* **18**: 1158

179 Appleton CT, Galloway JM, Gonzalez MS, Gaballa M and Basnight MA (1993) *J. Am. Coll. Cardiol.* **22**: 1972

180 Berger M, Bach M, Hecht SR and Van Tosh A (1992) *Am. J. Cardiol.* **69**: 562

181 Abdulla AM, Kavouras T, Rivas F and Stefadouros MA (1980) *JAMA* **243**: 1539

182 Askenazi J, Koenigsberg DI, Ziegler JH and Lesch M (1981) *N. Engl. J. Med.* **305**: 1566

183 Brigham KL, Kariman K, Harris TR, Snapper JR, Bernard GR and Young SL (1983) *J. Clin. Invest.* **72**(1): 339

184 Mancini MC, Borovetz HS, Griffith BP and Hardesty RL (1985) *J. Surg. Res.* **39**(4): 305

185 Rinaldo JE, Borovetz HS, Mancini MC, Hardesty RL and Griffith BP (1986) *Am. Rev. Respir. Dis.* **133**(6): 1006

186 Zelter M, Lipavsky A, Hoeffel JM and Murray JF (1984) *J. Appl. Physiol.* **56**(6): 1512

187 Matthay MA and Wiener-Kronish JP (1990) *Am. Rev. Respir. Dis.* **142**(6 Pt 1): 1250

188 Murray JF, Matthay MA, Luce JM and Flick MR (1988) *Am. Rev. Respir. Dis.* **138**: 720

189 Parker RE, Wickersham NE, Roselli RJ, Harris TR and Brigham KL (1986) *J. Appl. Physiol.* **60**(4): 1293

190 Grimbert FA, Parker JC and Taylor AE (1981) *J. Appl. Physiol.* **51**(2): 335

191 Matthay MA and Chatterjee K (1988) *Ann. Intern. Med.* **15109**(10): 826

192 Forrester JS, Diamond GA and Swan HJ

(1977) *Am. J. Cardiol.* **39**: 137

193 Anderson FL, McDonnell MA, Tsagaris TJ and Kuida H (1981) *Arch. Intern. Med.* **141**: 1207

194 Sprung CL, Long WM, Marcial EH, Schein RM, Parker RE, Shomer T and Brigham KL (1987) *Am. Rev. Respir. Dis.* **136**(4): 957

195 Guyton AC and Lindsey AW (1959) *Circ. Res.* **7**: 649

196 Harris TR, Bernard GR, Brigham KL, Higgins SB, Rinaldo JE, Borovetz HS, Sibbald WJ, Kariman K and Sprung CL (1990) *Am. Rev. Respir. Dis.* **141**(2): 272

197 Bernard GR, Artigas A, Brigham KL, Carlet J, Falke K, Hudson L, Lamy M, Legall JR, Morris A and Spragg R (1994) *Am. J. Respir. Crit. Care Med.* **149**: 818

198 Toivonen HJ and Catravas JD (1991) *J. Appl. Physiol.* **71**(6): 2244

199 Kaplan JD, Calandrino FS and Schuster DP (1991) *Am. Rev. Respir. Dis.* **143**(1): 150

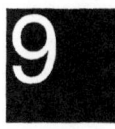

# 9 Neurogenic inflammation in the airways: Measurement of microvascular leakage

*M.G. Belvisi and*
*D.F. Rogers*

The role of sensory nerves in the acute inflammatory response was first demonstrated in the conjunctiva of rabbits and the skin of cats and humans. It is now known that sensory nerves mediate a local tissue response, termed 'neurogenic inflammation', in several somatic (e.g. skin and joints) and visceral (e.g. airways and urinary bladder) locations [1–3]. Neurogenic inflammation denotes the vasodilatation, increased vascular permeability, and plasma exudation (oedema) that follow sensory nerve stimulation (Fig. 9.1). This response appears to be mediated by local, or axon, reflexes and the peripheral release of neurotransmitter(s) because sensory nerves can mediate the phenomenon without being connected to the central nervous system. Because these nerves can subserve motor (efferent) functions as well as afferent functions, they may be considered to be 'sensory-efferent' nerves [4].

Neurogenic inflammation in the airways attracted interest in the early 1980s [5, 6]. Vascular permeability and plasma exudation in the respiratory tract of guinea pigs and rats was increased on stimulation of airway vagal sensory neurones, either by direct antidromic electrical stimulation of the vagus nerves or by chemicals that stimulate sensory nerve endings. The neurogenic inflammatory response is considered to be a non-adrenergic, non-cholinergic (NANC) neural response mediated via release of the tachykinins substance P (SP) and neurokinin A (NKA) from sensory nerve endings and the subsequent activation of $NK_1$ receptors on the endothelial cells [7]. Evidence for this hypothesis includes the observations that: 1) SP injected intravenously mimics the effect of vagal stimulation, 2) pretreatment of animals with capsaicin, which selectively degenerates tachykinin-containing unmyelinated sensory nerves, abolishes the effect of vagal stimulation, and 3) perhaps the most convincing evidence is that plasma extravasation evoked either by capsaicin or vagus nerve stimulation is inhibited by tachykinin $NK_1$ receptor antagonists [8, 9].

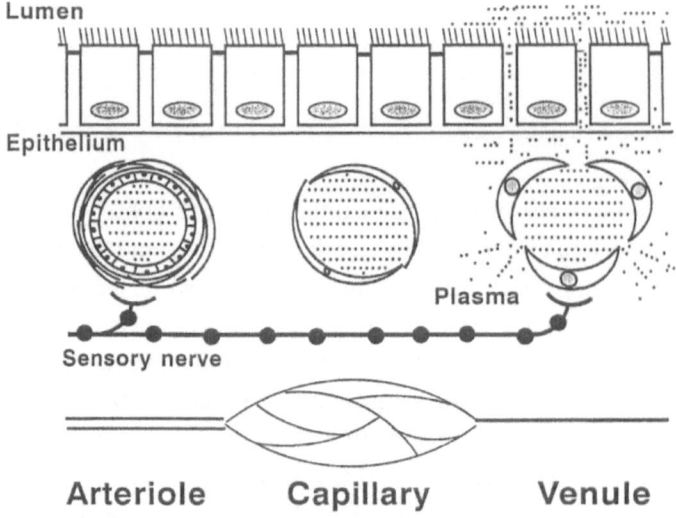

*Figure 9.1. Simplified schematic of proposed mechanism of neurogenic plasma exudation in the airways*

Arterioles and post-capillary venules are innervated by sensory nerves, whereas there is no evidence of similar capillary innervation. Activation of sensory nerves releases tachykinin neurotransmitters, for example substance P (SP), which interacts with tachykinin receptors on the venular endothelial cells to induce contraction. The resultant gaps formed between the cells allows outflow of plasma into the airway wall, causing tissue oedema, and subsequently passage of plasma into the airway lumen, which contributes to changes in the composition of airway surface liquid. Plasma leakage has not been demonstrated from arterioles or capillaries in the airways. Sensory neuropeptides, in particular SP and calcitonin gene-related peptide, may enhance leakage by inducing arteriolar vasodilatation and increasing blood flow to sites of leakage.

It has been well documented that electrical stimulation of the vagus nerve in rodents, as well as local stimulation of the nerve endings with irritants (e.g. cigarette smoke or formalin) or with inflammatory mediators (e.g. bradykinin or histamine), can cause extravasation of plasma proteins into the airway wall followed by a concomitant transudation of plasma into the airway lumen. Based on these observations it has been suggested that local neural reflexes involving the release of vasoactive tachykinins may contribute to airway inflammation and the pathophysiology of a number of airway diseases including asthma [10] and chronic coughing and sneezing [11]. However, although extravasation of plasma proteins and tissue oedema are fundamental components of the acute inflammatory response seen in the skin and nasal mucosa, the contribution of microvascular permeability in the airway mucosa to the pathogenesis of bronchial asthma is not yet clear. However, the demonstration of mucosal oedema and the presence of airway luminal exudates and mucus plugs in the bronchial lumen in *post mortem* studies in patients with severe asthma support a role for increased microvascular permeability in asthma [12].

This chapter is concerned with the experimental measurement of neurogenic microvascular leakage and plasma exudation in the airways. The three principal uses of these techniques are: 1) in the investigation of basic mechanisms underlying oedema formation in the airways (and luminal transudation), 2) in the testing of the effectiveness of tachykinin receptor antagonist drugs, and 3) in screening of novel drugs with inhibitory actions on sensory nerve activity.

## Material and equipment

A summary of the conditions of the experiments is given in Table 9.1. The following equipment is recommended for studies involving neurogenic plasma exudation, although not all equipment will be required for all types of experiment (*see* Section on *Methods* below).

- Heated blanket: Homeothermic System, Harvard Apparatus Ltd., Edenbridge, Kent, UK.
- Small animal ventilator: Harvard Apparatus, South Natick, Massachusettes, USA.
- Transducer for pulmonary pressure: Sensortechnics, Rugby, Warwickshire, UK.
- Transducer for blood pressure: Druck Ltd., Groby, Leicestershire, UK.
- Lectromed Multitrace 2: Ormed Ltd., Welwyn Garden City, Hertfordshire, UK.

*Table 9.1. Conditions for investigation of neurogenic airway plasma exudation*

| Conditions | Information |
|---|---|
| Species | Rats; 200–300 g |
| | Guinea pigs; 300–400 g |
| Body temperature maintenance | 38 °C |
| Blood gases (ventilated) | $PaO_2$ 114 mm Hg, $PaCO_2$ 37 mm Hg, $SaO_2$ 98 mm Hg (pH 7.4) |
| Criteria for quality of preparation | Good blood pressure trace Good pulmonary pressure trace (if used), with stable breathing mechanics (e.g. animal not breathing 'against' pump) Good venous cannulation (for administration of drugs) Exposed tissue of animal turns from brown to blue/brown after injection of Evans blue dye (indicating effective injection) |
| Time to set up experiment | 45 min |
| Duration of experiment once set up | 10–20 min |
| Useful papers describing technique | [15, 16, 36] |
| Experiments (animals) per day | [5–10] |
| Cost per experiment | £40 |

- Subminiature electrodes: Harvard Apparatus Ltd., Edenbridge, Kent, UK. These electrodes are designed so that the anode and cathode are set in plastic to maintain a constant distance between them. An adjustable plastic flange holds the nerve in place.
- Electrical stimulator: Model S88, Grass Instruments, Quincy, Massachusettes, USA.
- Glass fibre filter (for removal of particulate phase of cigarette smoke): Cambridge filter Corporation, Syracruse, New York, USA.
- Ultrasonic nebuliser (for administration of drug aerosols): model 2512, PulmoSonic, DeVilbiss Co, Philadelphia, USA.

# Methods

## Anaesthesia

Several anaesthetic regimes have been adopted for anaesthetising small laboratory animals in order to perform experiments involving the measurement of neurogenic plasma leakage (Tab. 9.2). Anaesthesia (with pentobarbitone sodium) rather than use of awake animals is recommended for use with cigarette smoke as a stimulant because it produces a greater increase in exudation and with less variability in response [6]. Urethane is a good general anaesthetic for the study of neural function in both central and peripheral nervous systems [13]. However, urethane anaesthesia has been found to reduce bronchiole-alveolar permeability to cigarette smoke [14], but no data are available for its effects on airway permeability. The authors use urethane on a regular basis and find it to give predictable anaesthesia with good increases in airway plasma exudation.

In rats, adequate depth of anaesthesia is determined by a lack of flexor response to pinching the toes. Our experience is that this is not sufficient

*Table 9.2. Anaesthetics*

| Species | Anaesthetic | Dose | Route |
|---|---|---|---|
| Rat | Sodium methohexital | 60 mg/kg | i.p. |
| Rat | Sodium pentobarbital | 40 mg/kg | i.p. |
| Guinea pig | Diazepam (premedication) followed by | 9 mg/kg | i.p. |
|  | Hypnorm[1] | 2.5 ml/kg | i.m.[2] |
| Guinea pig | Urethane | 2 g/kg[3] | i.p. |

*i.p., intraperitoneal; i.m., intramuscular; [1]0.315 mg fentanyl citrate and 10 mg fluanisone per ml solution. Note: Opioid drugs are highly effective at inhibiting neurogenic responses, including airway plasma exudation. Hypnorm, due to its opioid drug content, is therefore not a recommended anaesthetic for most investigations of airway neurogenic plasma exudation [16]. [2]Administered as a divided dose (of ~0.5 ml) into the medial aspect of each thigh. [3]8 ml/kg of a 25% (w/v) solution in 0.9% (w/v) saline.*

in guinea pigs and lack of a blink reflex in response to gentle touching of the cornea is more reliable.

## Surgery

Experimental set-ups are shown in Figure 9.2. Anaesthetised guinea pigs or rats are placed supine on a heated blanket to maintain body temperature (rectal) at 37 °C. Male animals have been used in most studies, although female animals can be used. For ease of subsequent cannulation and administration of drugs and solutions, it is preferable to have the animal's head facing towards the experimenter. It is not necessary to pin down the fore legs. However, if the position of the legs is interfering with the surgery, they can be tethered to adjacent supports via thread tied around the 'wrists.'

The fur covering the throat and chest is wetted thoroughly to limit subsequent contamination of the dissection and to reduce airborne contamination (with possible development of occupational allergy in sensitive individuals). Using a scalpel with a new blade or sharp scissors a midline incision through the skin is made from the chin to the just below the cranial tip of the sternum (the *manubrium*). The following procedures are best carried out using blunt dissection. This involves using forceps or blunt-ended scissors to gently prise apart muscle fibre layers. The forceps or scissors are pushed closed into the muscle mass and are then opened. The process is repeated until structures of interest become exposed. First, the subcutaneous muscles of the neck, principally the superficial cervical platysma, are parted in the mid-line. The exposed sternohyoideus muscles are then parted to reveal the ventral surface of the trachea. The sternohyoideus can be clamped apart if the time-course of 'blueing' of the trachea with plasma marker dyes is required. Fluid loss by the exposed tissue needs to be minimised and this can be achieved by covering with saline-dampened gauze or with an impervious membrane (e.g. Clingfilm).

Cervical jugular veins are used for the systemic administration of drugs, solutions and plasma markers (dyes or radiolabelled tracers). In our experiments, we use the right jugular vein, leaving the left side of the

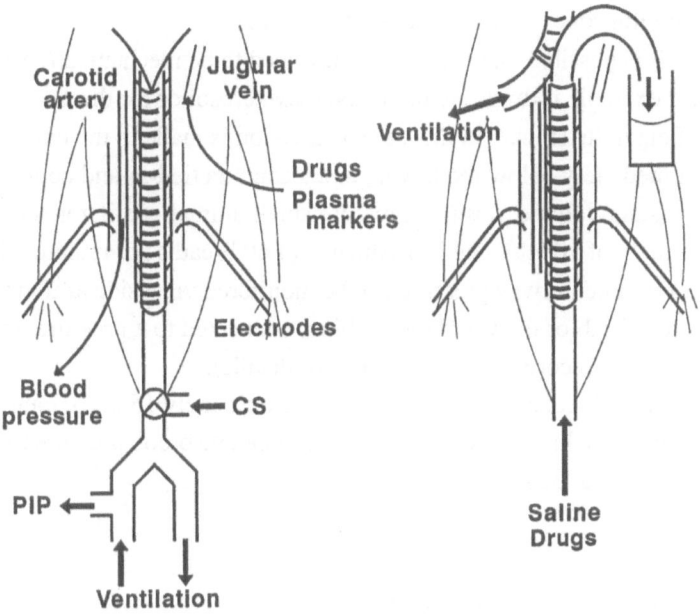

*Figure 9.2.* **In vivo** *preparations for measurement of airway neurogenic plasma exudation.*
*Anaesthetised small laboratory rodents is the preferred experimental set-up*

Left panel: Measurement of tissue exudate. The animal may or may not be ventilated. If ventilated, concomitant measurements of airway resistance can be made, for example pulmonary insufflation pressure (PIP). Drugs can be given by aerosol into the ventilation circuit. Cigarette smoke (CS) can be blown into the lungs via a side-port. Drug solutions and plasma markers, for example Evans blue dye, are administered via the jugular veins, and blood pressure is recorded from the carotid artery. The cervical vagus nerves are stimulated electrically via bipolar platinum electrodes. Right panel: Measurement of luminal transudation of plasma. An extrathoracic segment of the trachea is cannulated at either end and isolated in situ. The animal breathes either spontaneously or aided via a third cannula directed to the lungs. Venously administered plasma markers, for example radiolabelled albumin, appearing in the lumen are collected at unit time intervals in the tracheal superfusate. For details see [31, 37].

chest free for measurement of blood pressure via the carotid artery. Choice of side depends primarily on the siting of blood pressure recording equipment and on the 'handedness' of the experimenter. Drugs are usually injected into the vein via an indwelling cannula. Systemic blood pressure can be monitored from a cervical carotid artery via an indwelling Portex cannula, filled with heparin-saline (10 U/ml), linked to a pressure transducer and connected to a recorder.

It is possible that the animal may need to be mechanically ventilated, for example if drugs are to be given by aerosol or for the administration of cigarette smoke. In this case an incision is made in the upper trachea, immediately below the larynx, and a cannula tied-in and connected to a constant volume, positive pressure small animal ventilator set at a tidal volume of 10 ml/kg and a frequency of 60 breaths per minute (Tab. 9.1). If required, airway pressure can be monitored via a side arm in the expiratory limb of the ventilation tubing, connected to a pressure transducer and trace recorder (*see* Chapter 1 for details).

After induction of anaesthesia (approximately 15 min), total time for surgery, including production of an acceptable blood pressure trace, is of the order of 30 min.

## Experimental procedure

After completion of surgery, the experimental procedure can commence. Each animal in general gives one piece of data (i.e. n = 1). Consequently, animals have to be divided into "test" and control groups. For example, for the examination of a pharmaceutical compound which might inhibit neurogenic plasma exudation, at the simplest level there would need to be a four groups of animals: 1) prepared for sensory nerve stimulation (e.g. dissected and the vagus nerves placed over electrodes), given drug vehicle, but not stimulated ("sham" stimulation) (baseline vehicle control group), 2) as for 1 above but given drug (to determine effect of drug on baseline leakage), 3) drug vehicle and stimulated (response group), and 4) drug and stimulated. Additional groups could be examined, for example no drug or vehicle and sham stimulated (baseline control). This group may be required if the baseline was considered too high and the effect of the vehicle on leakage needed to be determined.

For these protocols, drug or vehicle is given at an appropriate time before stimulation (according to the kinetics of the drug, but generally of the order of 15–20 min). One minute before stimulation, the plasma marker (e.g. Evans blue dye) is injected i.v. A variety of stimuli can then be used to activate the sensory nerves.

### Direct electrical stimulation of the vagus nerve

The cervical vagus nerves are exposed by blunt dissection (*see* above), separated from the trachea and sectioned below the nodose ganglia at the level of the fifth tracheal cartilage ring in order to avoid simultaneously stimulating the central nervous system (CNS) when stimulating peripheral systems (herein, the airways). The caudal ends of the nerves are then fixed across the bipolar platinum electrodes which are connected to a double channel square wave stimulator. The electrical voltage, frequency and pulse width of the electrical stimulus and the time for which it is applied affect the magnitude of the exudative response. Parameters of 5 V, 7 Hz, 5 ms for 3 min are optimum for induction of significant leakage throughout the airways and with minimal effects on systemic blood pressure [15] (Fig. 9.3). The concern with blood pressure is twofold: 1) severe hypotension will kill the animal, and 2) changes in bronchial blood pressure, and hence blood flow, may affect leakage by altering flow to the sites of leakage.

Bilateral electrical stimulation of the vagus nerves in the guinea pig evokes plasma exudation into the larynx, trachea and bronchial tree as evidenced by colouration of the tissue with Evans blue dye [6, 15, 16] (Fig. 9.4). Furthermore, electrical stimulation of the vagus nerves in the rat evokes extravasation of Monastral blue from venules in specific regions of the larynx, trachea and mainstem bronchi. The increase in vascular leakage has a rapid onset and a short duration, beginning within 30 s of the start of vagal stimulation and lasting for 3–5 min. Most of the extravasated Monastral blue is trapped within the walls of postcapillary venules and collecting venules with a diameter of 10–80 µm. Arterioles, capillaries and venules larger than 80 µm have no endothelial gaps and so it would appear that postcapilliary venules are the principal sites of action of vasoactive substances. In addition to the leakage present within the airway structures, neurogenic stimulation induces a concomitant, in part atropine-sensitive, movement of plasma proteins into the airway

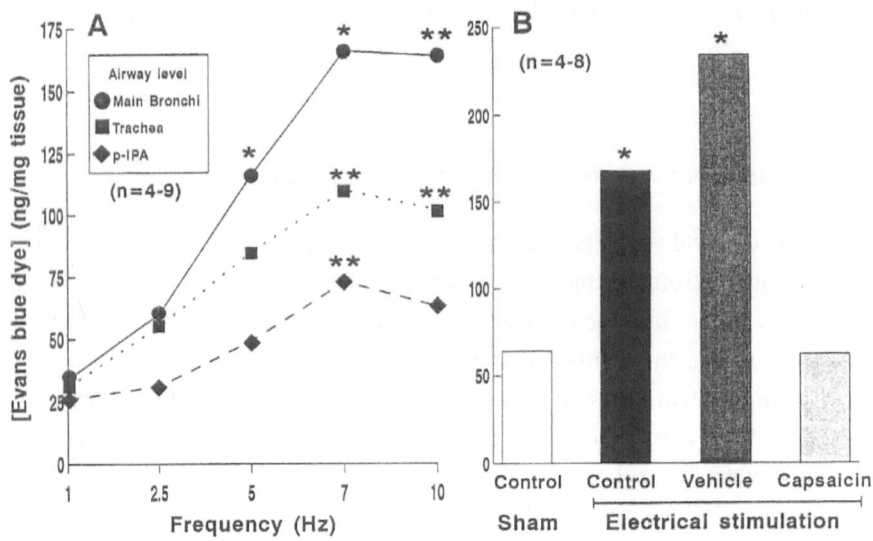

**Figure 9.3. Neurogenic plasma exudation in the airways demonstrated by direct bilateral electrical stimulation of the cervical vagus nerves in guinea pigs**
(See Fig. 9.2, left panel for experimental set-up). A: Frequency response curve of tissue content of the plasma marker Evans blue dye at different airway levels, with other electrical parameters held at 5 V, 5 msec for 5 min (p-IPA, proximal intrapulmonary airways; *$p < 0.05$, **$p < 0.01$ vs controls, equivalent to values at 1 Hz). B: Demonstration of involvement of sensory nerves in the exudative response in A. Electrical stimulation increases Evans blue dye content of the main bronchi (black bar) above sham stimulated values (open bar). Pretreatment of animals 1 week prior to the experiments with the vehicle for capsaicin has no effect on the stimulated exudative response, whereas degeneration of the nerves with capsaicin eliminates the response. *$p < 0.05$ vs sham control. Redrawn from data in [15].

lumen that has been determined by measuring the movement of radiolabelled albumin.

The increased leakage into airway tissues on nerve stimulation is not abolished by pretreatment of the animal with propranolol and atropine suggesting that the response is due to the release of a non-adrenergic, non-cholinergic (NANC) neurotransmitter(s). It is now clear that this nerve stimulation-induced oedema is due to the release of substance P and NKA from sensory nerve endings. Evidence that the neurogenic inflammatory response is mediated predominantly by the release of SP includes the observation that SP injected intravenously mimics the effect

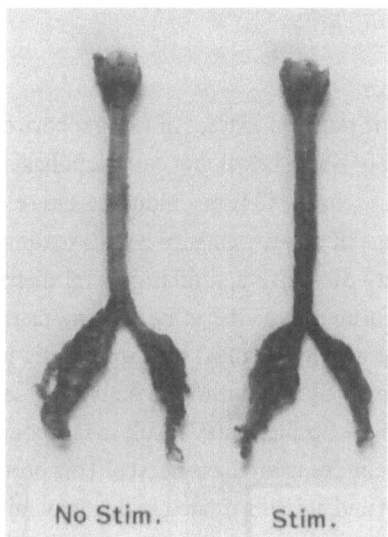

**Figure 9.4. Macroscopic visualisation of neurogenic plasma exudation in guinea pig airways**
*Animals were anaesthetised with urethane, pretreated with atropine and propranolol to eliminate cholinergic and adrenergic influences, and Evans blue dye was injected intravenously. Both cervical vagus nerves were either stimulated electrically (Stim.) or given a sham procedure (No stim.), and the animal perfused of intravascular dye. Photograph shows dorsal view of larynx, trachea, main bronchi and intrapulmonary airways which were exposed by scraping away parenchymal tissue. Tissue Evans blue content (shown in grey) was markedly greater in stimulated than in control airways.*

of vagal stimulation. Tachykinins are thought to elicit their functional effects via activation of neurokinin receptors of which three receptor subtypes have been proposed, $NK_1$, $NK_2$ and $NK_3$, based on receptor binding and biofunctional studies [7]. The neurokinin receptor/s involved in the nerve stimulation-induced airway oedema response have been characterised pharmacologically using receptor selective antagonists and been found to be predominantly of the $NK_1$ receptor subtype [9, 17]. Moreover, in peripheral guinea pig airways $NK_2$ receptors have also been implicated in the neurogenic plasma extravasation [18]. In addition to the direct action of tachykinins acting on the venular endothelium to increase vascular permeability, there are also indirect mechanisms involving mast cell activation and 5-HT release.

## Chemical stimulants

### Capsaicin

Capsaicin is the pungent extract of hot peppers of the *Capsicum* family. It has previously been shown that capsaicin has selective effects on peptide-containing sensory C-fibres inducing the release of SP from the peripheral endings of airway sensory nerves leading to increases in vascular permeability that have a similar general distribution to that of nerve stimulation. Furthermore, it has been demonstrated that plasma extravasation in the airways evoked by capsaicin is inhibited by an $NK_1$ receptor antagonist [8]. In addition to activating sensory nerves, systemic administration of capsaicin may result in temporary or permanent depletion of neuropeptides from these nerves. This process is termed capsaicin desensitisation and animals treated in this way fail to develop neurogenic inflammation upon sensory nerve stimulation (Fig. 9.5). In fact, prior to the development of neurokinin receptor antagonists, capsaicin pretreatment was used as a method of assessing the contribution of sensory nerve activation to a given response.

### Bradykinin

Bradykinin (BK) is an endogenous inflammatory nonapeptide which is generated either by cleavage of low molecular weight kininogen by tissue kallikrein or by activation of the plasma proteolytic cascade and is thought to be an important mediator in inflammatory airway diseases such as asthma. Bradykinin evokes plasma leakage in guinea pig and rodent airways [19]. Recent studies, using neurokinin receptor antagonists, have provided direct evidence that bradykinin-induced airway microvascular is, in part, mediated by activation of $NK_1$ receptors presumably through the release of SP and NKA [20].

### Cigarette smoke

Active or passive exposure to cigarette smoke is a common form of irritation to the respiratory tract mucosa in humans, and activates tracheobronchial primary afferent sensory nerves. Reflex bronchoconstriction observed upon cigarette-smoke exposure is mainly due to a particulate component of the smoke, while mucosal oedema, as evidenced by plas-

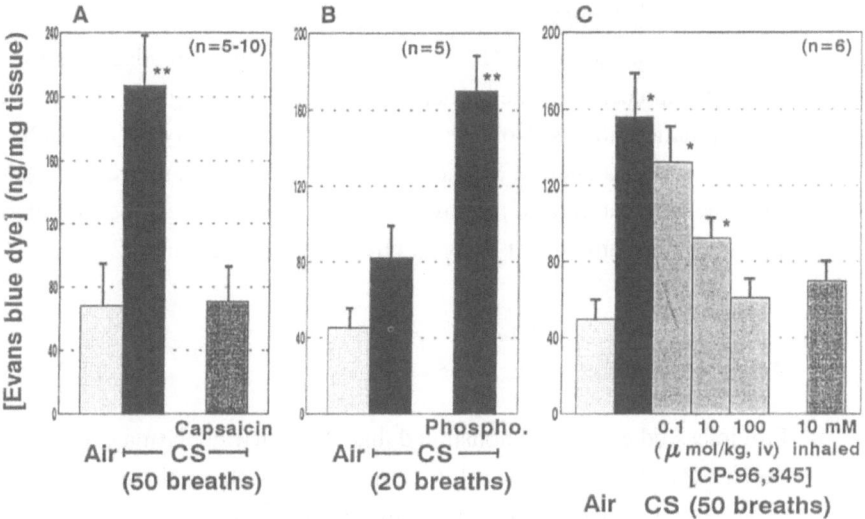

**Figure 9.5. Reflex neurogenic inflammation in guinea pig main bronchi in response to acute inhalation of cigarette smoke, CS**

(See Fig. 9.2, left panel for experimental set-up). A: Fifty tidal volumes (breaths) of CS increases tissue content of the plasma marker Evans blue dye ~3-fold above that induced by an equivalent air inhalation. The response is eliminated by degeneration of sensory nerves by pretreatment with capsaicin. B: Plasma exudation in response to a threshold administration of CS is potentiated by phosphoramidon (Phospho.), an inhibitor of the enzyme neutral endopeptidase which degrades substance P. C: CS-induced plasma exudation is inhibited in a dose-related manner by the tachykinin $NK_1$ receptor antagonist CP-96, 345 (iv: intravenous). The antagonist is also effective when given by inhalation as an aerosol. $^*p < 0.05$, $^{**}p < 0.01$ compared with air. N = number of animals per group. Redrawn from data in [24].

ma protein extravasation, is thought to be caused by hydroxyl radicals in the gas-vapour phase [21]. Many studies have documented that cigarette smoke evokes plasma extravasation in rat trachea via the release of tachykinins from C-fibre sensory nerve endings. Direct evidence, using the tachykinin receptor antagonists CP-96, 345, FR 113680 and FK 224, is now available demonstrating that cigarette-smoke-induced airway plasma exudation is mediated by stimulation of capsaicin-sensitive C-fibres and release of tachykinins [22–24] (Fig. 9.5).

## Sodium metabisulphite

Sodium metabisulphite (MBS) is often used as an antioxidant and preservative and can provoke bronchoconstriction and cough when inhaled by asthmatic patients. However, the mechanism underlying its mechanism of action is unclear. Studies in guinea pigs have demonstrated that MBS aerosol can induce microvascular leakage which can be inhibited by capsaicin pretreatment or by an $NK_1$ receptor antagonist [25].

## Other stimulants

Previous studies have demonstrated that acute airway plasma extravasation induced by hypertonic saline [26] or the late-phase of leakage in response to allergen challenge of sensitised animals nerves [27] is also due to activation of capsaicin-sensitive sensory nerves.

## Quantification

Assessment of plasma leakage usually relies on the measurement of extravasated albumin, using either radiolabelled albumin or dyes as intravascular markers. The majority of studies have used the diazo dye, Evans blue, as a marker of plasma extravasation which is a relatively safe and simple technique. Spectrophotometric measurements of the amount of dye extractable from the tissue being studied are used to quantify the plasma protein extravasation.

## Evans blue dye technique

Intravenous injection of Evans blue dye and its subsequent leakage into airway tissues has been used to quantify plasma exudation [5]. This technique relies upon the binding *in vivo* of the dye to plasma macromolecules, in particular albumin.

Evans blue (30 mg/kg: 30 mg/ml in saline and filtered to exclude 0.2 µm particles) is injected into a jugular vein 1 min before nerve stimulation (electrical or chemical). At the end of the stimulation the tissue content of dye is assessed after perfusing the systemic circulation with saline to remove intravascular dye. The left ventricle is incised, a blunt-ended 13-gauge needle is inserted into the ascending aorta, and the ventricles are cross-clamped. Spencer-Wells forceps are suitable for this. Blood is expelled from the incised right atrium at 100 mmHg pressure until the perfusate is clear (approximately 150 ml infused). Plasma exudation in a variety of airway tissues can be studied, including nasal mucosa, larynx, trachea, main bronchi and intrapulmonary airways [28]. Tissues of interest are carefully removed; the intrapulmonary airways can be exposed by gently scraping away the parenchyma with a blunt razor blade. The tissues are dried, either by 'blotting' with filter paper or in a freeze drier [29]. Freeze drying may reduce variability (Rogers, unpublished observation), although this has not been formally studied. The dry tissue is then weighed and the dye extracted in formamide at 37 °C for 16 h. Other protocols have been used, for example 50 °C for 24 h [30]; there is no formal evidence that any one is superior to another in its ability to extract the maximal amount of dye. The dye concentration can be determined colorimetrically or fluorimetrically. Colorimetry is performed at the absorbance maximum of 620 nm wavelength, and fluorimetry at an excitation wavelength of 620 nm (band width 10 nm) and an emisssion wavelength of 680 nm (band width 40 nm). In both cases, a tissue blank, incubated in formamide, needs to be run. Fluorimetry may be more sensitive and give lower values for the tissue blank than colorimetry [30]. Tissue content of Evans blue (ng/mg wet weight tissue) is calculated from standard curves of dye concentrations in the range (0.5 – 10 µg/ml).

There is a significant correlation between the tissue content of Evans blue dye and [125I]-labelled albumin in all airways studied, including the larynx, trachea, main bronchi and intrapulmonary airways [31]. However, there was only significant correlation for transudation (i.e. the passage of fluid into the airway lumen) of the two markers at high rates of plasma leakage, with the radiolabelled technique being more sensitive [31]. Furthermore, the Evans blue dye method does not reveal the precise location or the morphological basis of the permeability change, because the extravasated dye quickly diffuses away from the sites of leakage and is not visible by light and electron microscopy.

## Monastral dyes as tracers

This method is used when the parameters of interest are the specific blood vessels which have become 'leaky' in response to a stimulus, and the distribution within the airway of these sites of increased vascular permeability. In this way monastral dyes (monastral blue, red and green) have been used in microscopy studies to overcome the problems encountered with the rapid diffusion of extravasated tracers such as Evans blue. The monastral pigments have several advantages over dyes such as Evans blue as they are electron dense and are too large to cross the endothelium of tracheal blood vessels with normal permeability. The monastral pigments can cross the endothelium of abnormally permeable blood vessels, but most of the extravasated pigment is trapped by the basal lamina of these vessels, thereby labelling the sites of extravasation.

Monastral pigments can be prepared for use as tracers in the following way. A 3% suspension (w/v) of Monastral blue in 0.85% saline is dispersed in an ultrasonic bath for 3 min, passed through a 5 μM Millipore filter and then injected. The tracer is usually administered as a dose of 30 mg/kg in a volume of 1 ml/kg into a vein prior to the stimulus to evoke leakage.

## [$^{125}$I]-albumin

Plasma protein extravasation into both the airway wall and tracheobronchial fluid can be determined by using radiolabelled tracers [32, 33]. Intravenous injection of 3 μCi/kg [$^{125}$I]-albumin is undertaken a few minutes prior to application of the leakage stimulus. At the end of the experiment, the animal is killed and arterial blood samples obtained for determination of plasma [$^{125}$I]-albumin. The chest cavity is then opened and the more distal extra-pulmonary bronchial divisions sutured. A catheter (external diameter 1.8 mm) can then be inserted and tied into the top of the trachea. Tracheobronchial lavage can then be performed with five consecutive washes of 150 μl Hanks' balanced salt solution (HBSS). These lavages can be pooled and counted in a gamma counter for $^{125}$I-labelled albumin. Finally, for measurement of leakage into airway structures the tissues can be dissected and their radioactivity determined in the gamma counter. The tissues are then lyophilised and the dry weight determined. Plasma protein extravasation can then be determined by dividing the counts/min of $[^{125}I]$- albumin in the tissues or lavage samples by that in 1 μl plasma. Results are expressed as microlitres of plasma per mg dry weight tissue or per total lavage.

Radiolabelled fibrinogen may be superior over radiolabelled albumin as a sensitive marker of plasma extravasation [34, 35].

## Application

Airway inflammation is a characteristic feature of bronchial asthma, Indeed, increased microvascular permeability with exudation of plasma leading to tissue oedema may be present even in mild asthma. Furthermore, plasma exudation into the airways may be important in the pathogenesis of bronchial hyperresponsiveness. It has been hypothesised that epithelial damage may expose sensory C-fibre nerve endings to inflammatory mediators carried to the site in the exuded plasma. Stimulation of these nerve endings may result in a local axon reflex with antidromic conduction along afferent nerve collaterals and release of peptide neurotransmitters. Therefore, neurogenic mechanisms have been implicated in the pathophysiology of asthma [10]. Neurogenic mechanisms with the local release of neuropeptides leading to plasma extravasation, bronchoconstriction, and mucus secretion are an established phenomenon in rodent airways. If similar neurogenic mechanisms are present in human airways drugs which inhibit sensory nerve function may be useful in asthma therapy. The rodent models of airway microvascular leakage described in this chapter may therefore be rapid and easy assays which could be used to test compounds which may have anti-inflammatory activity in airway disease.

## Species differences

Most work on airway plasma exudation has been performed on small rodents, particularly rats and guinea pigs. In general, there are no notable differences between these two species in magnitude of response or distribution of leakage throughout the airways.

## Discussion

In small laboratory animals neurogenic inflammation induced by capsaicin or antidromic electrical stimulation of the vagus nerve mimics vascular permeability changes within the airways evoked by endogenous SP or certain irritants. Therefore, studies in which neurogenic plasma extravasation is utilised as a model of airway inflammation provides a convenient model to study the effect of anti-inflammatory agents which could be developed for the treatment of airway inflammatory conditions such as asthma. A variety of methods are available, and the choice of preparation will depend upon the question being posed. For example, the demands of rapid screening of potential tachykinin antagonists will be less than those of basic research into underlying mechanisms. At the simplest level, possibly for screening, vagal stimulation of unventilated animals using leakage of intravenous Evans blue dye, as the plasma marker, into the lower trachea and/or main bronchi will give a rapid indication (within minutes) of the efficacy of a drug. For more detailed work, particularly involving investigation of leakage into the airway lumen, radiolabelled plasma markers appear to be more precise, with monastral dyes useful in studies of localisation of leakage sites. Different techniques can be combined and are complimentary to each other. For example, use of monastral dyes and radiolabelled plasma markers could be used to study localisation and luminal leakage in the same preparation, although radiolabelled fibrinogen may be a useful single marker for both processes.

## Troubleshooting

### Difficulty in cannulating veins

Cannulating veins can be difficult because they tend to collapse when incised. If only a few injections are to be made (three or less), the vein need not be cannulated. Instead, the injection needle is passed through the *pectoralis major* muscle and into the vein. When the needle is withdrawn, the muscle provides a protection against bleeding.

## Difficulty in cannulating arteries

Arteries are easier to cannulate than veins because of their more rigid walls. However, problems can occur. It is, therefore, best to make the initial incision as distal as possible to the intended direction of insertion of the cannula (herein for the carotid artery, as far cranial as possible). If this insertion point fails, another can be made further along the artery.

## Poor blood pressure trace

Instead of a clear trace showing the pulse with a good separation between diastoly and systoly, the trace appears as a continuous line. This is usually due to a blockage which flushing with heparin-saline usually removes. The blockage may be due to the tip of the cannula pressing against the inside wall of the artery. Slightly withdrawing the cannula can help. However, if the blockage is tenacious, it may be due to endothelium stripped from the vessel as the cannula was inserted. This may require a new line to be established (*see* Section on *Difficulty with cannulating arteries*, above).

---

# Acknowledgements

The authors wish to thank the following for support: The Wellcome Trust, Fisons Pharmaceuticals (Loughborough, UK), and Pfizer Central Research (Sandwich, UK).

# References

1 McDonald DM (1988) *J. Neurocytol.* **17**: 583

2 McDonald DM, Mitchell RA, Gabella G and Haskell A (1988) *J. Neurocytol.* **17**: 605

3 Barnes PJ, Belvisi MG and Rogers DF (1990) *Trends Pharmacol. Sci.* **11**: 185

4 Maggi CA and Meli A (1988) *Gen. Pharmacol.* **19**: 1

5 Lundberg JM and Saria A (1982) *Acta Physiol. Scand.* **115**: 521

6 Lundberg JM, Brodin E and Saria A (1983) *Acta Physiol. Scand.* **119**: 243

7 Khawaja AM, Rogers DF (1996) *Cell Biol.* **28**: 721

8 Eglezos A, Giuliani S, Viti G and Maggi CA (1991) *Eur. J. Pharmacol.* **209**: 277

9 Lei Y-H, Barnes PJ and Rogers DF (1992) *Br. J. Pharmacol.* **105**: 261

10 Barnes PJ (1986) *Lancet* **1**: 242

11 Karlsson J-A (1993) *Thorax* **48**: 396

12 Dunnill MS (1960) *J. Clin. Pathol.* **13**: 27

13 Maggi CA and Meli A (1986) *Experientia* **42**: 109

14 Burns AR, Van Oostdam J, Walker DC and Hogg JC (1987) *J. Appl. Physiol.* **63**: 84

15 Belvisi MG, Barnes PJ and Rogers DF (1990) *J. Neurosci. Meth.* **32**: 159

16 Belvisi MG, Rogers DF and Barnes PJ (1989) *J. Appl. Physiol.* **66**: 268

17 Hirayama Y, Lei Y-H, Barnes PJ and Rogers DF (1993) *Br. J. Pharmacol.* **108**: 844

18 Tousignant C, Chan CC, Guevremont D, Brideau C, Hale JJ, Maccoss M and Rodger IW (1993) *Br. J. Pharmacol.* **108**: 383

19 Rogers DF, Dijk S and Barnes PJ (1990) *Br. J. Pharmacol.* **101**: 739

20 Sakamoto T, Barnes PJ and Chung KF (1993) *Eur. J. Pharmacol.* **231**: 31

21 Lei Y-H, Barnes PJ and Rogers DF (1996) *Br. J. Pharmacol.* **117**: 449

22 Delay-Goyet P and Lundberg JM (1991) *Eur. J. Pharmacol.* **203**: 157

23 Morimoto H, Yamashita M, Matsuda A, Miyake H and Fujii T (1992) *Eur. J. Pharmacol.* **224**: 1

24 Lei Y-H, Barnes PJ and Rogers DF (1995) *Am. J. Respir. Crit. Care Med.* **151**: 1752

25 Sakamoto T, Tsukagoshi H, Barnes PJ and Chung KF (1994) *Am. J. Crit. Care Med.* **149**: 387

26 Umeno E, McDonald DM and Nadel JA (1990) *J. Clin. Invest.* **85**: 1905

27 Bertrand C, Geppetti P, Baker J, Yamawaki I, Nadel JA (1993) *J. Immunol.* **150**: 1479

28 Evans TW, Rogers DF, Aursudkij B, Chung KF and Barnes PJ (1988) *Am. Rev. Respir. Dis.* **138**: 396

29 Lötvall JO, Elwood W, Tokuyama K, Barnes PJ and Chung KF (1991) *Clin. Sci.* **80**: 241

30 Saria A and Lundberg JM (1983) *J. Neurosci. Meth.* **8**: 41

31 Rogers DF, Boschetto P and Barnes PJ (1988) *J. Pharmacol. Meth.* **21**: 309

32 Didier A, Kowalski ML, Jay J and Kaliner MA. (1990) *Am. Rev. Respir. Dis.* **141**: 398

33 Erjefält I and Persson CGA (1989) *Am. Rev. Respir. Dis.* **2**: 93

34 Pedersen KE, Rigby PJ, Self and Goldie RG (1991) *Br. J. Pharmacol.* **104**: 128

35 Tousignant C, Chan CC, Young D, Guevremont D and Rodger IW (1993) *Canad. J. Physiol. Pharmacol.* **71**: 506

36 Lundberg JM, Brodin E, Hua X and Saria A (1984) *Acta Physiol. Scand.* **120**: 217

37 Rogers DF, Alton EWFW, Aursudkij B, Boschetto P, Dewar A and Barnes PJ (1990) *J. Physiol.* **431**: 643

# 10 Intravital microscopy: Surface lung vessels and interstitial pressure

*D. Negrini*

Over the last 15 years our laboratory has been studying the mechanisms involved in establishing and controlling water and solute exchanges in the pleuro-pulmonary interstitial tissues that are schematically depicted in Figure 10.1. Pleuro-pulmonary fluid turnover involves several compartments (the parietal pleural interstitium, the systemic capillaries, the pleural space, the pulmonary interstitium and the visceral capillaries, the parietal lymphatic network draining the pleural space and the pulmonary lymphatics) and takes place across four membranes (the endothelium of systemic and visceral capillaries, the parietal and visceral mesothelia).

Pulmonary interstitial tissue is peculiar in that it fulfills two main functions. On one hand, it is responsible for the mechanical behavior of the lung in that it provides tensile strength and elastic recoil; on the other, interstitial fluid content determines the thickness of the alveolo-capillary membrane modulating gas exchange. In turn, hydration of the extracellular matrix depends upon microvascular to interstitial net filtration pressure gradient, endothelial permeability to fluid and solutes, interstitial tissue compliance and lymphatic removal. Interaction among these mechanisms may lead to either a dehydrated lung tissue in physiological conditions or to pulmonary edema when one or more of these factors change.

Interstitial fluid pressure is a key parameter in interstitial space physiology; indeed, it depends upon both the degree of tissue hydration and the interstitial compliance, i.e. the mechanical behavior of tissue matrix. The methods proposed in the present article were developed to measure interstitial fluid pressure in physiological and pathophysiological conditions with a non-invasive technique. The experimental approach implies the exposure, in spontaneously breathing rabbits, of a portion of parietal pleura (intact parietal pleural window) to visualize the pulmonary superficial structures by maintaining the lung phys-

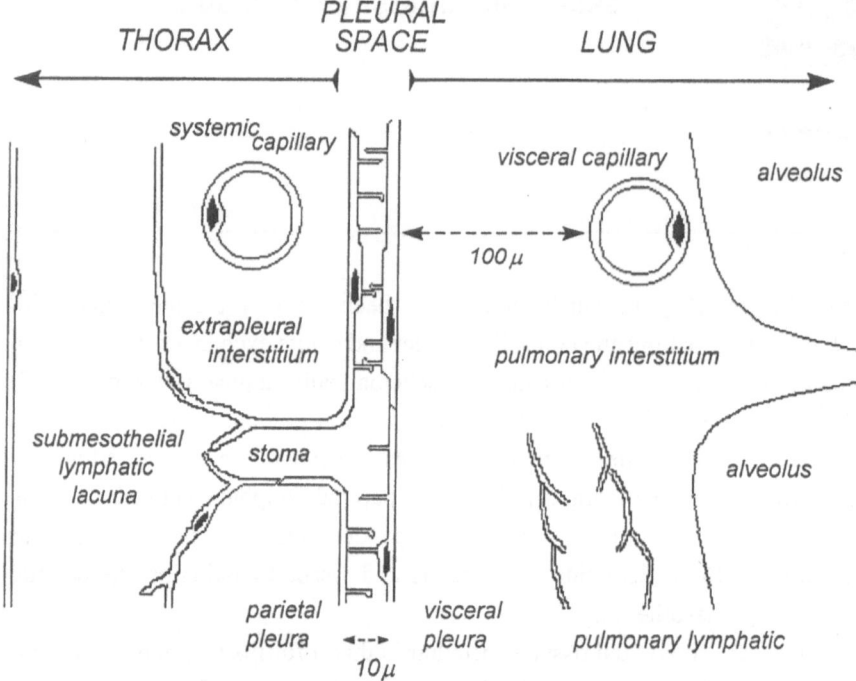

*Figure 10.1 Schematic drawing of the pleuro-pulmonary compartments, including the parietal thoracic side, the pleural space and the pulmonary parenchyma*

iologically expanded at zero alveolar pressure and negative intrapleural pressure. Micropuncture through the intact parietal and visceral pleura allows non-invasive recordings of hydraulic pressures in the pulmonary superficial microvasculature and interstitial space.

The great advantage of these methods is that it avoids opening of pleural spaces and re-expansion of the collapsed lungs at positive alveolar pressure. Furthermore, since in rabbits the pleural spaces are anatomically separated at the anteromedial mediastinum, pulmonary vascular pressures and cardiac output can be measured without collapsing the lungs. Thus preparation of the intact pleural window in rabbits allows: a) micropuncture of pulmonary interstitium and microvasculature leaving intact the lung-chest wall mechanical coupling and the pulmonary and systemic circulation; b) full control of the cardiovascular variables; c) imaging of the microvascular unit, in the intact lung.

The intact parietal pleural window approach leaves unaffected the cardiac activity, a factor implying unavoidable tissue movement and great difficulties in micropuncturing the pulmonary superficial structures. However, the benefits gained by preserving the physiological mechanical and vascular conditions surely overcome such a disadvantage.

## Material and equipment

Non invasive measurements of hydraulic pressure in the pleuro-pulmonary compartments on the *in situ* lung surface are gathered via the servo-nulling pressure measuring system (Instrumentation for Physiology and Medicine, San Diego, CA). This device implies use of glass micropipettes filled with 0.5–2 M NaCl solution; when the pipette is inserted in fluids with smaller molarity, as body fluids or saline solution, the interface between the iperosmotic fluid in the pipette and the iso-osmotic fluid outside moves and the electrical resistance of the pipette changes. The sensitivity of the pressure signal is inversely proportional to the molarity of the fluid in the pipette. The null-balancing feedback generates a counter-pressure that keeps the interface at a stationary position and that is equal to the unknown pressure. The servo-null system consists of a main amplifier, a preamplifier box and a liner motor pump that converts voltage to pressure; the latter is measured through a pressure transducer (Gould P23 XL) and conveyed to a thermic oscillograph (Gould 6600) (Fig. 10.2).

### Pipette preparation

Pipettes are made from borosylicate glass capillaries (Corning Glass Works, Corning NY, OD 1.0 mm, ID 0.78 mm). The first step of pipette preparation consists in cleaning for 24 h in a bath of 2 N nitric or chromic acid; Then, capillaries are washed in flowing water for ≈12 h, rinsed with distilled water and dried in an oven at 70 °C. Subsequently, capillaries are siliconized in a bath of liquid silicon (Sigma Cote) for 1 day

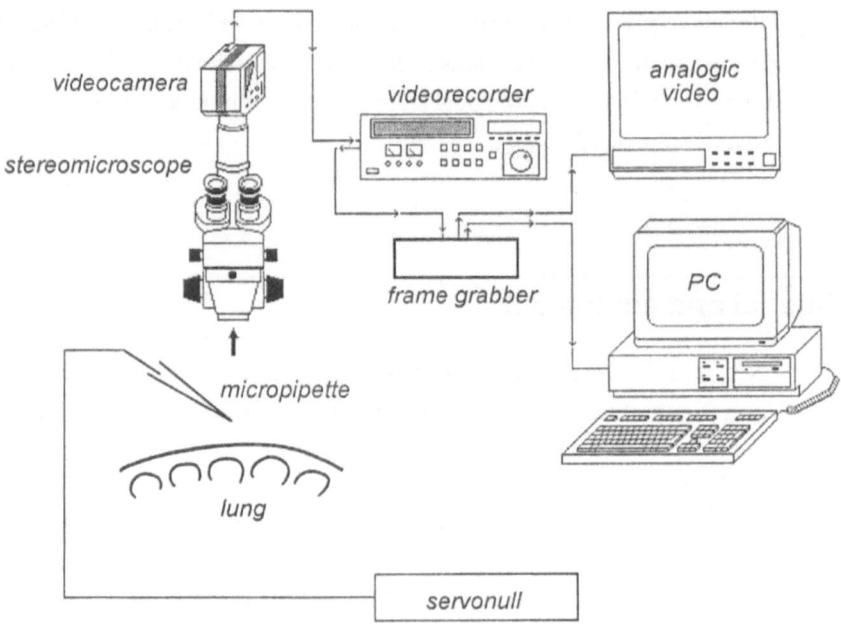

**Figure 10.2 Schematic representation of the instrumentation required to micropuncture the lung surface**

and finally dried out in the oven. Pipette tip is shaped in a capillary puller (Model PC-84 Sachs-Flaming Type, Sutter Instrument Company, San Rafael, CA), programmed to model pipettes with tapes 200–300 μm long and tip diameter of 1–3 μm. Pipette dimension are checked under a calibrated optic microscope (Nikon, SE, Tokyo, Japan) at magnifications of ×10, ×40 and ×400. The tip is subsequently sharpened for ≈5–7 min under stereomicroscopic view (SMZ-10, Nikon, Tokyo, Japan) on the diamond grinding plate of a rotating beveler (K.T. Brown Type Microelectrode Beveler, Model BV-10, Sutter Instruments Company, San Rafael, CA); the best incidence angle to bevel sharp pipettes is ≈30 degrees. For final cleaning, nitrogen is flown through the pipette tip sequentially immersed in: a) an acid mixture of 10% nitric acid, 10% chloridric acid and 80% distilled water; b) distilled water and, finally c) acetone, to allow quick evaporation of distilled water and complete drying of the pipette. Given their dimensions and fragility, extreme care is required in pipettes handling and storing: they may be fixed horizontally and parallel to each other to a support of wax in a covered glass box, or placed vertically in a covered box filled with small glass spheres.

Prior to their use the pipettes have to be rinsed again as described above. Then, via a flexible stainless steel needle, the pipette is filled with 0.5–2 M NaCl hyperosmotic solution containing 0.2 mg/ml of lissamine green (Sigma Chemical, Italia) filtered through a 0.2 μm millipore filter. The pipette is then secured in its allocation at one port of the metal holder (Instrumentation for Physiology and Medicine, San Diego, CA) filled with hyperosmotic NaCl solution through a 150 PE plastic tubing connected at the other port of the holder. The latter is moved to a Lucite box where the pipette tip is immersed just under the surface of a saline solution pool; the air cavity of the Lucite box is connected to a 20 ml plastic syringe and to a water manometer to set the pressure in the Lucite box and calibrate the pressure response of the pipette. Tubing from the pipette holder is then linked via a stainless steel male-male connector and a plastic tubing to a motor-driven pressure head, filled with mineral oil. Air at the pipette tip is pushed out by simply pressuring the fluid in the pipette with a syringe.

The electrical circuit is then closed by connecting the pipette holder to the preamplifier box. If the electrical circuit of the servo-null is closed, the pipette records a stable pressure value that corresponds to the atmospheric pressure recorded at the saline pool surface; this is regarded as the zero reference pressure of the system. Via the syringe connected to the Lucite box and to the manometer, the pipette is calibrated by imposing step changes of ±5 cm $H_2O$ in the Lucite box; pipettes displaying a non linear calibration in the pressure range −30 to 30 cm $H_2O$ are not reliable for interstitial or microvascular pressure measurements. After calibration the pipette is moved in a three dimensional hydraulic micromanipulator (Joystick Micromanipulator MO-188 or MO-109, Narishighe, Tokyo, Japan). The micromanipulator allows course and fine movements in the x-y-z directions to move the pipette close to the insertion point; a fourth movement is used to drive the pipette into the tissue in steps of 5 μm each.

Systemic arterial, central venous, pulmonary arterial and left atrial pressures are recorded via saline filled catheters inserted into the carotid artery, the jugular vein, the pulmonary artery and the left atrium, respectively. The catheters are linked via three-way stopcocks to physiological pressure transducers (4-327-I Transamerica Delaval) that convey their signals to an oscillograph (Gould 6000).

---

# Methods

## Surgery

The experiments are performed on rabbits anesthetized with an anesthetic cocktail composed of urethane diluted at 25% in saline solution plus pentobarbital sodium (10 mg/ml of urethane solution). To induce anesthesia, 2.5 ml per kg body weight of the anesthetic cocktail is given in an ear vein. The initial dose of anesthetic induces a superficial anesthesia with no suppression of corneal reflexes; deep and stable anesthesia is achieved by adding boluses of $\approx 0.5$ ml of anesthetic over time, checking the anesthesia level on the basis of the disappearance of the corneal reflexes. This phase may be critical, because a slight anesthetic overdose may abolish spontaneous breathing and cause death of the animal, if not promptly passively ventilated. For this reason, the first surgical step after anesthesia induction consists in tracheotomy and tracheal cannulation with a T-cannula. This facilitates spontaneous breathing, easily allows ventilation if needed and provides a tracheal access for oxygen flow during micropuncture (as explained in details below). The animal is left to breath spontaneously through the tracheal cannula during the whole surgical preparation. During micropuncture, the animal must be paralyzed to avoid respiratory movements; in this phase arousal from anesthesia is signaled by a sudden increase in heart rate.

Cannulation of the right or left carotid artery guarantees a pathway to add further anesthetic, to withdraw arterial blood samples for arterial blood gas analysis and allows a continuous recording of arterial systemic pressure. The carotid artery is cannulated with a plastic tube (100 PE) with blunted tip inserted into the proximal end of the artery. A jugular vein can be exposed by carefully resecting the superficial tissue on the lateral ventral portion of the throat. After legation of all collateral veins, the jugular vein is cannulated with a saline filled plastic or silicon tubing (200 PE); the venous line may provide useful for continuous recording of central venous pressure or to infuse liquids or drugs into the pulmonary circulation. The carotid and the jugular catheters are connected via a luer connector to a plastic three-way stopcock. In case pressure measurements are needed the catheters lines are connected via saline filled tubing to physiological pressure transducers (Model 4-327-I, Transamerical Delaval) plugged into the thermal oscillograph.

The respiratory system of rabbits differs from that of other mammalian species in that the right and left lungs are enclosed in distinct pleural sacs completely separated along the medio-ventral line. Thus it is possible to reach the heart and cannulate the pulmonary artery and the left atrium without collapsing the lungs; this allows us to measure the actual pressure drop across the pulmonary circulation throughout the whole experimental period maintaining the mechanical and functional integrity of the respiratory system and of the systemic and pulmonary circulation. The surgical approach requires resection of the skin and the external intercostal muscles on ventral portion of the thorax; with the animal lying supine, the exposed sternum is split with a longitudinal midsternal thoracotomy running from the manubrium to the xiphoid process. Bone bleeding is limited by spraying bone wax on the cut edges (Ethicon Ldt., W810 A, UK) or by cauterization with a heated blade. The edges of the thoracotomy are pulled apart via a retractor with short blunt teeth that is left in place during cannulation of pulmonary artery and left atrium. The mediastinal tissues covering the ventral surface of the heart are carefully retracted laterally on both sides, leaving uncovered the ventral medial surface of the pericardium, which is cut medially with sharp scissors to reach the surface of the heart. During this phase attention must be paid in order to avoid damage to the pleurae which lay either lateral and caudal to the heart.

## *Cannulation of left atrium and pulmonary artery*

The left atrial and pulmonary arterial plastic catheters (200 PE) have a blunt flat tip with a flange of about 1.5–2 mm; the flange is made by melting the tip of the catheter over a weak flame and then pressing the soft tip against a cold flat surface. The left atrium, which in the supine rabbits lays laterally below the heart is pulled out gently with a blunt forceps and a silk thread with a terminal curved needle (Sterile suture 6-0, BV-1, Ethicon Ltd., UK) is sewed in the let atrium wall to form a ring around the forceps. Using sharp scissors, an incision is made in the atrium wall inscribed into the thread circle and the saline-filled catheter tip is quickly inserted into the hole; the suture thread is securely tightened around the catheter flange and fixed with a double knot.

Similarly, after sewing a ring of silk suture thread (Sterile suture 4-0, RB-1, Ethicon Ltd., UK) on the right ventricle surface, a saline-filled blunt catheter is inserted through a deep incision (2–4 mm wide) made into the right ventricular cavity; the thread is immediately tightened around the flange and the catheter is gently pushed cranially to reach the pulmonary artery. The left atrial and pulmonary arterial catheters are rinsed with saline solution and connected via three-way stopcocks to the physiological pressure transducers.

Cardiac output is measured directly by securing an ultrasound flowmeter (Transonic System, Inc., model T201, Ithaca, NY; probe type 6SB102) around either the pulmonary artery or the ascendant aorta; After carefully removing all tissue surrounding the vessels, the probe is wrapped around the vessel and secured by a small screw. Important steps to obtain a good recording throughout all the experiment are: 1) to choose an adequate probe, with size only slightly larger than the vessel diameter; 2) to get rid of all tissues surrounding the vessels; 3) to spray a continuous layer of ultrasonic gel (Acquasonic 100, Ultrasonic Transmission Gel, Parker Laboratories, Orange, NJ) between the outer vessel and inner probe surfaces. The probe is then plugged into the flowmeter that displays the recorded flow value on a digital screen.

At this stage the general surgical preparation is completed (time required: about 1 h), the chest retractor is removed and the animal is turned laterally to prepare the pleural windows.

## Preparation of the intact parietal pleural window

On one side of the chest two or more intercostal spaces can be prepared
for transpleural pressure recordings. With the animal laying supine or
slightly lateral, the external and the internal intercostal muscles on one
side of the chest are removed over most of the chosen intercostal space
to expose the endothoracic fascia. Preparation of the intact parietal pleural window is performed through a stereomicroscope (Stereomicroscope
model SMZ-2 T, Nikon) connected to a color videocamera (model TK-
885E, JVC) and to a color video monitor (multisystem RGB, model TM-
150 PSN-K, JVC); the screen of the monitor is calibrated in order to
measure the caliper of the visualized pulmonary structures. The endothoracic fascia is then removed over areas of about 0.2–0.3 cm$^2$, leaving
only the extreme thin layer of the parietal pleura, which, being almost
transparent, allows a clear view of the anatomical structures of the lung
surface through the intact pleural space. Removal of the endothoracic
fascia must be performed with a thin iridectomy forceps by carefully
stripping the endothoracic fibers that runs perpendicular to the length of
the ribs. This final phase is particularly delicate and requires much attention to avoid rupture of the very thin mesothelium with consequent pneumothorax and lung collapse; if this happens the experiment is over. Not
more than two to three windows may be prepared in a single intercostal
space.

A satisfactory range of stereomicroscope magnification is ×60–×100,
with a total magnification on the video screen of about ×120–×200, resulting in a video image such as the one shown in Figure 10.3. The alveoli and the pulmonary microvasculature on the lung surface, including arterioles, venules and capillaries, can be clearly recognized; furthermore, the perivascular interstitial space surrounding the larger surface vessels can be visually identified as a continuous clear border
around the larger surface vessels. The thickness of the parietal and visceral mesothelia and of the pleural liquid does not allow us to identify
arterioles and venules judging from the bloodstream flow direction. The
distinction can be made by injecting a small bolus of a dye solution
(0.5 ml of lissamin green or Evans blue) directly into the pulmonary artery; the vessel on the monitor screen is an arteriole if the dye flows from

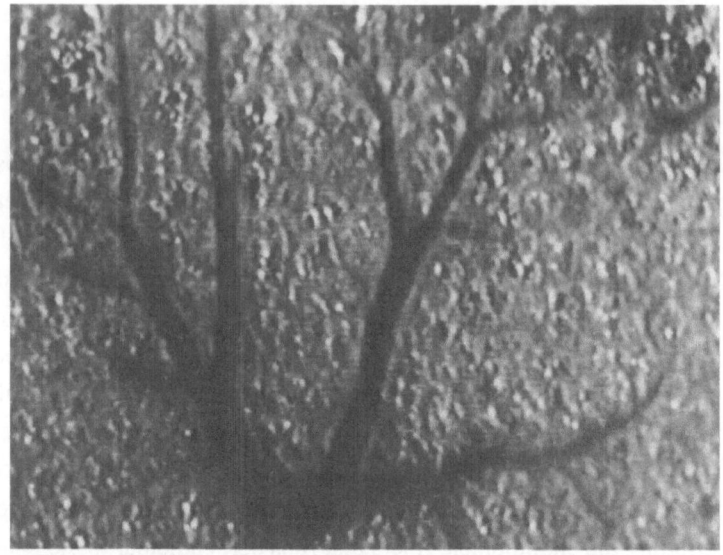

*Figure 10.3 Stereomicroscopic image of the lung surface observed through the intact parietal pleural window (×60)*

the larger toward the smaller feeding branching and a venule if it flows in the opposite direction.

### Video imaging analysis

Images from the stereomicroscope are sent to a video tape recorder (Panasonic AG-7355) and stored for later imaging analysis. Images chosen for later analysis are digitalized with a frame grabber and Imaging Technology PCVISIONplus 512, Woburn, MA) with a resolution 512×512 pixels and 256 gray levels (8 bits for pixel) installed on a personal computer (Hewlett-Packard PC Vectra 486/33VL) equipped with image processing software (Biomedical OPTIMAS v.4.02, Optimas Corporation; Edmonton, WA). At the magnification used, actual pixel dimension are 5.5×3.7 µm.

The time required for preparation of each pleural window is about 30 min. Further details are given in Table 10.1.

# Experimental procedure

In general, one major problem of the micropuncture technique is tissue motion that can easily break the thin and delicate glass pipette tip at any time during pipette insertion or withdrawal from the tissue and/or dislocate the pipette during pressure recording. In particular, when micropuncturing the lung enclosed in the intact chest wall, sources of tissue motion are respiratory movements and heart beating. Spontaneous ventilation is stopped prior to micropuncturing by paralyzing the animal with 0.2 ml/Kg of pancuronium bromide given intravenously. During micropuncture the animal is oxygenated with 50% humidified oxygen delivered intratracheally via a small plastic catheter (90 PE, 5–6 cm long) inserted at one port of the tracheal T-cannula; the other port is left open to the atmosphere to allow oxygen flow recirculation. Between two consecutive micropuncture phases the animal is mechanically ventilated at a frequency of 20 breaths/min and a tidal volume of $\approx 20$ ml (Mechanical ventilator model 6025, Biological Research Apparatus, Ugo Basile, Comerio, Italy).

Micropuncture is usually performed with the animal lying supine or in a slightly left lateral decubitus, according to the position of the pleural window chosen for micropuncture. The pipette holder is seated in a three-direction micromanipulator and the pipette tip is immersed in a saline pool prepared next to the pleural window and grounded to the animal. The pressure value recorded at the saline pool surface is the atmospheric pressure and is regarded as the zero of the system; hence, the position of the oscillograph pen must correspond to the zero value that is usually placed the center of the tracer. Once the zero pressure value is set, the pipette is driven into the tissue; insertion of the pipette through the parietal pleura is made easier by using a large incidence angle (45–70°) in order to minimize pleural indentation caused by the pipette tip pushing against the pleura itself [3]. In case the pipette is properly inserted into the target tissue, the electrical contact of the servo-null system is estabilished and a good pressure tracer is recorded immediately after pipette insertion. Criteria for acceptance of the pipette pressure recordings are as follows: a) the electrical zero on with-

Table 10.1 Details of the experimental and surgical set up

| Conditions | Facts |
|---|---|
| Species | Adult (1.8–2.5 Kg) or newborn rabbits |
| Mechanical ventilation (between micropunture phases): tidal volume | 20–25 ml (adult) |
| respiratory frequency | 20–22 cycles/min |
| Oxygen flow outflow pressure (during micropuncture) | 1 cm H₂O |
| Time to set up the experiment | 30 min |
| Duration of surgical preparation | 1 h |
| Time for pleural window preparation | 20–30 min each |
| Duration of micropuncture phase | Up to 6–7 h |
| Criteria for quality of preparation | Integer pleural spaces; no pneumeothorax |
| Experiments/day/unit | 1 |

drawal of the pipette has to be unchanged compared to pre-insertion position; b) the recording has to be stable for at least 2–3 min; c) repeated measurements from the same region have to yield values within ±1 cm H₂O. Only 30–40% of the trials result in a good pressure recording. After the recording is completed the pipette is rapidly withdrawn and immediately immersed in the saline pool; if the zero of the servo-null system is unaltered, the pipette tip is still perfect and the recording can be considered valid, whereas if the zero has moved from the original position, the electrical characteristics of the pipette-servonull system have changed with respect to the pre-insertion zero conditions; this means that the pipette tip is broken or plugged and the recording must be disregarded since the pipette calibration is not reliable any more.

## Application

Micropuncture performed through the intact parietal pleural window has been developed in our laboratory to measure, with minimal distortion, the hydraulic pressure in the pleuro-pulmonary compartments, with the aim of gaining new insights on the mechanisms of filtration and absorption of liquid in these complex interstitial systems under physiological conditions. Indeed, hydraulic pressure is a key parameter in the simple equation describing the net pressure gradient ($\Delta P_{net}$) acting between any two compartments separated by a membrane:

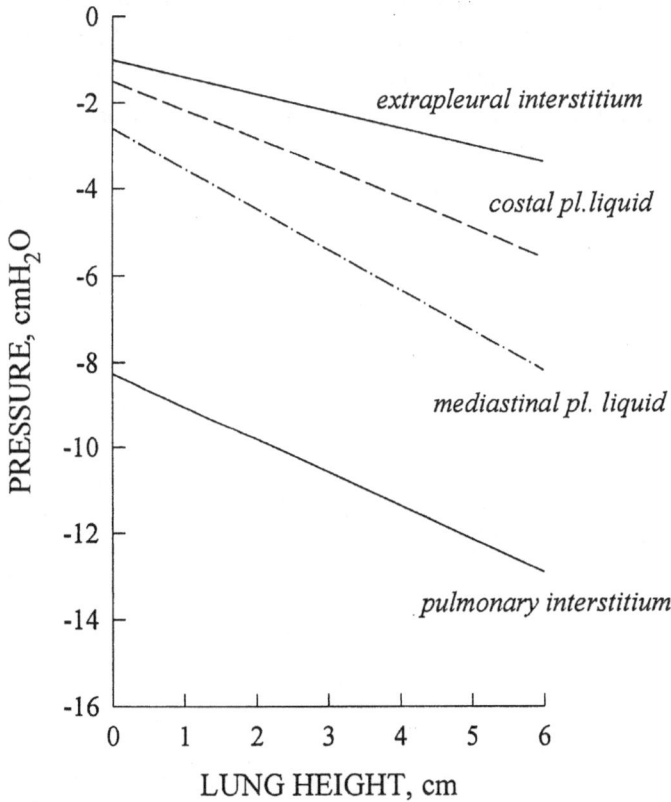

Figure 10.4 Hydraulic pressures in the pleural liquid, the parietal extrapleural and the pulmonary interstitium as a function of lung height. Pleural liquid pressures are more subatmospheric in the mediastinal region compared to the costal ones [12]

$\Delta P_{net} = \Delta P_h - \sigma \Delta \pi$, where $\Delta P_h$, $\Delta \pi$ and $\sigma$ are the transmembrane hydraulic and colloidosmotic pressure gradients and the reflection coefficient of the membrane for total proteins, respectively.

### Physiological conditions

Micropuncture measurements gathered in physiological condition [1, 2] reveal that pulmonary interstitial pressure ($P_{ip}$) is significantly more subatmospheric then pleural liquid pressure ($P_{liq}$) at any lung height (Fig. 10.4); both $P_{ip}$ and $P_{liq}$ decrease with increasing lung height by about 0.7 cmH$_2$O/cm [1, 2], being $\approx -11$ and $-5$ cmH$_2$O respectively, at the right atrium level (60% lung height in supine animal, indifferent point of the circulatory system). As shown in Figure 10.4, the extrapleural parietal interstitial pressure ($P_{epl}$) values also decreases with lung height by $\approx 0.4$ cmH$_2$O/cm, being approximately $-2$ cmH$_2$O at right atrial level [2–4].

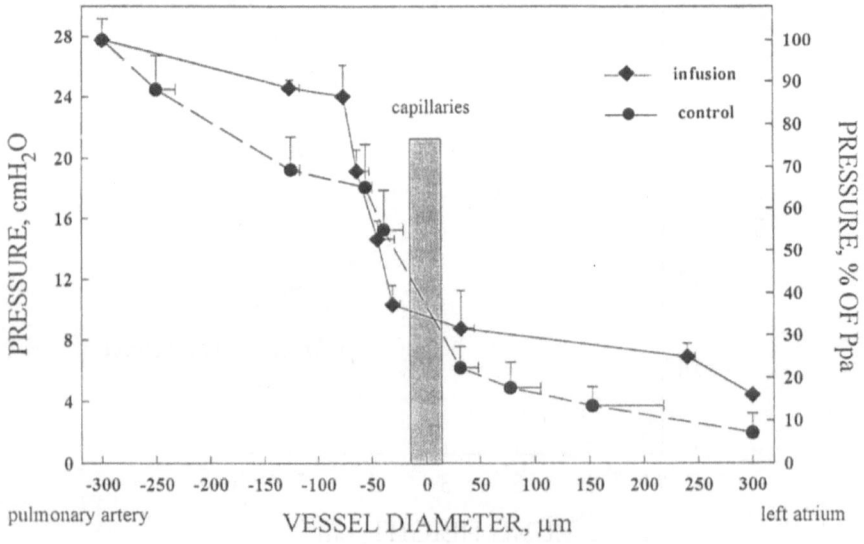

**Figure 10.5 Pulmonary vascular pressure profile under control conditions (filled circles, broken line) and during development of pulmonary edema (filled diamonds, continuous line)**
*On the right Y-axis, data are expressed as percentage of pulmonary arterial pressure.*

The intact parietal pleural window technique allowed us to provide the first description of the pressure profile in the pulmonary vascular bed under zone-3 condition with intact circulatory and respiratory systems [5]. As shown in Figure 10.5 (filled circle, dashed line) in physiological conditions the main resistive segment of the pulmonary circulation is provided by the smallest vessels, from 60 μm diameter arterioles to 60 μm diameter venules and the estimated functional capillary pressure ($P_{cap}$) is as low as ≈ 10 cm $H_2O$ [5]. During transition towards hydraulic pulmonary edema induced via intravenous saline infusion, total pulmonary vascular resistance remains essentially unchanged [6], whereas segmental resistances are greatly modified (Fig. 10.5, filled diamonds, solid line), with significant increase in precapillary flow resistances and/or capillary recruitment. These responses to saline loading favor an intrinsic control of $P_{cap}$, that is basically unchanged with regard to control conditions.

Transmembrane $\Delta P_{net}$ can be reckoned from hydraulic and colloidosmotic pressure in all pleural compartments and by knowing the protein reflection coefficient of the pulmonary and systemic endothelia and of the mesothelia separating the pleuro-pulmonary compartments (Fig. 10.6). In physiological condition, $\Delta P_{net}$ at mid heart level sustains fluid movement from the systemic capillary supplying

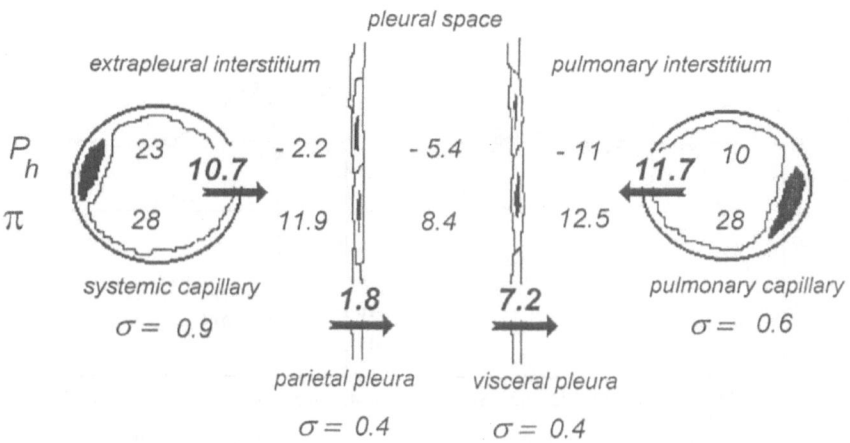

**Figure 10.6 Hydraulic ($P_h$) and colloidosmotic pressures (π) and net pressure gradients (arrows) acting in the pleuro-pulmonary compartments**
Pressures are in cm $H_2O$

the parietal pleural tissue into the surrounding extrapleural interstitium. The pleural space contains a very small amount of fluid ($\approx 0.3$ ml/kg body weight, 7), whose volume is set through a tight control of the interaction of the filtration/reabsorption mechanisms [8]; in physiological conditions filtration is minimized via a very small pressure gradient (only $\approx 1$ cm $H_2O$) and a low permeability of the parietal mesothelium [9–11].

Data included in Figure 10.6 also indicate that the low $P_{ip}$ value forces fluid out of the capillaries into the pulmonary interstitium with a rather large $\Delta P_{net}$. In terms of fluid and solute turnover in the pleuro-pulmonary compartments, this finding has the following important functional implications: a) under physiological conditions pulmonary capillaries provide net fluid filtration and not net reabsorption, as previously suggested on the basis of the low pulmonary capillary functional pressure; b) a direct consequence of point a) is that pleural liquid cannot eventually be drained in the pulmonary capillaries; c) the main mechanism involved in draining interstitial fluid and thus setting and maintaining a subatmospheric pressure values in the pleuro-pulmonary compartments is the lymphatic system. This conclusion is consistent with a bulk of experimental results obtained in our laboratory, demonstrating the ability of the lymphatic system to generate negative pressures in the pleural [12, 13] and peritoneal [14] cavities

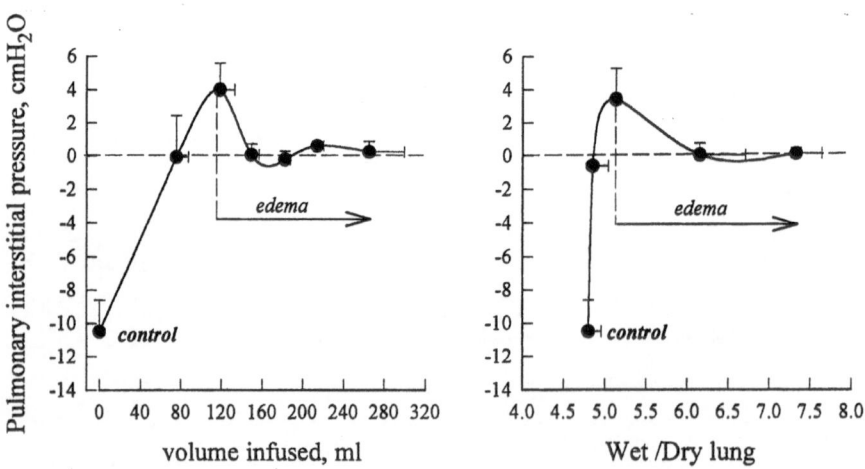

Figure 10.7 Pulmonary interstitial pressure (P_ip) plotted as a function of the saline volume infused (left panel) and as a function of wet weight to dry weight ratio (right panel) during development of pulmonary edema

and to efficiently modulate its drainage flow in response to conditions of increased filtration [8, 13, 14].

## Transition to edema

The intact parietal pleural window preparation allowed us to measure $P_{ip}$ in conditions of altered lung fluid balance, namely in the transition phase from physiological condition to pulmonary edema [15, 16]. Data reported in Figure 10.7 (left panel) show that during progressive development of pulmonary edema, $P_{ip}$ initially increases from the physiological control value ($\approx -10$ cm $H_2O$, *see* also Fig. 10.4) to $+10$ cm $H_2O$; this phase is characterized by a very low pulmonary interstitial tissue compliance, as also suggested by the steep slope of the relationship presented on the right panel of Figure 10.7, showing $P_{ip}$ data plotted as a function of the lung wet weight to dry weight ratio. On further increasing pulmonary tissue hydration, tissue compliance increases, causing $P_{ip}$ to drop towards atmospheric pressure. The low compliant behavior of the normal lung tissue justifies the difficult clinical discovery of pulmonary edema, which becomes detectable only in the late stage, when interstitial tissue has lost its buffer capability (high compliant phase in Fig. 10.7, right panel) and pulmonary parenchyma and, eventually, alveolar spaces are already flooded.

## Lung fluid balance in the newborn

The micropuncture technique has been successfully applied in the newborn lung to study the transition from the liquid filled to the aerated condition in term and preterm animals [17, 18]. At birth, interstitial pulmonary pressure in term rabbits rises as results of alveolar fluid reabsorption. The increase in interstitial pressure is a key factor to generate a pressure gradient favoring fluid drainage into pulmonary capillaries and critically depends upon a low compliance of the interstitial tissue matrix. The crucial phase of luminal fluid reabsorption lasts about 3 h, but it takes about 30 days for the lung to turn into the adult state that is characterized by a rather dehydrated interstitium. In premature rabbits no increase in interstitial pressure was observed after birth, reflecting either a poor reabsorption of alveolar fluid and/or a rather high compliance of the interstitial matrix due to

267

incomplete matrix development. As a result, in the premature rabbit the lung remained in a condition of chronic edema.

## Mechanical behavior of interstitial matrix

With a biochemical study of matrix macromolecules in control and edematous lungs, we have attempted to establish a link between the mechanical behavior of pulmonary tissue matrix and the interstitial pressures changes during edema development. The initial step of this investigation has focused on proteoglycans, high molecular weight matrix macromolecules characterized by the presence of highly hydrophylic anionic sites and by the ability to bond with other matrix components, like collagen. Data suggest that the physiological proteoglycans interactions are mostly unaltered in the early low compliant phase of transition to edema (Fig. 10.7); severe pulmonary edema occurs in conjunction with rupture and/or disarrangement of the high molecular weight proteoglycans chains.

## Video image analysis of the superficial lung structures

The intact parietal pleural technique allows acquisition of steromicroscopic video images of the intact *in situ* lung surface. The images are then digitalized and analyzed to determine the geometry of microvessels ranging in diameter from 30 to 200 µm and of the perimicrovascular interstitial spaces with thickness varying from 10 to 150 µm. [19]. This approach may be applied to evaluate, in the intact lung, fluid movements between the vascular and perimicrovascular compartment, to study pulmonary microvascular reactivity to drugs in normal or altered functional conditions or to describe the geometry of the superficial pulmonary vascular tree.

In summary, the intact parietal pleural window may be applied to all fields of pulmonary research that require visualization of the surface structures and measurements of interstitial and vascular pressures with a very careful assessment of the physiological control conditions. This advantage cannot be provided by other techniques implying experimental perturbations of the lung-chest wall coupling and/or the systemic and pulmonary circulation.

## Species differences

The general model of fluid exchange in the pleuro-pulmonary compartments basically applies to all mammalian species. However, data collected on newborn and adult mammals reveal that there are noticeable age and size related differences; indeed, in all mammalian species considered, pleural liquid pressure, volume and protein concentration decrease with increasing age and size [4, 7]. On considering transpleural fluid filtration and reabsorption mechanisms, these findings suggest that, on increasing body size and/or age: a) filtration pressure gradients are reduced [4]; b) mesothelial and possibly endothelial permeability to water and solute are also reduced [11]; c) lymphatic removal is enhanced [4, 7].

The allometric adaptation of interstitial fluid turnover is a fascinating issue that deserves to be further investigated, particularly in the mammalian lung. However, notwithstanding our interest in comparative aspects of the pleuro-pulmonary fluid balance, so far micropuncture of the intact lung surface through the intact parietal pleural window have been performed exclusively in adult and newborn rabbits. In fact, as addressed earlier, rabbits have separated pleural spaces that allow simultaneous recording of pulmonary vascular pressures and cardiac output by simultaneously preserving the integrity of the pleural sacs. Another important factor to take into account when choosing the mammalian species for micropuncture is the entity of lung tissue motion: indeed, strong tissue movements due to cardiac oscillations do not allow pipette insertion in lungs of animals larger than rabbits and with a more powerful cardiac stroke, like dogs or sheep. Finally, the thickness of the pleural membranes has to be considered: to reach the pulmonary interstitium or microvasculature, the pipette tip is driven across the parietal and visceral pleura. Rabbits, like dogs and cats, have thin pleurae, with an average thickness (including the submesothelial interstitial layer) of 20–30 µm on the parietal side and up to about 100 µm on the visceral one. Larger species, like sheep and pigs, have thick pleurae, and even in dogs, with thin pleurae, a rather thick submesothelial interstitium makes it difficult pipette insertion. At the other extreme, mammalian species smaller than rabbits have very narrow intercostal spaces, in which preparation of a pleural window may be very difficult. Furthermore, rabbits are among the cheapest and easiest to handle of laboratory mammals.

## Discussion

The first direct measurement of pulmonary interstitial pressure has been achieved by hollow capsules chronically implanted in the lung parenchyma [20]; after an initial inflammatory phase, the capsule is entrapped by solid tissue and the capsule is filled with fluid which is assumed to be at the same pressure of the surrounding interstitial fluid. Pulmonary interstitial pressure has also been derived by measuring the absorption pressure in lung segments filled with Tyrode's solution [21]. Both these techniques are very invasive, they may cause inflammation, and necessarily imply disrupture of the original lung-chest wall mechanical coupling.

The micropuncture technique so far represents the less invasive approach to measure interstitial fluid pressure. In particular, the present intact parietal pleural window has represented a principal improvement to micropunture applied in pulmonary research, leading to the first description of lung fluid exchange between pulmonary microvasculature and surrounding interstitial space in physiological condition and during the early transition phase towards development of pulmonary edema in the intact lung. An alternate experimental model is the widely used isolated-perfused lung preparation (*see* Chapter 2). This technique offers, with respect to our intact preparation, certain advantages: a) pulmonary blood flow, upstream and downstream vascular pressures are set by the investigator and may be changed throughout the experiment; b) micropuncture measurements of interstitial and microvascular pressures may be extended to the whole lung surface; c) micropuncture is greatly facilitated by a weak tissue movement; d) drug administrations and their effect on the pulmonary system are better controlled in the perfusion circuit; e) finally, measurements of permeability coefficients of the pulmonary endothelium can be performed. For all these benefits the isolated-perfused lung has been widely and profitably used since at least 20 years in pulmonary research. However, when dealing with the lung fluid balance, the technique may presents some drawbacks: a) the mechanical lung-chest wall coupling is completely disrupted; b) in most instances lungs are inflated at positive alveolar pressure, rather than being expanded at zero alveolar and negative intrapleural pressures, as in physiological condition. Points a) and b) also apply to experiments performed with intact pulmonary vascular perfusion, but open thorax [22]. From the mechanical standpoint there is a major difference between the condition in which lungs are expanded in the intact chest wall at physiological subatmospheric intrapleural pressure ($P_{pl}$) and alveolar pressure ($P_{alv}$) close to zero (condition A), and the opposite case with lungs isolated or expanded in the open chest at positive $P_{alv}$ and atmospheric $P_{pl}$ (condition B). In fact, when the lung is physiologically expanded in condition A the pulmonary interstitium is subjected to a tensile stress, whereas in condition B it undergoes a compressive stress [2]. As a result, at a given transpulmonary pressure, $P_{ip}$ differs substantially, being more subatmospheric in condition A than in condition B; $P_{ip}$ data gathered in condition B can be roughly compared to data obtained at the same transpulmonary pressure in physiological condition A only after subtracting $P_{alv}$ from the $P_{ip}$ value data, as: $P_{ipA} = P_{ipB} - P_{alvB}$. For example, if $P_{ipB} = -1$ cm $H_2O$ with lungs expanded in the open chest at $P_{alvB} = 7$ cm $H_2O$, an approximate correction for comparison to physiological state might be: $P_{ipA} = (-1-(7)$ cm $H_2O = -8$ cm $H_2O$; c) in the isolated-perfused lung pulmonary vascular and alveolar pressures are not physiological, but necessarily set by the investigator; d) use of vasodilator is often required to facilitate low pressure perfusion; e) handling of the lung and long exposure to ambient air may damage the lung surface; f) pulmonary lymphatic drainage is abolished, a very important factor to be considered when dealing with fluid homeostasis. Hence, when dealing with pulmonary tissue mechanics and/or fluid balance the isolated perfused preparation does not mirror the physiological conditions, but actually implies a certain degree of interstitial edema.

The intact parietal pleural window technique described in the present article has been developed to overcome the isolated-perfused lung disadvantages and to allow least invasive measurements of pulmonary microvascular and interstitial pressure values in the lung physiologically expanded in the pleural space and with intact vascular perfusion. The present surgical approach, unlike others that imply implantation of an artificial pleural membrane after opening the chest [23], leaves the pleural membranes intact and simultaneously allows recordings of pulmonary vascular pressures and cardiac output throughout the whole experiment.

---

# Troubleshooting

## Technical problems

A common pitfall that hinders calibration and use of a pipette is the lack of electrical continuity due to air bubbles in the tubing connecting the pipette to the motor driven pump. Small air bubbles may form at tubing connections, in the pipette holder or at the pipette tip. Frequent sources of air bubbles are irregularities of the glass capillary perimeter or broken glass fragments in the pipette holder; when this is the case the pipette has to be removed from the holder and the whole connection steps have to repeated after careful cleaning of the holder. Another cause of electrical discontinuity is a broken pipette tip or a poor beveler, in which case the pipette must be replaced with a new one.

## General drawbacks of the micropuncture technique

a) One of the major criticisms against the micropuncture technique is the difficulty in precisely identifying the pipette tip position, which cannot be visualized when the pipette tip is in the tissue. A reliable way to ascertain where the pipette is recording from may be to figure the depth (D) of the pipette tip into the tissue according to the simple equation: $D = M \cdot \cos\alpha$, where M is the micromanipulator displacement in the direction of insertion and $\alpha$ is the indentation angle. The thickness of the parietal pleura, the pleural space and of the visceral pleura is $\approx 30$, 10 and 30 µm, respectively; thus, for example, to reach the pulmonary interstitium the pipette tip has to be at least 80–100 µm deep. Micropuncture of the lung surface vessels and of the perimicrovascular interstitial space is made easier by the fact that these compartments are large enough to follow pipette positioning on the video screen.

b) A stable positive or negative off scale of pressure recording after pipette insertion into the tissue might signify that the pipette is pushing against the tissue or it has been plugged by the tissue itself; a positive off scale may also depend upon lack of electrical continuity (clearly detectable on the preamplifier screen) that occurs when the pipette tip is exposed to air rather than to fluid, namely, when the pipette tip is in an alveolus. All these deficiencies are usually solved by gently withdrawing or moving the pipette by a few microns. c) The most frequent reason of failure in pressure recording is by and large the quality of the pipette. A good pipette with a thin, sharp tip may be used for several measurements, whereas an imperfect tip causes difficulty during calibration, insertion and recording.

## Micropuncture through the intact parietal pleural window

The main problems to solve when micropuncturing the lung superficial structures in our animal preparation are tissue movement and the thickness of the parietal and visceral pleura, as already addressed in the *Species Differences* section. Since in our preparation the animal is paralyzed, the unique source of tissue movement is heart beating, the strength of which may be quite variable from animal to animal, also depending upon heart rate. This problem may be at least partly overcome by preparing the pleural windows in the caudal intercostal spaces, as far as possible from the heart to reduce the impact of heart contraction on the lung tissue; in addition, a low heart frequency makes the recording much easier.

Another source of tissue movements is a progressive recovery of breathing movements due to a decreased concentration of the paralyzing drug in the blood; this problem may be easily overcome by addition of the drug. Finally, to prevent atelectasis of pulmonary parenchyma, it is important to ventilate the lung between consecutive micropuncture phases.

## References

1  Miserocchi G, Negrini D and Gonano C (1990) *J. Appl. Physiol.* **69**: 2168
2  Miserocchi G, Negrini D and Gonano C (1991) *J. Appl. Physiol.* **71**: 1967
3  Miserocchi G, Kelly S and Negrini D (1988) *J. Appl. Physiol.* **65**: 555
4  Negrini D and Miserocchi G (1989) *J. Appl. Physiol.* **67**: 1967
5  Negrini D, Gonano C and Miserocchi G (1992) *J. Appl. Physiol.* **72**: 332
6  Negrini D (1995) *Microcirculation* **2**: 173
7  Miserocchi G, Negrini D and Mortola J.P (1984) *J. Appl. Physiol.* **56**: 1151
8  Miserocchi G, Venturoli D, Negrini D and Del Fabbro M (1993) *J. Appl. Physiol.* **75**: 1798
9  Negrini D, Townsley MI and Taylor AE (1990) *J. Appl. Physiol.* **69**: 438
10  Negrini D, Reed RK and Miserocchi G (1991) *J. Appl. Physiol.* **71**: 2543
11  Negrini D, Venturoli M, Townsley MI and Reed RK (1994) *J. Appl. Physiol.* **76**: 627

12  Miserocchi G, Nakamura T, Mariani E and Negrini D (1981) *Resp. Physiol.* **46**: 61

13  Miserocchi G and Negrini D (1986) *J. Appl. Physiol.* **61**: 325

14  Miserocchi G, Negrini D, Mukenge S, Turconi P and Del Fabbro M (1989) *J. Appl. Physiol.* **66**: 1579

15  Miserocchi G, Negrini D, Del Fabbro M and Venturoli (1993) *J. Appl. Physiol.* **74**: 1171

16  Negrini D, Passi A, De Luca G and Miserocchi G (1996) *Am. J. Physiol.* **270** (*Heart Circul. Physiol.* **39**): H2000

17  Miserocchi G, Haxhiu-Poskurica B and Del Fabbro M (1994) *J. Appl. Physiol.* **77**: 2260

18  Miserocchi G, Haxhiu-Poskurica B and Del Fabbro M and Crisafulli B (1995) *Resp. Physiol.* **102**: 239

19  Venturoli D, Crisafulli B, Del Fabbro M, Negrini D and Miserocchi G (1995) *Microcirculation* **2**: 27

20  Meyer BJ, Meyer A and Guyton AC (1968) *Circul. Res.* **22**: 263

21  Parker JC, Allison RC and Taylor AE (1981) *J. Appl. Physiol.* **51**: 911

22  Bhattacharya S, Glucksberg MR and Bhattacharya J (1989) *Circul. Res.* **64**: 167

23  Wagner WW (1969) *J. Appl. Physiol.* **26**: 375

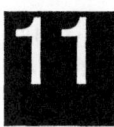

# 11 Lymphatics

*R.E. Drake and*
*J.C. Gabel*

Lymphatic vessels play a critical role in the lung because they remove excess fluid and protein from the lung tissue. Fluid and protein continuously filter from the lung microvessels, and if it were not for the lymphaic vessels, this filtrate would accumulate within the lung [20, 39]. Investigators may learn much about the lymphatic system by studying the flow characteristics of cannulated lymphatic vessels. In addition, cannulated lympatics are a powerful tool in studies of lung microvascular permeability [36]. Most estimates of microvascular permeability require some measure of 1) microvascular filtration rate and 2) filtrate protein concentration. Because the lymphatics drain microvascular filtrate from the lung tissue, investigators may estimate filtration rate from the lymph flow rate and filtrate protein concentration may be estimated from lymph protein concentration.

Although lymphatic vessels can provide valuable information about the lung, there are some serious problems that investigators may encounter with lymphatics. For instance, cannulas placed into lymphatic vessels change the lymph flow rate and the lymph protein concentration may be increased or decreased as lymph passes through lymph nodes. Investigators who do not consider these and other problems are likely to misinterpret their data.

## Basic physiology of the lymphatic system

A network of tiny lymphatic vessels drains fluid from the lung tissue spaces to nodes located near the lung. After the fluid percolates through the nodes, it enters one of several postnodal lymphatic vessels which usually drain to one of the body's main lymph trunks (the thoracic duct or the right lymph duct). From there the lymph empties into veins within the neck.

Because the lung tissue fluid pressure is less than neck vein pressure, lymphatic vessels must pump lymph fluid up a pressure gradient. Two mechanisms are responsible for this pumping. First, lymphatic vessels are intermittently compressed during normal respiration. In the lung, the lymphatics run within the peribronchiolar and perivascular spaces and the pressure in those spaces varies with respiration. Outside the lung, the lymphatics are exposed to the changes in pleural pressure during respiration. When the lymphatics are compressed, fluid is forced forward toward the neck veins; retrograde flow is prevented by one-way valves. When the pressure surrounding the lymphatics is reduced, the valves allow fluid to fill the lymphatics from the tissue space. Thus the lymphatics are "primed and ready" for the next compression.

The second pumping mechanism involves the smooth muscle within the postnodal lymphatic vessel walls. This muscle contracts rhythmically and thus drives lymph forward through the lymphatics [12, 17, 34]. If the pressure within the lymphatic is increased, the contraction rate and force of contraction are increased [24]. This increased pumping is important to allow the lymphatic vessels to increase their flow rate. For instance, if the lung becomes edematous, excess fluid will flow into the lymphatics. The contraction frequency and stroke volume of the stretched lymphatic vessels is increased and that helps the lymphatics to remove the excess tissue fluid. Increased pumping is also important in allowing the lymphatic vessels to maintain normal lymph flow when the pressure within the neck veins is increased. That is, increases in neck vein pressure cause an increase in intralymphatic pressure. The increased lymphatic pressure causes increased lymphatic pumping which, in turn, may compensate for the increased pressure at the outflow to the lymphatics [14, 17, 24]. Although the smooth muscle pump provides an important mechanism to increase lymph flow from edematous tissues or to compensate for increased neck vein pressure, it is overwhelmed by very high flow rates or by high neck vein pressures [6]. Furthermore, the pump cannot drive high flow rates against high outflow pressures.

Hydraulic resistance to fluid flow through the tissue spaces and lymphatic vessels is also important to lymph flow. Tissue fluid flow into the lymphatics probably depends on the hydraulic resistance to flow through the tissue matrix near the entrance to the lymphatics. Once within the lymphatic vessels, the lymph fluid must flow through the resistance of the lymphatic vessels and nodes. When the lung becomes edematous, the hydraulic resistance of the swollen tissue matrix is decreased and the lymphatic vessels become dilated. Consequently, the resistance to lymph flow may be decreased substantially [6, 7].

Although most investigators consider the lymphatics as a system to remove edema fluid from the lung tissue, lymph flow seems to depend more on microvascular filtration rate than on edema fluid volume [15]. For instance, when investigators increased microvascular filtration rate enough to cause edema, lymph flow rate increased substantially. However, if the filtration rate is reduced to baseline after the edema has formed, the lymph flow will return to near baseline within a few minutes even though the lungs remain edematous. The reason is that edema fluid accumulates at sites remote to the terminal lymphatics.

## Methods

Investigators have cannulated lung lymphatics in several species of animals [34], but almost all studies are now done with dogs or sheep. In the 1930s to 1950s investigators collected lymph from the right lymph duct in dogs. Although the right lymph duct is easy to cannulate, it contains considerable lymph from nonpulmonary tissues [23]. More recently, investigators have cannulated the relatively large tracheobronchial lymphatic vessels which run at the hilus of the left lung [23, 28]. Generally, investigators open the left chest between the fifth and sixth ribs and retract the left lung to expose the hilus. Usually a tracheobronchial lymphatic is located within the connective tissue 1–2 cm, below the hilus of the upper left lung lobe. The vessels may be identified by injecting dye into the lung just below the visceral pleura or into a node at the lung hilus. Tracheobronchial lymphatics are ~1–2 mm in diameter and they drain from the hilus towards the neck. We use silk suture to ligate the vessels and they become distended with lymph upstream of the ligature. We carefully strip the connective tissue from the vessel upstream of the ligature, use an 18-gauge needle to make a hole in the vessel wall, and cannulate the vessel with 0.965 mm O.D. (PE50) polyethylene tubing or 1.2 mm O.D. silastic tubing. We tie the lymphatic vessel around the cannula (and thus secure the cannula) with silk suture. The baseline lymph flow from cannulated tracheobronchial lymphatics varies considerably from vessel to vessel, but the average flow is ~ 10 µl/min.

Tracheobronchial lymphatics drain ~ 25% of the total lung tissue [29], but it is difficult to determine the specific lung regions drained by a given tracheobronchial lymphatic. We have cannulated hilar lymphatic vessels which drain directly from the lower left lung lobe in dogs [7]. These vessels are much smaller than tracheobronchial lymphatics and we must use very small tubing for the cannulation (0.61 mm O.D.). The baseline flow rate from cannulated hilar lymphatics is usually ~ 1.0 µl/min.

Tracheobronchial and hilar lymphatic vessels have proven very useful for acute studies in dogs, however it is difficult to maintain delicate lymphatic cannulas in awake dogs. Consequently investigators have performed only acute experiments with tracheobronchial or hilar lymphatics in dogs. In contrast, many investigators have successfully maintained chronic lung lymph cannulas in sheep.

Staub et al. [33] described the sheep lung lymph preparation. Briefly, investigators anesthetize the sheep and open the right chest. They cannulate an efferent from the large caudal mediastinal lymph node (CMN) and ligate any other visible efferent vessels [21]. Some investigators cannulate the thoracic duct downstream of the CMN efferent-thoracic duct junction. Then they ligate the thoracic duct upstream of the junction. To minimize systemic lymph flow to the CMN, investigators ligate and resect the tail of the node at the lower border of the right pulmonary ligament. Although the investigator may use the sheep for acute studies, investigators usually tunnel the cannula through the chest wall, close the chest, and allow the sheep to recover. With this preparation, investigators have collected lung lymph for a month or more in awake sheep. The cannulated lymphatic vessel drains ~ 70% of the total lung tissue and baseline lymph flow from awake sheep is ~ 100 µl/min.

Although the lymph collected from sheep was first thought to be pure (or nearly pure) lung lymph, there is now anatomical and physiological evidence of nonpulmonary lymph contamination [5, 11, 32]. The main source of nonpulmonary lymph is via diaphragmatic lymph vessels. These vessels drain fluid from the abdominal space and liver. Although investigators disagree about the amount of nonpulmonary lymph in the sheep preparation [5, 11, 32] diaphragmatic lymph flow is substantially increased by anything that causes excess fluid filtration within the abdominal cavity. Roos et al. were able to eliminate most of the diaphragmatic lymph flow to the CMN by carefully cauterizing the surface of the diaphragm [32]. However their technique does not eliminate all of the diaphragmatic contamination and it does not account for nonpulmonary lymph flow from lymphatics draining other tissues (the chest wall and esophagus). We have developed a technique to virtually isolate the CMN from any nonpulmonary lymph flow in acutely prepared sheep [8]. However this technique has not been used to prepare sheep for chronic studies. Some investigators have cannulated prenodal lung lymphatics in sheep, but the technique is difficult.

## Common technical problems

Frequently investigators cannot find a lymphatic vessel. To identify prenodal lymphatics, we recommend that investigators inject Evans blue dye into the lung tissue just below the visceral pleura. Usually the dye readily enters subpleural lymphatics and it can be seen in hilar lymphatics within 5–10 min. To identify postnodal lymphatics, the dye should be injected directly into the node. The disadvantage of injecting dye into the lung or node is that it may cause bleeding into the lymph. Because of this problem, we do not recommend dye injections unless the investigator cannot locate a lymphatics without it. Sometimes the lumen of the cannula is obstructed by a valve and the flow rate is irregular or intermittent. (In well cannulated lymphatics in anesthetized, mechanically ventilated animals, lymph usually surges forward with each cycle of ventilation.) This problem can be corrected by advancing the cannula through the valve or withdrawing it from the valve. Another common problem is lymph clotting within the cannula. Clotting is often a problem with chronic cannulas – particularly in the first few days after surgery. During that time the lymph usually contains some blood and presumably contains more clotting factors than normal lymph. To suppress clotting, some investigators coat the cannulas with heparin [33]. Sometimes the investigator may dislodge a clot by injecting 0.1–0.4 ml of fluid into the cannula, then aspirating. However it is risky to inject fluid through a lymphatic cannula because the lymphatic valves prevent fluid from flowing past the first lymphatic segment. Thus, if investigators inject too much fluid, the lymphatic may burst. Some investigators have used streptokinase to clear clots from lymph cannulas and they have been able to maintain lymph flow for up to 18 weeks in sheep [38].

## Lymph flow rate measurement

Most investigators determine lymph flow rate ($\dot{Q}_L$) by placing the free end of the lymphatic cannula into a pipette or graduated tube and measuring the volume collected in a given time [6, 15, 28]. Although this technique will yield the flow from the cannulated vessel, the cannula itself may influence the flow rate. Thus the flow from a cannulated lymphatic may not equal the flow through the same vessel if it had not been cannulated [6]. This is because the cannula influences the outflow pressure to the lymphatic vessel. Normally the outflow pressure to the lung lymphatics is the pressure within the neck veins (or the pressure within the large lymphatic trunk at the outflow of the lung lymphatics). For a cannulated lymphatic the outflow pressure is the pressure within the lymphatic at the tip of the cannula. That pressure is determined by the height of the outflow end of the cannula plus the product of the cannula resistance times lymph flow rate.

The solid curves in Figure 11.1 show flow *vs.* outflow pressure relationships for lung lymphatics in an awake sheep [6]. At baseline, increases in outflow pressure to ~ 15 cm $H_2O$ cause no decrease in lymph flow. This is because increases in lymphatic pumping compensate for increases in outflow pressure over this range of outflow pressures. For outflow pressures > 15 cm $H_2O$ the pump fails and lymph flow decreased. There is no plateau for the flow *vs.* pressure relationship for the lung with high microvascular filtration rate because the high lymph flow rates overwhelm the pump [14]. (The flow rate from the tissue spaces into the lymphatic is greater than the product of lymphatic stroke volume times contraction frequency.)

For uncannulated lymphatics, the outflow pressure is the pressure in the neck veins. This is illustrated by the open circles in Figure 11.1 where

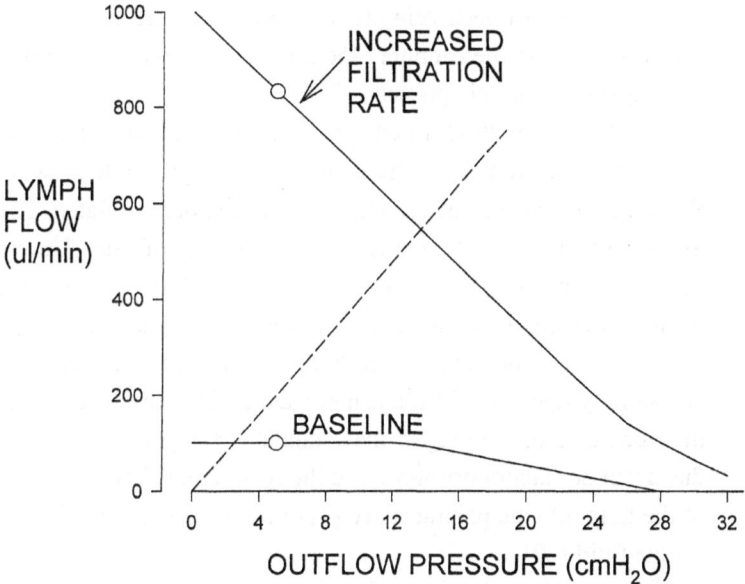

**Figure 11.1.**
*Solid curves represent the flow rate vs. outflow pressure relationships for a lymphatic vessel. Open circles show the flow rates with outflow pressure = 5 cm H₂O (normal neck vein pressure). Dashed line is the flow vs. pressure relationship for a typical cannula. Intersections of dashed line and solid curves indicate the flow rate from the vessel if it were cannulated.*

we have assumed neck vein pressure = 5 cm $H_2O$. For the baseline flow *vs.* outflow pressure relationship, flow = 100 μl/min and for the relationship from the edematous lung, flow = 820 μl/min

The dashed line in Figure 11.1 represents the flow *vs.* pressure characteristics of a cannula with resistance = 0.025 cm $H_2O$/μl/min and the outflow end of the cannula placed at zero height. We believe that cannula resistance and position are typical for previous experiments. The cannula line crosses the baseline flow *vs.* outflow pressure relationship at 100 μl/min. Thus, due to the plateau in the baseline flow *vs.* outflow pressure relationship, the flow from the cannulated vessel is the same as the flow from the vessel against neck vein pressure (open circle). However, the cannula line crosses the flow $vs.$ outflow pressure relationship for the edematous lung at flow $= 550$ $\mu$l/min. Thus, for the edematous lung, the flow from the cannula is much less than the 820 $\mu$l/min flow from the lymphatic against neck vein pressure. Also the percent increase in estimated flow from the cannula (450%) is much less than the increase in flow against neck vein pressure (720%).

For the lung with elevated filtration rate in Figure 11.1, 270 $\mu$l/min less lymph flowed from the cannulated lymphatic than would have flowed through the same lymphatic if it were not cannulated. There is no evidence that slowed lymph flow slows the rate of fluid filtration from the lung microvessels. Thus the reduced lymph flow caused by the lymph cannula represents an imbalance between fluid filtration and lymph flow. In some sheep, the reduction in lymph flow may be matched by an increase in lymph flow from uncannulated lymphatic vessels which drain the same area of the lung as the cannulated lymphatic. In addition, studies from our laboratory show that the lymph may flow from the surface of the lung into the pleural space [4] or it may accumulate in the lung as edema fluid [20].

The example of Figure 11.1 is for a lymphatic with an active postnodal smooth muscle pump. For anesthetized animals in which the pump is inhibited or for lymphatics cannulated near the node (before the postnodal lymphatic pump), the baseline flow $vs.$ outflow pressure plateau may be absent. In that case, the baseline flow from the cannula may not equal the baseline flow against venous pressure.

## Lymph protein concentration

Investigators usually assume that lymph protein concentration $(C_L)$ equals the protein concentration of microvascular filtrate. However, the composition of lymph may be altered as the lymph passes through lymph nodes. Lung lymph nodes are perfused by the systemic blood circulation and the blood capillaries may absorb fluid from the lymph or filter fluid into the lymph [2, 31]. The absorption/filtration state of the node blood capillaries depends on the balance in hydrostatic and protein osmotic pressures across the capillary membrane. Thus a high capillary hydro-static pressure will cause fluid to filter from the blood into the lymph and thereby dilute the lymph [1]. Conversely high plasma protein osmotic pressure may cause fluid absorption from the blood capillaries into the lymph and thereby increase the lymph protein concentration. If the net pressure within the blood capillaries (capillary hydrostatic pressure minus protein osmotic pressure) is equal to the net pressure in the lymph then there may be no fluid movement across the membrane and $C_L$ may not change within the node. The changes in $C_L$ within the node are dependent on the amount of time that the lymph is in the node [2]. If lymph flow is relatively slow, then the lymph composition may be changed significantly as the lymph passes through the node. On the other hand, with a rapid lymph flow, there may not be enough time for significant change in $C_L$.

Trauma to a node or agents which increase microvascular permeability may cause fluid and protein to leak from the node blood capillaries directly into the lymph. For instance, endotoxin infused IV into sheep causes blood capillaries to leak fluid and protein into the lymph [3].

Tissue protein washout is another factor which may affect $C_L$. As filtrate passes from the microvessels to the lymphatics, it must pass through the lung interstitial space. The interstitial space contains several grams of protein sequestered within the tissue matrix. Although there is probably a slow exchange of protein between the interstitial matrix and the filtrate, there is no net protein exchange and the concentration of protein in the initial lymphatics probably equals the filtrate protein concentration. However, in many studies the filtrate protein concentration is altered. Consequently the equilibrium between interstitial protein and filtered protein is upset and protein may diffuse from (or be washed from) the interstitial matrix and into the lymph. Then the lymph protein concentration will exceed the filtrate protein concentration until the excess protein is cleared from the interstitial matrix.

Parker et al. [30] have shown that it may take > 24 h to wash interstitial protein from the lungs of sheep. Parker and his associates increased pulmonary capillary pressure in their sheep and collected lung lymph for ~ 24 h. Figure 11.2 shows our interpretation of their findings. Increases in pulmonary capillary pressure cause an immediate decrease in filtrate

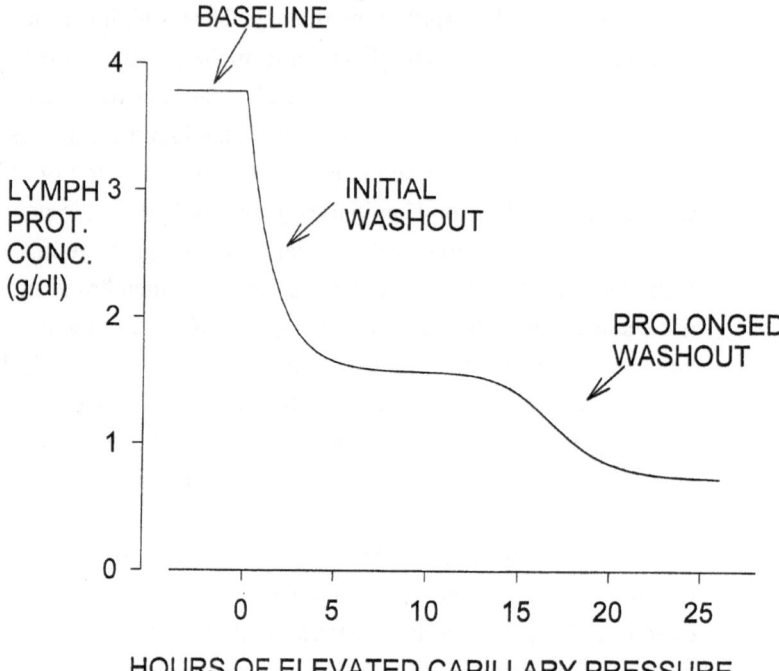

*Figure 11.2. Estimated time course of protein concentration in lymph after an increase in microvascular filtration rate.*

protein concentration and $C_L$ should slowly decrease as protein is cleared from the lung. As shown in Figure 11.2, $C_L$ decreased to an apparent plateau within 4 h after Parker et al. increased microvascular pressure. We believe this initial $C_L$ decrease was due to protein clearance from the interstitial free fluid spaces and from the lymphatic vessels and node. After ~14 h. $C_L$ began to decrease further and Parker et al. speculated this $C_L$ decrease was due to the clearance of protein from the interstitial matrix. If they were correct, then the $C_L$ between 4–14 h was the sum of the filtrate protein concentration plus the concentration of protein washed from the interstitial matrix. Presumably, after ~24 h, $C_L$ = the filtrate protein concentration. A recent study from our laboratory supports Parker et al. because it shows that after 4 h of increased microvascular filtration rate in sheep, $C_L$ is ~1.0 g/dl higher than filtrate protein concentration [8].

## Discussion

Cannulated lymphatics are one of the best tools we have to study lung fluid balance and microvascular permeability. However investigators must choose the best animal model for the study they plan. For lymphatic studies in which it is important to use awake animals, the sheep preparation (or the closely related goat preparation, [35]) is the only choice now available. Because investigators can allow the sheep to recover from the surgery, the sheep are presumably "normal" at the time of experiments. Another important advantage is that sheep seem to respond to many pathologic agents in a similar manner to humans [38]. For instance, *E. coli* endotoxin infusion into sheep causes a response similar to the adult respiratory distress syndrome in humans. In spite of the advantages of the sheep lymph preparation investigators must consider the possible influence of nonpulmonary lymph contamination. Lymph from nonpulmonary tissues could be a disaster in experiments in which the systemic microcirculation is affected. Any agent or procedure which increases fluid filtration into the abdominal cavity is likely to increase diaphragmatic lymph flow to the sheep caudal mediastinal lymph node [10]. Investigators collecting CMN lymph may misinterpret the increased lymph flow and assume lung lymph flow has increased.

The main advantage of the dog preparation is the purity of the lymph. Although it is usually impossible to trace tracheobronchial lymphatics to their origin, most investigators believe that these lymphatics contain pure lung lymph [22, 29]. Lymph from hilar lymphatics is certainly pure lung lymph because the tiny hilar lymphatics drain directly from the lung tissue and they can be cannulated before they enter a node. The disadvantage of the dog preparation is that it must be used with anesthetized, acutely prepared dogs. The lungs may be injured during the preparation and the data may be abnormal due to an increased microvascular permeability. Another disadvantage of acute preparations is that the lymphatic smooth muscle pump is usually inhibited in anesthetized, acutely prepared animals [34].

The cannula artifact is a serious problem in any study in which the investigator draws conclusions from lymph flow rate data. The key to accounting for the cannula problem is to cause the same pressure within the cannulated lymphatic as in the lymphatic before it was cannulated. Then the flow from the cannulated lymphatic should equal the flow through the same lympatic if it had not been cannulated [14]. For lymphatic vessels cannulated near the neck veins the normal intralymphatic pressure is nearly equal to neck vein pressure [13]. Thus investigators may account for the cannula artifact by using a low resistance cannula and placing the cannula outflow end at a height equal to the neck vein pressure. Then the pressure at the outflow to the cannulated lymphatic should equal the neck vein pressure. For prenodal lymphatics or postnodal lymphatics cannulated far from the neck veins the normal pressure at the cannulation site may be more or less than neck vein pressure. In that case there is no simple technique to account for the cannula artifact and we refer readers to previous publications [14].

Lymph flow rate is particularly important in studies in which investigators must estimate the microvascular filtration rate. The law of mass balance dictates that total lung lymph flow must equal filtration rate if 1) the lung fluid volume is stable and 2) there is no nonlymphatic exit by which fluid may leave the lungs. These conditions are probably true at baseline and with moderate increases in microvascular filtration rate. However, at high filtration rates, the lymphatic drainage system is overwhelmed and fluid collects within the lung tissue. Furthermore, in edematous lungs, fluid may flow through the pleural surface of the lungs and into the chest cavity. Thus, at high filtration rates, lymph flow rate may be much less than microvascular filtration rate.

Investigators have used two other techniques (besides lymph flow rate) to estimate microvascular filtration rate (*see* Chapter 8). First, filtration rate can be estimated from the rate of lung weight gain [7, 26]. We believe this is an excellent technique, however it can be misleading due to changes in lung blood volume. Furthermore, increases in lung fluid per unit time are equal to the difference in filtration rate minus lymph flow rate. Thus the increase in lung fluid should equal the filtered fluid volume only if investigators obstruct the lymphatics. Investigators have also estimated microvascular filtration from increases in red blood cell concentration as blood passes through the lungs [27]. So far this technique has been used only in isolated lungs.

The exchange of fluid or protein within a lymph node is a problem because it may cause investigators to incorrectly estimate filtrate protein concentration from lymph protein concentration. The best solution to this problem is to use prenodal lymph. Unfortunately prenodal lymphatics are difficult to cannulate. Another possible solution is to ligate or resect the blood circulation to the node. With blood flow stopped, there can be no fluid or protein exchange across the capillary walls. At high lymph flow rates lymph composition is changed very little within nodes and investigators may take advantage of this by causing a high lymph flow rate [2].

Tissue protein washout is a difficult problem because tissue protein may be cleared through the lymphatics along with filtered protein. Consequently investigators may overestimate filtrate concentration from the lymph protein concentration. One solution may be to tag plasma protein at the beginning of an experiment. That way filtered protein would be tagged but protein washed from the tissue space would contain no tag. Investigators could then calculate the filtrate protein concentration from the concentration of tagged protein in the lymph.

Nonlymphatic techniques to assess microvascular protein transport involve radiolabeled protein [16, 18]. The label may be detected with counters placed outside the animal or the lungs may be removed and analyzed for labeled protein.

In summary, cannulated lymphatics can be used to assess lymph vessel function, microvascular filtration rate or microvascular filtrate protein concentration. However it is important to chose the best animal preparation for a specific study. Furthermore, investigators must be aware of the potential problems caused by the cannula artifact and the possibility that lymph protein concentration may not equal filtrate protein concentration.

## Acknowledgements

The work in this chapter was supported by National Institutes of Health Grants DK-41859 and HL-49424.

## References

1  Adair TH and Guyton AC (1983) *Am. J. Physiol.* **245**: H616

2  Adair TH, Moffatt DS, Paulsen AW and Guyton (1982) *Am. J. Physiol.* **243**: H351

3  Adair TH, Montani JP and Guyton AC (1984) *J. Appl. Physiol.* **57**: 1597

4  Allen SJ, Laine GA, Drake RE and Gabel JC (1988) *Am. J. Physiol.* **255**: H492

5  Demling RH and Gunther R (1982) *Lymphology.* **15**: 163

6  Drake R, Giesler M, Laine G, Gabel J and Hansen T J (1985) *Appl. Physiol.* **58**: 70

7  Drake RE, Scott RL and Gabel JC (1983) *Am. J. Physiol.* **14**: H125

8  Drake RE, Dhother S, Oppenlander VM and Gabel JC (1996) *Lymphology* **29**: 112

9  Drake RE, Allen SJ, Katz J, Gabel JC and Laine GA (1986) *Am. J. Physiol.* **251**: H1090

10  Drake RE, Allen SJ, Gabel JC, Katz J and Laine GA (1987) *J. Appl. Physiol.* **62**: 706

11  Drake RE, Adair T, Traber D and JC Gabel (1981) *Am. J. Physiol.* **241**: H354

12  Elias RM, Johnston MG, Hayashi A and Nelson W (1987) *Am. J. Physiol.* **253**: H1349

13  Gabel JC and Drake RE (1992) *J. Appl. Physiol.* **73**: 654

14  Gallagher H, Garewal D, Drake RE and JC Gabel (1993) *Lymphology* **26**: 56

15  Gee MH and Spath JA Jr. (1980) *Circulation Research* **46**: 796

16  Gorin AB, Weidner WJ and Demling RH (1978) *J. Appl. Physiol.* **45**: 225

17  Johnston MG and Feuer C (1983) *J. Pharm. Exper. Therap.* **226**: 603

18  Kern DF, Levitt D and Wangensteen D (1983) *Am. J. Physiol.* **245**: H229-H236

19  Koike K, Albertine KH and Staub NC (1986) *J. Appl. Physiol.* **60**: 80

20  Laine GA, Allen SJ, Katz J, Gabel JC and RE Drake (1986) *J. Appl. Physiol.* **61**: 1634

21  Landolt CC, Matthay MA and Staub NC (1981) *J. Appl. Physiol.* **50**: 1372

22  Leeds SE, Teleszky LB, Uhley HN, Russell S and FR Elevitch (1982) *Surg. Gynecol. Obst.* **155**: 225

23  Martin DJ, Parker JC and Taylor AE (1983) *J. Appl. Physiol.* **54**: 199

24  McHale NG and Roddie IC (1976) *J. Physiol.* **261**: 255

25  McHale NG, Roddie IC and Thornbury KD (1980) *J. Physiol.* **309**: 461

26  Mitzner W and Sylvester JT (1986) *J. Appl. Physiol.* **61**: 1830

27  Oppenheimer L, Unruh HW, Skoog C and Goldberg HS (1983) *J. Appl. Physiol.* **54**: 64

28  Parker JC, Falgout HJ, Parker RE and Granger DN (1979) *Circ. Res.* **45**: 440

29  Parker JC, Crain M, Grimbert F, Rutili G and Taylor AE (1981) *J. Appl. Physiol.* **51**: 1268

30  Parker RE, Roselli RJ and Brigham KL (1985) *J. Appl. Physiol.* **58**: 869

31  Quin JW and Shannon AD (1977) *J. Physiol.* **264**: 307

32  Roos PJ, Wiener-Kronish JP, Albertine KH and Staub NC (1983) *J. Appl. Physiol.* **55**: 996

33  Staub NC (1975) *J. Surg. Res.* **19**: 315

34  Staub NC (1974) *Physiol. Rev.* **54**: 678

35  Stothert JC Jr. (1981) *J. Appl. Physiol.* **51**: 226

36  Taylor AE and Granger DN (1984) Exchange of macromolecules across the microcirculation. In: *Handbook of Physiology. The Cardiovascular System. Microcirculation.* Bethesda MD, *Am. Physiol. Soc.*, Sect. 2, Vol IV, Part 1, Chap. 11, p. 467

37  Townsley MI, McClure DE and Weidner WJ (1984) *J. Appl. Physiol.* **56**: 857

38  Traber DL, Adams T, Henriksen N, Traber LD and Thomson PD (1983) *J. Appl. Physiol.* **54**: 1167

39  Zarins CK, Rice CL, Smith DE and John DA (1976) *Surg. Forum-American College*, **S27**: 257

# Airway liquid

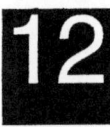

# Evaluation of secretory and transport processes which determine the composition of airway surface liquid

*R.H. Scott, M. Acevedo*
*and A. Griffin*

Airway surface liquid has complex physical and biochemical properties, which are suited to protect the airways from damage caused by infections and irritation by particles in inhaled air. Airway epithelial cells and gland cells (serous and mucous cells) secrete and transport materials such as lysozyme, antiproteases, sulphated proteoglycans, hyaluronic acid, mucins, ions and water which determine the chemical composition and the physical properties of the mucus gel lining the airways. The quantities and nature of the transported and secreted components of airway surface liquid can be detrimentally changed as a feature of several airway diseases. Thus from a therapeutic angle there is a need to understand the control mechanisms which ultimately determine the resistance and health of the airways. *In vitro* animal models provide some useful approaches for investigations into cellular mechanisms of transport and secretion. Electrophysiological techniques are very valuable for studying ion transport across the surface epithelium. Additionally, cell cultures can offer a solution to overcome problems with access to gland cells [1–3]. Cell culture combined with electrophysiological techniques can extend functional studies to the single cell level and allow detailed evaluation of the mechanisms of action of pharmacological agents. In this chapter, some of the practical aspects and limitations of studying certain secretory and transport events which regulate the formation of airway surface liquid are outlined.

# Methods

## Studies using isolated trachea

### The ferret isolated whole trachea in vitro preparation

Structurally the ferret trachea differs from human trachea in that the ferret epithelial cell layer contains no nerve fibres and few or no goblet cells, the mucus secretion being derived from submucosal gland cells (4). However, with respect to other characteristics including the viscoelasticity and transportability of secreted mucus, human and ferret trachea are similar [5]. As an experimental model the ferret trachea preparation allows a number of measurements such as smooth muscle tone, composition of airway surface liquid, albumin and ion transport to be studied in parallel. Anaesthetized (intraperitoneal injection of sodium

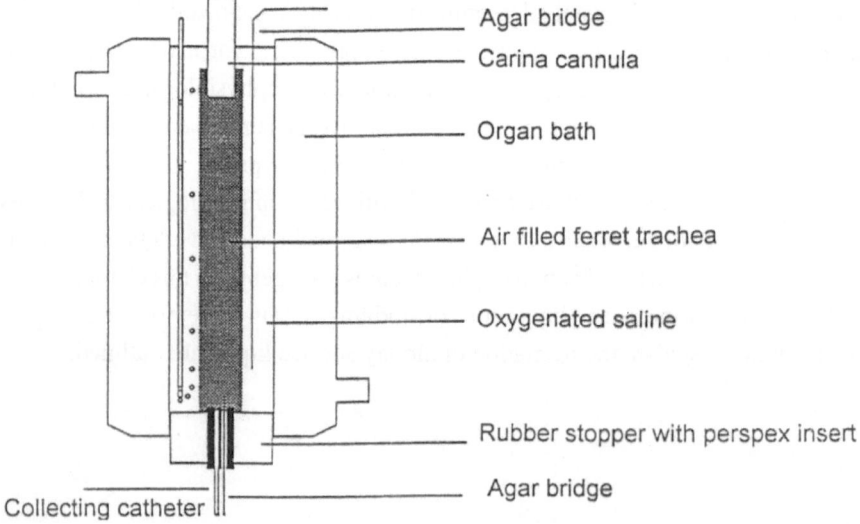

Agar bridge
Carina cannula
Organ bath
Air filled ferret trachea
Oxygenated saline
Rubber stopper with perspex insert
Agar bridge
Collecting catheter

*Figure 12.1 Diagram showing the air-filled ferret trachea supported in an organ bath with water jacket*
The trachea is inverted, so that the laryngeal end is at the bottom of the organ bath and the caudal end at the top of the organ bath.

pentobarbitone, 50 mg·kg$^{-1}$) female ferrets (Mustela putorius), either the polecat or albino strains aged between 6 and 12 months and weighing 0.75–1.5 kg should be used. Expose the trachea and then cannulate just below the larynx and attach to a perspex conical collecting well (narrowing perspex cannula), which is inserted into a rubber cork (Fig. 12.1). The ferret can then be killed by cardiac puncture and injection of sodium pentobarbitone (50 mg·kg$^{-1}$) into the heart. Open the thoracic cavity down the midline and open the ribcage to expose the full length of the trachea. The trachea should be cut just above the carina and removed from the thoracic cavity, cleared of connective tissue and cannulated with a 50 mm length of polythene tubing (Portex, ID 2 mm, OD 3.5 mm) at the carina end. Place the preparation laryngeal end down, in a water jacketed glass organ bath which is connected to a Churchill laboratory thermocirculator and maintain at 37 °C. The trachea should be continuously bathed in Krebs-Henseleit buffer, (containing in mM: NaCl, 120; KCl, 4.7; CaCl$_2$, 2.4; MgSO$_4$·7 H$_2$O, 0.6; NaHCO$_3$, 24.9; KH$_2$PO$_4$, 1.2; glucose, 5.6 and gassed with 95% O$_2$ and 5%CO$_2$) on the submucosal side only, so that the trachea lumen remains air-filled (Fig. 12.1).

## Protocol for stimulating secretions

The secretagogues, methacholine and phenylephrine produce concentration-dependent increases in lysozyme and albumin outputs from the ferret trachea [6]. After a 30-min equilibrium period in which the trachea is bathed in Krebs-Henseleit only, application of 20 µM methacholine (Sigma) or 100 µM phenylephrine (Sigma) produces 70% of the respective maximum responses for lysozyme and albumin outputs [6]. Tracheal secretions are carried by gravity and epithelial ciliary activity to the laryngeal cannula, where they pool during the 30-min collection time periods. The secretions can be withdrawn into polyethylene catheters (Portex ID 0.5 mm, OD 1.0 mm) which are inserted into the laryngeal perspex cannula. After each 30-min collection period the Krebs-Henseleit buffer surrounding the trachea is replaced with fresh buffer containing the secretagogue. Tracheal secretion samples are taken every 30 min, the catheters should be sealed with bone wax (Ethicon) and stored at −20 °C until re-

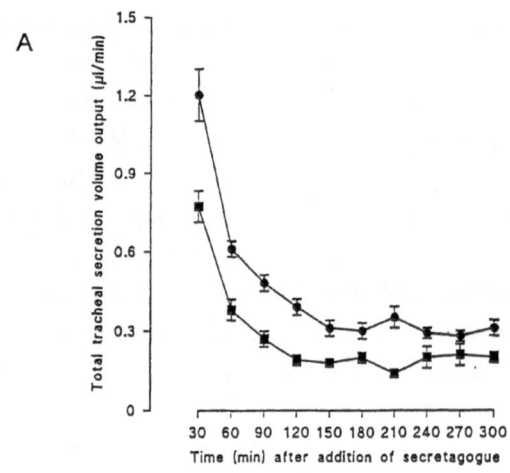

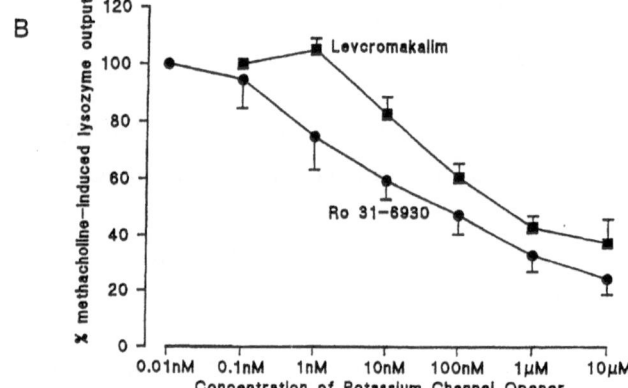

**Figure 12.2**

*(A) Time course of the effects of 20 µM methacholine (●) and 100 µM phenylephrine (■) on total tra-*
*cheal secretion volume output from the ferret isolated whole trachea* in vitro

*The graph shows the initial increase in volume output which declines to a stable output in the main-*
*tained presence of the secretagogues. Points represent the means of four determinations, vertical bars*
*represent standard error of the mean. (B) Potassium channel openers attenuate maintained secre-*
*tagogue-induced lysozyme output from the ferret isolated whole trachea* in vitro*. Graph shows the ef-*
*fect of the levcromakalim (■) and Ro 31-6930 (●) on maintained lysozyme output produced by 20 µM*
*methacholine. Data represents the means of 4–10 determinations, vertical bars give the standard er-*
*ror of the mean values.*

quired. Steady maintained secretion output is observed typically after 2
to 3 h (Fig. 12.2 A). The ferret whole trachea *in vitro* preparation has been

shown to be viable for up to 6 h since the potential difference across the trachea is maintained, baseline levels of secretion are low but uniform, ciliary beating and mucociliary transport are observed and the epithelium remains intact [7]. Lysozyme activity and albumin levels are usually analysed within 48 h of completing the experiment, but storage at −20 °C for up to 6 months has previously been shown not to change the enzymatic activity of lysozyme in the samples [6]. When defrosted, the secretions can be washed out of the catheters into Eppendorf vials with 1 ml of double distilled, deionized water and dried, (the dry weight of airway surface liquid is approximately 2% of its volume). The collected secretions should be sonicated to break up solidified components of the secretions. The total volumes of secretions can be established by assessing the differences between the weights of the dried and secretion filled catheters. Basal secretion over 30 min is typically <0.1 µl; this is worth checking as it shows that no hypersecretion is taking place. The maintained secretion induced by secretagogues over 30 min is 6–12 µl [8]. The actions of pharmacological agents on secretagogue- induced lysozyme and albumin output from the *in vitro* ferret air filled trachea can be investigated. Three different potassium channel openers (Ro 31-6930, levcromakalim and pinacidil; 100 pM to 10 µM) attenuate maintained secretagogue- induced secretion over the 30-min stimulation periods in a consistent and dose-dependent manner [8] (Fig. 12.2B).

## Assay for lysozyme

The concentration of lysozyme in each of the tracheal secretion samples is measured using a modified turbidimetric assay [9]. The modified assay [6] relies on the ability of lysozyme to disrupt the cell wall of the bacterium Micrococcus lysodeikticus causing a fall in the optical density of the sample (measured at 450 nm). A suspension of 0.3 mg·ml$^{-1}$ M.lysodeikticus (Sigma) in 1.5 ml of phosphate buffer (50 mM, pH 7.4) containing 1 mg·ml$^{-1}$ sodium azide (Sigma) and 1 mg·ml$^{-1}$ bovine serum albumin (Sigma) should be prepared. The concentration and output of lysozyme is established by incubating 20 µl of the sample in the M. lysodeikticus suspension; values for each sample can be calculated from a standard curve (hen egg white lysozyme). No basal lysozyme secretion can usually be detected, but typical values for secretagogue-evoked lysozyme secretion for whole ferret trachea are at peak over 400 ng·min$^{-1}$, and maintained stable levels are 88 to 130 ng·min$^{-1}$ [8].

## Albumin transport

To investigate the effect of drugs on the active transport of albumin across the ferret trachea, bovine serum albumin (BSA) is added to the buffer bathing the submucosal surface of the trachea at a concentration of 4 mg·ml$^{-1}$. Fluorescein isothiocyanate (FITC) labelled BSA (Sigma) at a concentration of 40 µg·ml$^{-1}$ is also added to the buffer as a marker and enables estimation of the total albumin in the tracheal secretion samples. The fluorescence of the samples is measured with a luminescence spectrometer using excitation and emission wavelengths of 550 nm and 490 nm, respectively. The fluorescent albumin concentration of the tracheal secretion samples is estimated from a standard curve (fluorescence *versus* concentration (25 ng·ml$^{-1}$ to 3 µg·ml$^{-1}$) of fluorescent BSA). The total concentration of the albumin in the samples is obtained by multiplying the fluorescent albumin concentration by the ratio of unlabelled to labelled albumin used in the experiments. The intraluminal fluorescent BSA concentration is not a consequence of the fluorescent label being broken off or transferred and therefore the fluorescence of the samples provides an accurate indication of the total albumin concentration [10]. Depending on the secretagogue used, maintained albumin output varies from 32 to 98 ng·min$^{-1}$.

## Measurement of potential difference across the tracheal wall

The electrical potential difference (PD) across the ferret tracheal wall provides an indication of the function and condition of the tracheal epithelium. The PD is governed by the degree of ion transport across the epithelium and the electrical conductance across the epithelium, which is mainly determined by the paracellular pathways. The PD across the ferret tracheal wall is assessed continuously throughout the duration of the experiment and recorded 5 min prior to the removal of airway surface liquid samples. PD is measured with two calomel reference electrodes (BDH), which are filled with 3.8 M KCl and placed in beakers containing 3.8 M KCl. An electrical connection with the *in vitro* trachea is achieved with two agar bridges, one placed on the submucosal side in the Krebs-Henseleit buffer and the other inserted into a second hole in the laryngeal perspex cannula. The agar bridges are made of polyethylene tubing (Portex ID 0.5 mm, OD 1.0 mm) filled with 3.8 M KCl in 2.5% w/v agar solution. Output from the two electrodes is passed into a high input impedance buffer amplifier and displayed on a digital voltmeter. A typical value of 8 mV with the lumen being negative with respect to the submucosal side is recorded for a healthy *in vitro* ferret trachea. Values vary with species, and are sensitive to drug application, for example platelet-activating factor (PAF), methacholine and phenylephrine [11].

## Ion transport across the airways

*Measurement of the ionic composition of periciliary fluid*

Airway epithelia regulate the volume and ionic composition of airway surface fluid. The depth of the fluid layer needs to be maintained for effective mucociliary clearance. The ionic composition is very important for mucus hydration, viscoelastic properties of the mucus, ciliary beating and functioning of the immune system in the lung. The ionic composition of the fluid has been difficult to determine due to its small volume, the variable contamination with cellular and bacterial debris, and the variable contribution of mucus. Recently, methods have been developed for the study of the composition of the airway fluid in *in vitro* preparations. Whole tracheal secretions have been collected from the ferret tracheal preparation [7] and the electrolyte composition assessed by atomic absorption spectrophotometry. A different approach is to collect fluid samples on filter paper strips after equilibration with the airway fluid. This method for isolated tracheal mucosa studies has been developed and used with X-ray analysis to determine electrolyte composition of the collected fluid [12]. Ion- selective microelectrodes have also been used to measure ion composition of the airway fluid in an *in vitro* guinea pig tracheal preparation [13]. Airway cultured monolayers have also been used to collect samples of the airway surface fluid in capillary tubes after long incubations, and ionic composition has been measured [14].

## Electrophysiological methods used in the investigation of ion transport in the airways. Measurement of short-circuit current ($I_{SC}$) and transepithelial resistance ($R_T$)

Airway epithelia have the capability for $Cl^-$ secretion and $Na^+$ absorption [15]. Both processes are active and electrogenic, and therefore carry an electrical current. The electrogenic nature of $Cl^-$ secretion and $Na^+$ absorption makes them amenable to study using electrophysiological techniques. Short-circuit current ($I_{SC}$) and transepithelial resistance ($R_T$) provide good information on these processes. We use sheep tracheal epithelium [16], because sheep and human trachea do not differ greatly in terms of structure, development, secretory cells and ion transport. Tracheas are immersed in a solution containing (in mM) 118 NaCl, 6 KCl, 2 $CaCl_2$, 1 $MgCl_2$, 5 Hepes, 6 glucose, 40 mannitol, pH 7.4. and transported to the lab. The cartilage from the posterior border is trimmed, the trachea is cut open by a longitudinal incision along the anterior border and kept immersed in the above solution at room temperature. To dissect the mucosa from underlying layers, the tissue is pinned down on a dissecting board, mucosa facing upwards. Under a stereomicroscope the mucosa is dissected from the underlying muscle by pulling it free with fine tip forceps while cutting the strands of tissue between the muscle layer and the mucosa with fine tip scissors. It is important to avoid pulling the mucosa too hard when isolating it, as this will result in damage. Damage to the tissue causes a low electrical transepithelial resistance and we reject any tissue with $R_T$ lower than 100 $\Omega \cdot cm^{-2}$.

The dissected mucosa is mounted as a flat sheet between two half chambers which allow separate control of mucosal and serosal bathing media. We use the perspex chambers (WPI, model CHM1). We clamp between the chambers an area of mucosa larger than 1 $cm^2$ to minimize the influence of easily damaged tissue at the edge of the preparation. The solutions bathing each side of the tissue are recirculated and oxygenated using bubble lifts. The solutions are kept at 37 °C by circulating water through the water jackets using a circulator. Two pairs of Ag/AgCl are connected to both sides of the tissue through 1 M KCl/agar bridges. One pair of electrodes is used to measure transepithelial potential, and the other to pass current. A dual voltage clamp amplifier (WPI, DVC-100) is used. This system allows continuous measurement of $I_{SC}$ and $R_T$ for two pieces of tissue at a time. The transepithelial voltage is clamped at zero and the current applied for this ($I_{SC}$) is measured. At regular intervals the voltage is changed to a different value ($V_2$, usually 1 or 2 mV), and the current applied for this is measured ($I_{V2}$). $R_T$ can then be calculated from Ohm's law, as: $R_T = V_2 / (I_{V2} - I_{SC})$.

Before mounting the tissue the series electrical resistance (resistance of the solutions, bridges) has to be measured, to compensate for the voltage drop across the solution during short-circuiting. The system used allows automatic series resistance compensation. When bathed in the presence of bicarbonate and $CO_2$, $I_{SC}$ across this tissue is approximately 60 A·cm$^{-2}$, whereas $R_T$ has an approximate value of 200 $\Omega$·cm$^{-2}$. The main components of $I_{SC}$ are a Na$^+$ current and a Cl$^-$ current. The Na$^+$ current can be blocked by adding amiloride (100 µM) to the mucosal bathing solution, whereas the Cl$^-$ current can be inhibited by applying loop diuretics such as bumetanide (10 µM) or frusemide (100 µM) to the serosal bathing medium. This technique is suitable when flat, large pieces of epithelium can be obtained. For distal airways this is not possible, and other methods are required. The determination of $I_{SC}$ in smaller airways has been described by the application of cable analysis [17, 18], and information on ion transport can also be gained from transepithelial potential measurements [19].

## Acid/base transport

Acid/base transport has been evaluated by measuring pH of the secretions collected from the isolated ferret trachea [7] and after 24 h incubation from cultured monolayers from human airway cells [14]. We have used isolated sheep trachea in order to monitor acid/base transport with a pH-stat method to assess movement of acid/base across whole trachea from sheep [20]. Tracheas are immersed in buffer containing (in mM) 118 NaCl, 6 KCl, 2 CaCl$_2$, 1 MgCl$_2$, 5 Hepes, 6 glucose, 40 mannitol, pH 7.4. In the lab, surrounding connective tissue is removed, and as much cartilage as possible from the posterior side of the trachea. Removal of this cartilage improves the oxygenation of the tissue and allows the trachea to be bent easily. The trachea is then bent into a U-shaped pouch, and the two open ends held together by a haemostat. The tracheal lumen is filled with poorly buffered solution (containing (in mM) 118 NaCl, 6 KCl, 2 CaCl$_2$, 1 MgCl$_2$, 1 Hepes, 6 glucose, 48 mannitol; buffering capacity at pH 7.2, 685 nmol.pH unit$^{-1}$). The trachea is immersed in solution with the same composition, taking care that the open ends are above the level of solution, in order to prevent mixing of the lumenal and serosal solutions (Fig. 12.3). The external solution is energetically bubbled with 100% O$_2$. A peristaltic pump is connected to either end of the tracheal lumen via polythene tubing. The solution in the lumen is recirculated by these means at a rate of approximately 100 ml·min$^{-1}$. A pH electrode is introduced into the tracheal lumen. The whole system is kept in an incubator at 37 °C.

Once the measured pH is stable (6.2 ± 0.1, n = 12), aliquots of NaOH (usually 10–20 µl of 0.1 M NaOH) are added to bring the lumenal solution pH to 7.2. The lumenal pH is maintained at this value, and the amount of NaOH added together with the time interval between additions is recorded. At the end of the experiment the trachea is cut open along its longitudinal border, and its area is measured in order to be able to express secretion as a function of area. Acid secretion (J$_H$) is calculated as the amount of NaOH added divided by the time interval between additions and the surface area of the trachea. In a set of control experiments we measured transepithelial potential across the preparation by the method described above in order to assess its viability. The values we obtained, of 12.6 ± 1.9 mV (n = 8), are no different from those obtained in isolated epithelial sheets from the same tissue (12.4 mV), suggesting a normal epithelial function during the experiments [16]. Under the conditions used, the trachea secretes acid towards the lumen. Acid secretion decays with time (Fig. 12.4 A, B). The decay in time can be fitted with a

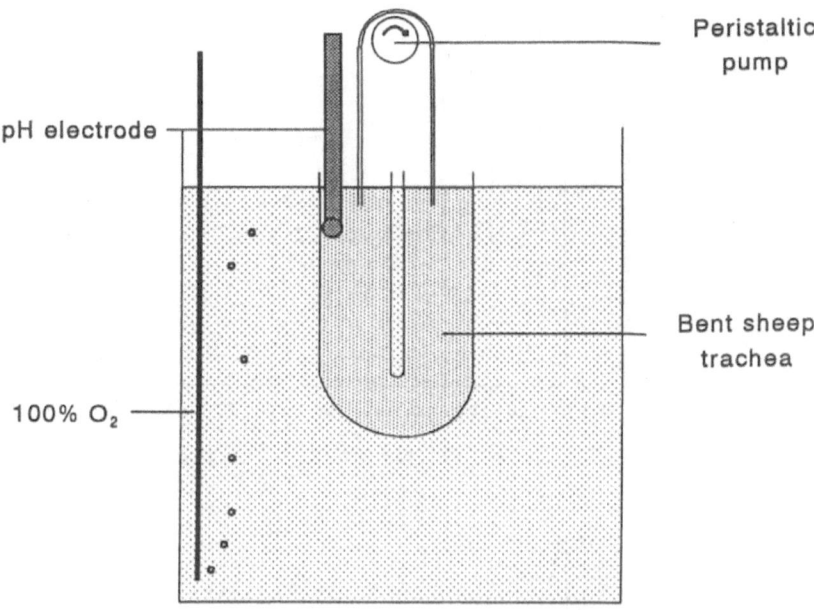

**Figure 12.3 Schematic diagram of the system used in pH stat experiments**
*The open ends of the trachea were kept above the level of the solution to avoid serosal and mucosal bathing media from mixing with each other. The mucosal bathing solution was mixed continuously with the help of a peristaltic pump.*

logarithmic function: $J_H = a - (b \times \ln(t))$, where a and b are the fitting co-efficients and t is the time in minutes. In our studies, under control conditions, the value for a was $19.4 \pm 1.1$ and the value for b $1.45 \pm 0.1$ (n=32). The variability of $J_H$ rates is quite considerable between tissues. In order to evaluate the effect of drugs, it is best to have a measure of value for $J_H$ before drug application. This is complicated by the fact that $J_H$ is decaying in time, and waiting to get a steady-state $J_H$ value is probably not advisable, since it is possible that the tissue deteriorates with time. It is possible to measure acid transport for 40 min under control conditions and then add the drug and continue monitoring. To account for the time decay, the results obtained after drug addition are compared to those expected for the control. Expected values are obtained from the non-linear regression analysis using data before drug application. We de-

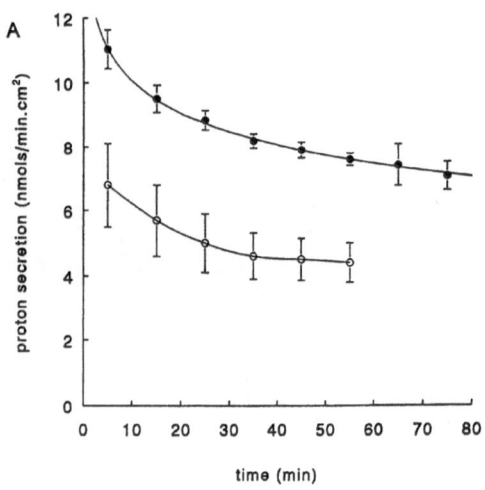

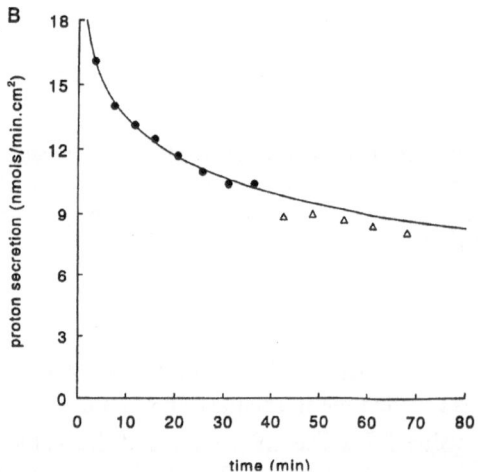

**Figure 12.4 These figures show the type of results obtained from the pH stat technique**
In (A) the time dependency of acid secretion in sheep trachea under control conditions is shown. Each point represents mean±SEM of six experiments obtained under control conditions (●) or in tracheas incubated in the absence of sodium (○). The lines are the best fits of these points to a logarithmic function. (B) Shows the results for an individual experiment. Under control conditions (●) acid secretion followed a logarithmic decay. (△) After 40 min, Bafilomycin A₁ was added (0.1 μM) and acid secretion was recorded for 30 min. It can be seen that acid secretion was smaller than predicted from the trend under control conditions. This effect, although small, was consistently seen in sheep tracheas.

monstrated in pilot experiments that, in the absence of drugs, data obtained during 40 min under control conditions allow an accurate prediction of the rate of acid transport at a time 20 min later. An example of the effect of bafilomycin $A_1$ (a proton pump blocker) is shown in Figure 12.4B.

## Acid/base transport across cell membranes of isolated tracheocytes

Transport of acid/base across the cell membrane of airway epithelial cells can be evaluated by monitoring changes in intracellular pH ($pH_i$). If the intracellular buffering capacity ($\beta_I$) is known, the rate of change in $pH_i$ ($dpH_i/dt$) after a pH challenge can be used to calculate acid/base flux across the membrane. $pH_i$ can be measured with fluorescent indicators [21], and this method has been applied in airway epithelial cells from nasal [22] and alveolar [23] origin. The $pH_i$ and buffering capacity [24] can be measured in ciliated epithelial cells from trachea. Tracheas are cut open, and mucosal strips are obtained by quick dissection. The strips are then washed with isolation solution (containing 118 NaCl, 6 KCl, 2 $CaCl_2$, 1 $MgCl_2$, 5 Hepes, 6 glucose, 40 mannitol, pH 7.4) and then with a solution similar to the isolation solution, but without $Ca^{2+}$ and $Mg^{2+}$, and containing 2 mM EGTA. Following this, the strips are incubated in $Ca^{2+}$, $Mg^{2+}$-free solution for 30 min at 37 °C. The solution is then discarded, and the strips are then incubated in isolation solution containing 5 mM DTT and 400 units·ml$^{-1}$ of collagenase (CLS3, Lorne Worthington) in a plastic flask.

This incubation takes place at 37 °C for 1 h in a shaking bath at a low shaking setting. At the end of the incubation, the collagenase containing solution is discarded (it contains a high percentage of dead cells), and the strips are resuspended in ice-cold isolation solution containing 1–2 µg·ml$^{-1}$ of DNase type I from bovine pancreas (Sigma). This is now shaken vigorously, and the resulting cell suspension is filtered through 100 µm nylon gauze. The filtered cell suspension is then centrifuged at approximately 100 g for 5–10 min, and the pellet is washed two to three times by resuspending in ice-cold isolation solution containing 1–2 µg·ml$^{-1}$ of DNase, to remove collagenase and DTT. Using this method we obtain an average of 5.3 million cells per trachea with 80% viability (estimated by Trypan blue exclusion). The cells are then attached to glass coverslips coated with poly-lysine. For $pH_i$ measurements the cells are first loaded with the pH sensitive dye. A small volume of isolating solution containing 10 µM BCECF/AM (2',7'-bis-(2-carboxyethyl)-5-(and -6) carboxyfluorescein, acetomethyl ester (Molecular Probes Inc.), prepared by adding BCECF/AM from a 10 mM stock in DMSO) is added to the cells. This is incubated at 37 °C for 30 min. After the incubation, the coverslip is rinsed with BCECF/AM-free isolation solution. The coverslip is mounted in an incubation chamber (Intracel), perfused continuously and kept at 37 °C on the stage of the fluorescence microscope.

For the fluorescence measurements we use a deltascan system (Photon Technology International). The excitation wavelengths are 445 and 490 nm and the emission 510 nm. We select a ciliated cell which shows ciliary activity and then reduce the field to cover the area occupied by the cell and fluorescence is measured for it. A background reading is done previously and subtracted from the cell fluorescence values. For $pH_i$ measurements, the ratio of fluorescence emitted at 490 and 445 is calculated ($F_{490}/F_{445}$), this ratio is a function of $pH_i$. The signal is calibrated for each cell at the end of the experiment as previously described [25]. It has been reported that nigericin becomes adsorbed to plastic, and is difficult to wash away [26], and this can affect the following cell under study so we discard the tubing used for perfusion after each calibration.

## Culture of ovine tracheal submucosal gland cells

### Preparation and characterisation

At the single cell level cell culture can be used to overcome problems with access and cell isolation. Trachea were transported to the lab in ice-cooled Dulbecco's phosphate buffered saline (Sigma). The sheep preparation is similar to human trachea, is also large and gives a good cell yield. In a sterile environment the tracheas are opened longitudinally through the smooth muscle band, pinned out on a sterile dissection base and then rinsed with sterile Hank's balanced salt solution (Sigma), containing 20 mM HEPES buffer (pH 7.4), 100 $\mu g \cdot ml^{-1}$ streptomycin (Gibco), 100 $U \cdot ml^{-1}$ penicillin (Gibco), 2.5 $\mu g \cdot ml^{-1}$ amphotericin B (Gibco) and 100 $\mu g \cdot ml^{-1}$ gentamycin (Sigma) to remove residual mucus and debris. The lumenal surface is then rubbed vigorously with sterile cotton gauze to remove the surface epithelial layer of the trachea. The gland-containing submucosal layer is dissected from the tracheal cartilage, minced with fine scissors and placed in fresh Hank's balanced salt solution (HBSS). The culture method used is based on a previously described technique [2]. The submucosa is enzymatically dissociated over a 12-h period in HBSS containing 500 $U \cdot ml^{-1}$ collagenase type IV (Sigma), 6 $U \cdot ml^{-1}$ elastase (Sigma), 200 $U \cdot ml^{-1}$ hyaluronidase (Sigma) and 10 $U \cdot ml^{-1}$ deoxyribonuclease (Sigma), in addition to the antibiotics. The preparation should be maintained at 22 °C in a heated shaker water bath.

The resultant mixture of dissociated cells and tissue fragments is left to stand for 5 min so that large tissue fragments settle out and the supernatant containing dissociated cells can be drawn off. A pellet of cells is obtained by centrifugation at 2000 rpm (200 g) for 10 min. The pellet is then resuspended in 1:1 Dulbecco's Modified Eagle's Medium to Ham's Nutrient Mixture F-12 (DMEM/HF12) (Sigma) supplemented with antibiotics, 5 $\mu M$ L-glutamine (Sigma) and 10% fetal calf serum (Gibco). Cell viability is measured using trypan blue exclusion and the cell number is estimated using a haemacytometer. The cells are plated at a density of approximately $1 \times 106 \, cm^{-2}$ onto collagen-coated glass coverslips in sterile $35 \times 10$ mm tissue culture dishes or six-well cell culture plates. The cells are bathed with 2 ml of DMEM/HF12 and refed every 48 h with fresh cell culture medium. The culture dishes are incubated at 37 °C in humidified air containing 5% $CO_2$ in an incubator.

## Methods for studying the effects of secretagogues on lysozyme release from cultured ovine trachea submucosal gland cells

After at least 14 days submucosal gland cell cultures reach confluence and they then can be used for studying the effects of secretagogues. Culture medium is removed and the monolayer of cultured cells is washed twice with gassed (95% $O_2$ and 5% $CO_2$) Krebs-Henseleit buffer. Krebs-Henseleit buffer (2 ml) is added to each culture well and left in contact for 30 min at 37 °C after which 1 ml of the Krebs-Henseleit buffer is removed for lysozyme analysis. This control period is repeated for another 30 min before introduction of secretagogues (methacholine (20 μM), phenylephrine (100 μM) and substance P (10 μM)). The secretagogues are in contact with the cultured cells for three 30-min periods; at the end of each period, 1 ml of buffer is taken for lysozyme analysis. Values for lysozyme release from mature cultures are typically around 100 ng·ml$^{-1}$ over two 30-min periods and this is enhanced by up to more than 300% by secretagogues [27]. A final 30 min control collection (Krebs-Henseleit buffer only) is performed for each culture well, during this period lysozyme release is reduced (30 ng·ml$^{-1}$). The 1 ml samples are freeze-dried to concentrate the lysozyme and then resuspended in 100 μl of distilled water before being assayed for lysozyme.

To assess the relationship between the time in culture and the release of lysozyme from the cultured ovine trachea submucosal gland cells samples were taken from the cell cultures that were 24 or 48 h old and 1 or 2 weeks old. The protocol used is different to that described above because of the small amounts of material released from young cultures. The culture medium is removed, replaced with 2 ml of fresh culture medium and the culture dishes are returned to the incubator. After 24 h the culture medium is removed and a lysozyme assay performed on that sample. Secretagogues are left in contact with the cell cultures for the whole of this 24-h period. A problem that arises from the long collection periods is that it may result in an underestimation of release because the kinetics of secretagogue action remains to be investigated. However, no basal or secretagogue induced lysozyme release (<0.5 ng·ml$^{-1}$) is observed in the first 5 days in culture. After 10 and 20 days in culture basal lysozyme secretion was 106 ng per well and 184 ng per well respectively and this level was increased by secretagogues by 25–86% [28].

## Electrophysiology

The whole cell variant of the patch clamp technique [29] can be used to record currents activated in cultured ovine tracheal submucosal gland cells. As with lysozyme release mature cultures (7–21 days in culture) of submucosal gland cells should be used for electrophysiology. Borosilicate glass capillary tubing has been used in our work for the fabrication of all low resistance (5–10 M$\Omega$) glass patch pipettes. The cells remain viable for up to 4 h with regular changes of the extracellular recording medium.

The constituents of the recording and patch pipette solutions depend on what current is being studied [27, 28], voltage-activated K$^+$ currents (Fig. 12.5 A, B) and Ca$^{2+}$- activated Cl$^-$ currents (Fig. 12.6] have been identified. At room temperature (20–25 °C), seal resistances between the patch pipette and the cell membrane in excess of 1 G$\Omega$ are readily achieved before entering the whole-cell recording configuration. Holding the cell membrane potential at –70 mV prevents voltage- activated K$^+$ current inactivation and allows maximum availability of K$^+$ channels. Voltage steps to potentials positive to –30 mV result in activation of voltage-activated K$^+$ currents which are sensitive to TEA and 4-aminopyridine. These currents can be activated every 10 s and have a net current amplitude of about 0.45 nA at +30 mV.

The whole cell patch clamp technique can be used in conjunction with intracellular flash photolysis to photorelease materials inside cells [30]. The photolabile caged compounds to be photolysed are included in the patch pipette solution and once the whole-cell configuration is achieved, the patch pipette solution and the intracellular environment equilibrate within 5 min. Photolysis of caged compounds inside cells can be achieved with a short flash (1 ms) of intense near ultra-violet light (8–20 mJ·mm$^{-1}$) from a xenon flash lamp (XF-10, Hi-Tech Scientific) focused onto the target cell [28]. The actions of the intracellular photolysis of caged Ca$^{2+}$ (DM-nitrophen) and caged InsP$_3$, (Calbiochem.) have been studied [28]. DM-nitrophen (4.0 mM) and CaCl$_2$ (2 mM) are included in CsCl-based patch pipette solution, which contained no MgCl$_2$ or EGTA. Caged InsP$_3$ can be included in the standard CsCl-based patch pipette solution at a concentration of 100 µM.

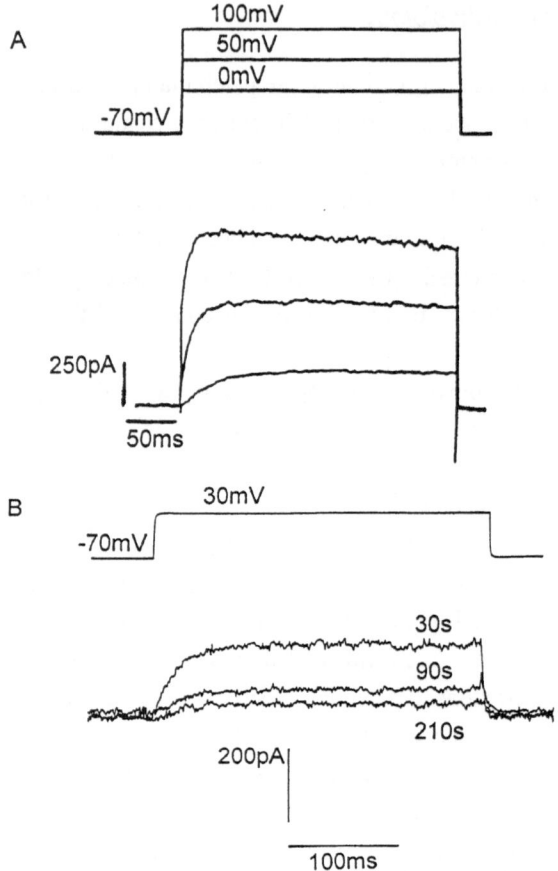

**Figure 12.5 Voltage-activated K⁺ currents evoked from ovine cultured submucosal gland cells**
*(A) Net outward voltage-activated K⁺ currents recorded from cultured submucosal gland cell maintained in culture for 14 days. The traces show the voltage step commands and the progressively larger K⁺ currents activated by voltage step commands to 0 mV, 50 mV and 100 mV, from a holding potential of −70 mV. (B) The action of caesium chloride on the voltage-activated K⁺ currents observed in cultured airway submucosal gland cells. Traces show the time-dependent effect of caesium chloride-based patch solution on the voltage-activated K⁺ current. The currents were activated by 300 ms depolarizing step commands to +30 mV from a holding potential of −70 mV, and evoked within 30 s of achieving the whole cell configuration, and after 90 s and 210 s. Note the marked decline in current.*

The quantum yield for caged InsP₃ is 0.65 and is similar to that for caged ATP, which is 0.63 [30]. A 200 V flash produces 11% photolysis of caged ATP in our system used [31], a 200 V flash would be expected

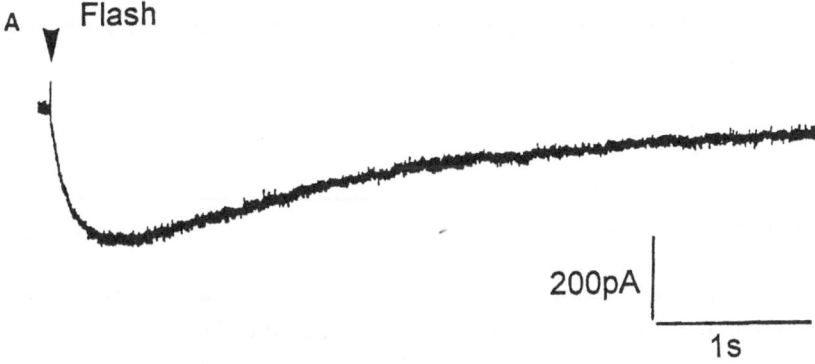

A ▼ Flash

200pA

1s

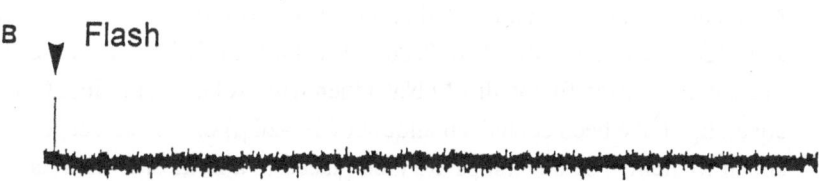

B ▼ Flash

**Figure 12.6**
*(A) Typical response to intracellular flash photolysis of DM-nitrophen, which activates a transient inward*
*$Ca^{2+}$-activated $Cl^-$ current in cultured tracheal submucosal gland cells. The cell was loaded with (4 mM)*
*DM-nitrophen in CsCl-based patch pipette solution, containing 2 mM $CaCl_2$, which was allowed to equi-*
*librate for 5 min. (B) Control, no response to the flash photolysis of DM-nitrophen occurs when the cell*
*was loaded with (4 mM) DM-nitrophen in CsCl-based patch pipette solution containing no added $CaCl_2$.*
*The cells were held at −70 mV, and a 200 V flash of intense near UV light applied at the points marked*
*by the arrow heads (note upward rapid flash artifacts) in both cases.*

to photorelease about 10 μM InsP₃ under our conditions. The photorelease of $Ca^{2+}$ from the calcium chelator DM-nitrophen in cultured submucosal gland cells evokes transient inward $Ca^{2+}$- activated $Cl^-$ currents
of between −0.3 and −0.9 nA at −90 mV [28] (Fig. 12.6). For a control,
cultured submucosal gland cells are loaded with CsCl-based intracellular patch pipette solution containing DM-nitrophen but with no added
$CaCl_2$. Photolysis of DM-nitrophen without $Ca^{2+}$ present fails to evoke
any inward or outward current responses (Fig. 12.6). Intracellular photo-

lysis of InsP$_3$ can also evoke modest and inconsistent inward currents which have proved difficult to work on in cultured submucosal gland cells.

## Troubleshooting

1) Commercially available enzymes used in cell dissociation are often quite variable in their activity. It is worth noting that some batches work better than others; it is convenient to test several lots with respect to suitable incubation times, and once one has been chosen, to use it consistently.

2) Procedure for coating coverslips with poly-D-lysine:
   Coverslips (Borosilicate glass round coverslips, 24 mm diameter, thickness No 1), are treated by adding 10 µl of an aqueous solution of 10% poly-D-lysine (Hydrobromide, Mol. Wt. 70000–150000) and left for 1 min. Coverslips are then rinsed first with 1 M NaCl then with isolation solution. Once the coverslips have been coated, an aliquot of 10–20 µl of the cell suspension is added to them. The coverslips are then placed in a Petri dish with its cover, and left in the fridge overnight.

## Conclusions

In conclusion *in vitro* animal model preparations (ferret and sheep trachea) can be selected which are of relevance to human airway physiology and pharmacology. Problems with obtaining stable base line recordings of secretions can be encountered with isolated trachea. But these difficulties can be limited by making comparisons with standard curves which compensate for time-dependent decreases in secretion or allowing several hours and repeated stimulating before studying submaximal but consistent responses. Cell culture offers good access to cells of interest, however it is apparent that the submucosal gland cells after isolation need at least a week in culture before they express functional ion channels and secrete lysozyme. Additionally, the cultured submucosal gland-like cells only contain a modest amount of lysozyme compared with cells in the *in vi-*

*vo* situation, and it has been suggested that they may take on an intermediate phenotype, expressing properties of other epithelial cell types. So some caution is necessary in the interpretation of results, nevertheless cultured preparations do provide a powerful tool and new opportunities to investigate aspects of cellular physiology at the single cell and subcellular levels.

## Acknowledgements

RHS and AG thank Roche Products Ltd UK for financial support and Mr P. Gater for his constructive comments. MA thanks The Wellcome Trust for support.

## References

1  Benali R, Dupuit F, Jacquot J, Fuchey C, Hinnrasky J, Ploton D and Puchelle E (1989) *Biol. Cell* **66**: 263

2  Sommerhoff CP and Finkbeiner WE (1990) *Am. J. Resp. Cell Molec. Biol.* **2**: 41

3  Tournier JM, Merten M, Meckler Y, Hinnrasky J, Fuchey C and Puchelle E (1990) *Am. Rev. Resp. Dis.* **141**: 1280

4  Robinson NP, Venning L, Kyle H and Widdicombe JG (1986) *J. Anat.* **145**: 173

5  De Sanctis GT, Rubin BK, Ramirez O and King M (1993) *Europ. Resp. J.* **6**: 76

6  Webber SE and Widdicombe JG (1987) *Brit. J. Pharmacol.* **91**: 139

7  Robinson NP, Kyle H, Webber SE and Widdicombe JG (1989) *J. Appl. Physiol.* **66**: 2129

8  Griffin A (1995) *Eur. J. Pharmacol.* **280**: 317

9  Lorenz TH, Korst DR, Simpson JF and Musser MJ (1957) *J. Lab. Clin. Med.* **49**: 145

10 Webber SE and Widdicombe JG (1989) *J. Physiol.* **408**: 457

11 Webber SE, Morikawa T and Widdicombe JG (1987) *Brit. J. Pharmacol.* **105**: 223

12 Joris L and Quinton PM (1992) *Am. J. Physiol.* **263**: L243

13 Rashmoune H and Shephard KL (1995) *J. Appl. Physiol.* **78**: 2020

14 Smith JJ and Welsh MJ (1993) *J. Clin. Invest.* **91**: 1590

15 Noone PG, Olivier KN and Knowles MR (1994) *Ann. Rev. Med.* **45**: 412

16 Acevedo M (1994) *Pflügers Arch.* **427**: 543

17 Ballard ST and Taylor AE (1994) *Am. J. Physiol.* **267**: L79

18 Croxton TL (1993) *Am. J. Physiol.* **265**: L38

19 Al-Bazzaz FQ (1994) *Am. J. Physiol.* **267**: L193

20 Acevedo M and Steele LW (1993) *Exp. Physiol.* **78**: 383

21 Rink TS, Tsien RY and Pozzan T (1982) *J. Cell Biol.* **95**: 189

22 Paradiso AM (1992) *Am. J. Physiol.* **262**: L757

23  Lubman RL and Crandall ED (1992) *Am. J. Physiol.* **262**: L1

24  Boyarski G, Ganz MB, Sterzel RB and Boron WF (1988) *Am. J. Physiol.* **255**: C844

25  Thomas JA, Buchsbaum RN, Zimniak A and Racker E (1979) *Biochemistry* **18**: 2210

26  Richmond P and Vaughan-Jones RD (1993) *J. Physiol.* **467**: 277P

27  Griffin A and Scott RH (1994) *Resp. Physiol.* **96**: 297

28  Griffin A, Newman TM and Scott RH (1996) *Exp. Physiol.* **81**: 27

29  Hamill OP, Marty A, Neher E, Sakmann B and Sigworth FJ (1981) *Pflügers Arch.* **391**: 85

30  Gurney AM (1994) Flash Photolysis of Caged Compounds. In: *Microelectrode Techniques, the Plymouth Workshop Handbook*, Ogden D (ed.), p. 389, The Company of Biologists Ltd, Cambridge

31  Currie KPM, Wootton JF and Scott RH (1995) *J. Physiol.* **482**: 291

# 13 Bronchoalveolar lavage

*U. Wagner and*
*P. von Wichert*

Bronchoalveolar lavage (BAL) is a method that allows the recovery of both cellular and noncellular components from the epithelial fluid lining the respiratory tract and differs from bronchial washings, which refer to the aspiration of either secretions or small amounts of instilled saline from large airways. BAL is accomplished by infusing a physiological salt solution through the bronchoscope and then recovering the infused solution together with the epithelial lining fluid (ELF) [1, 2]. Diagnostic BAL has to be differentiated from therapeutic BAL with the need of larger volumes (up to 10 to 20 l), performed through a double lumen tube that selectively catheterizes a major bronchus. The latter procedures are used periodically in patients with alveolar proteinosis and occasionally in subjects with cystic fibrosis or in those with special inhaled particles or noxious gas exposure, however, the indications for massive, whole lung lavage under general anaesthesia are few [2]. Generally, BAL is done in conjunction with fiberoptic bronchoscopy.

## Methods

### Endoscopic techniques of BAL in man

BAL, although a powerful diagnostic tool, is not yet internationally standardized, so that results of different investigators often lack comparability. Thus, there are efforts of a variety of national pulmonary societies to achieve international standardization. The following recommendations are given based on the guidelines of European Society of Pneumology [3] and the American Thoracic Society [4].

BAL is performed predominantly (in about 93% of centers) [3] under local anaesthesia with a flexible fiberscope. Thus, BAL performed under general anaesthesia appears to yield similar results. It is also possible to carry out BAL in patients with an oral or nasotracheal tube in position by inserting the fiberscope through the tube, provided the diameter is greater than 6 mm, thus faciliating adequate spontaneuous or mechanical ventilation. Most centers use a standard size fiberscope with a sucking channel of about 2 mm. Although small diameter fiberscopes allow sampling in more distal segments of the bronchial system, the risk of bronchial collapse increases. On the other hand, when using large diameter fiberscopes, the instrument cannot be advanced as far and more bronchial constituents are found in the fluid recovered. Optimal recovery is accomplished by occluding the bronchial lumen with the bronchoscope. Therefore the tip of the instrument has to be advanced into a bronchial segment until wedge position is reached. Mechanical lesion of the segment intubated resulting from inadequate handling should be carefully avoided. For the same reason coughing should be prevented because it can cause trauma, contamination with blood and loss of instilled fluid.

## Premedication

Generally atropine is used (keeping in mind contraindications such as glaucoma, cardial disorders, etc.) to minimize vasovagally induced bradycardia as well as to decrease airway secretion. As far as the influence of atropine on the yield of BAL is concerned, it was shown that in atropine pretreated patients a higher BAL-return is achieved compared to a control group. The effect of atropine on the composition of the noncellular components of BAL remains unclear [5].

Additionally, some investigators use sedating compounds such as diazepam or meperidine. Because of possible influences on spontaneous breathing, however, these drugs cannot be generally recommended. Some centres use antitussive drugs such as hydrocodone to reduce coughing and thus increasing comfort of the patient. Because of side-effects, however, also these drugs cannot be generally recommended.

## Local anaesthesia

Local anaesthesia is usually accomplished by local application of lidocaine: In the first step as spray aerosol for treatment of nasal, oral, pharyngeal and laryngeal area, and in the second step by direct instillation *via* the bronchoscope for anaesthesia of the vocal cords, trachea and bronchi. Excess lidocaine in the segment lavaged should be removed prior to instillation of the lavage fluid, since it may influence cell viability [3].

## Site of lavage

In localized disease the involved segment should be lavaged. Little information exists, however, as to the appopriate site of BAL in patients with diffuse lung disease.The right middle lobe or the lingula has been most commonly used [6]; occasionally, a lateral or anterior segment of the lower lobe is used. Because the bronchoscope wedges in fourth or fifth order bronchi, it has been estimated that approximately 1.5 or 3% of the lung and approximately a million alveoli are sampled. This should provide material that reflects the diffuse process involving the lower respiratory tract, including the alveolar structure. Some centers, however, routinely sample two or three different areas, because of reports of marked heterogeneity in the inflammatory and immune process involving various parts of the lower respiratory tract in diffuse interstitial diseases [7, 8].

## Fluid used to perform lavage

The fluid used to perform bronchoalveolar lavage must be a pyrogen-free saline solution (isotonic 0.9% NaC1, suitable for intravenous use). Lavage fluid should be warmed to body temperature (37 °C) because it causes less cough and bronchospasm, less deterioration of lung function and, therefore, a better fluid recovery and increased cell yield of BAL in comparison to instillations of fluid at room temperature [9, 10]. However, most groups when performing BAL for diagnostic or research purposes have used fluid at room temperature.

## Methods to instil and recover the fluid

BAL is usually performed with sterile buffered or unbuffered saline. Saline fluid is instilled through the working channel of the fiberoptic bronchoscope as a bolus with a syringe (the method usually employed), or by hydrostatic flow from a reservoir [11]. The fluid is usually recovered with the help of a suction trap to which mechanical suction is applied, or is allowed to drain out under gravity [12], or is aspirated manually using the attached syringe [11]. When using mechanical suction (and hand suction) attention must be paid to ensure that excessive negative pressure is not applied in order to avoid collapse of airways beyond the tip of the bronchoscope (which would impede fluid return), or trauma to the mucosal surface of the bronchus, causing bleeding and appearance of erythrocytes in the lavage. Negative pressure of 25–100 mm Hg from normal clinical suction apparatus is usually appropriate. Occasionally, in patients with destructive lung disease, a few deep breaths can help the flow of fluid and increase the return volumes [11, 13]. After each instillation, the recovered fluid is collected in the syringe, in a sterile suction flask, in a plastic specimen trap, or in a siliconized vessel. The adhesion of macrophages to the walls must be avoided in order to prevent loss or activation of mononuclear cells. Therefore unsiliconized glass materials should not be used.

## Volumes of fluid to be used

The greatest technical variation in carrying out bronchoalveolar lavage relates to the volume of fluid used. The volume infused by investigators usually range from about 100 ml to about 300 ml in each lung segment or subsegment lavaged. Much of the data on bronchoalveolar lavage cells and secretions derives from lavage performed with aliquots of 20 ml and a total lavage volume of 100 ml. Other research groups, however, believe that 50–100 ml boluses, with a total volume of 300 ml are more appropriate, enabling more cells and proteins to be recovered for research purposes. In this context, the total number of cells collected seems to correlate with the volume of fluid instilled and recovered, especially when instilled lavage volumes are between 100 and 300 ml [14]. It has been demonstrated in nonsmokers that the proportion of alveolar cells in each bolus, when lavaged at the same site, was roughly uniform [15]. Data on proportions of bronchoalveolar cells reported by various groups performing lavage with different amounts of saline suggest that, at least in normals, the information about cell types obtained in volumes of 100–250 ml is comparable. Smaller volumes of instilled fluid carry the risk that a more "bronchial" washing component dominates the cellular picture. In this case, the BAL cells are more likely to be characterized by the presence of increased numbers of neutrophils, particularly in the first two aliquots [16, 17].

The yield of cells is significantly dependent on the condition of the prealveolar airways. Recovery of fluid in the case of obstructive disorders of the airways may be markedly attenuated for example in chronic bronchitis [18], and asthma [16] and the recovered cells may show higher concentrations of neutrophils. Thus, the recovery of BAL fluid exerts an influence and seems to be responsible for the considerable intersubject variability seen in a study [19].

The problem of quantification of non-cellular components of the lavage fluid is addressed below.

Although bronchoalveolar lavage is a safe technique, the incidence and importance of the side-effects appear different using small *versus* large lavage volumes. It has been demonstrated that patients receiving small volumes had only minor reduction of vital capacity, which returned to baseline within 24 h, and all other parameters were unchanged. In contrast, there was significant, although reversible, reduction in several functional parameters within 30 min after a large volume lavage [20]. It is unclear how long the instilled fluid must remain in the lung segment before being aspirated. A small delay of a few seconds, allowing the patient to breathe one or two times, may result in a better mixing in the lung segment between saline and cellular and non-cellular components of the alveolar surfaces. Lavage fluid is probably absorbed across the alveolar surfaces which suggests not waiting too long before retrieving it [21, 22].

## Recovery

The fluid volume recovered from BAL usually is 40–70% of the volume instilled [23]. In COPD and emphysema recovery might be less than 30% due to airway instability. Decreased recovery volumes were also reported in elderly patients and smokers. The minimum recovery should not be less than 25 ml.

## Should the first aliquot of lavage be processed separately?

Several investigators have carried out cell differential analysis on sequential aliquots of the recovered lavage fluid. When using sequential boluses of 60 ml it has been demonstrated that in nonsmokers the proportions of alveolar cells in each bolus are roughly uniform [15]. However, in smokers the first "wash" is different from all subsequent boluses [23]. Characteristics of the first bolus are the relatively high proportion of epithelial cells and polymorphonuclear leucocytes and fewer macrophages, suggesting a more "bronchial" than "alveolar" sampling. Using small volumes, however, the percentage of fluid returned from the first "wash" and the number of cells recovered is generally low. In the absence of airway inflammation, the cellular and acellular components contribute little to the total lavage and, therefore, have only a small influence on the overall results. In contrast, when the subjects undergoing bronchoalveolar lavage have a disorder affecting the bronchial portion of the airways, or if there are obvious signs of bronchial inflammation at bronchoscopy, then the analysis can be heavily influenced by the contribution of the bronchial airways and the same investigators then recommend that the first sample of bronchoalveolar lavage should be collected and analysed separately [2, 17, 23]. Other investigators believe that such samples are useful indicators of bronchial inflammation, but consider it unlikely that alveolar components can be accurately differentiated in those cases.

## Handling of the harvested lavage material

### Mucus filtration

Many investigators consider that the bronchoalveolar fluid must be strained through a sterile gauze to trap large mucous particles [13, 21]. Nylon mesh or a very loose single-layer mesh of cotton gauze is usually appropriate and, especially in smokers and patients with bronchial inflammation prevents mixture of the mucous particle with the cell pellet after centrifugation. The process of straining the recovered fluid, even through a single layer of cotton gauze, may cause loss of cells and other components of the lavage; however, the full effect has not yet been clearly investigated. Other workers consider that filtration should be avoided for routine diagnostic purposes because of the risk of loss of cells and other components and instead they remove the surface layer of mucus after the first centrifugation of the lavage sample [25]. Filtration of BAL fluid preferentially removes bronchial epithelial cells (reduction from 10 to 6% [23]) and, therefore, should be avoided if changes in this cell type may be of importance [16].

Timely handling of lavage specimens is most important if the cells are to be cultured or if labile substances are to be measured. For the usual clinically important protein measurements (e.g., albumin and the immunoglobulins) and for cell quantification and differential cell counts, delays of up to 4 h can be tolerated without loss of clinically important information. When the fluid is to be stored for future use, preservation at −80 °C is ideal. However, most compounds in BAL fluid can tolerate storage at −20 °C without degrading.

As soon as the fluid arrives in the laboratory, patient identification information, the lobes lavaged, and the volume of saline instilled and recovered from each site are recorded. The first returned aliquot (the "bronchial" sample) and the last four returned aliquots (the "alveolar" samples) are separately pooled, and the cells in the unprocessed fluid are counted with a hemacytometer. The cell count must be done before the cells are washed because with each washing, 15% to 20% of the cells are lost. After the cells have been counted, the percentage of viable cells may be determined using trypan blue or erythrosin dye. These stains are excluded by living cells but stain dead cells.

Before cells are processed for cytologic examination, mucus in the specimen is removed, for two elementary reasons: the mucus would otherwise obscure the cells, and the cellular content of the mucus can differ remarkably from the cellular content of the fluid phase of the lavage specimen. For the alveolar sample, filtration of the cell-rich fluid through a single layer of sterilized nylon gauze ordinarily suffices to remove excessive mucus and does not alter cell counts or differentials. For the bronchial sample, filtering through a single layer of gauze removes the majority of the mucus, but sufficient mucus may remain in the fluid to interfere with the cytologic preparations. For the bronchial sample, therefore, after the cells are counted they are centrifuged (1200 rpm, 5 min) and resuspended in 10 ml of Hank's balanced salt solution (HBSS). The remaining excess mucus is removed with the decanted cell-poor, supernatant lavage fluid. The cells in the bronchial lavage fluid sample are again counted prior to the preparation of slides for cytologic examination.

Some standard methods subjectively considered important by the authors because they are easily carried out and of major importance in routine diagnostics, are explained in detail (while other methods are only mentioned in brief):

### Conventional stains

### Membrane filters [26]
Membrane filters for Papanicolaou staining are prepared in a standard manner.
1) Soak the cellulose membrane filter in 95% ethanol and place it on a sintered glass filter attached to a vacuum flask.
2) Wash the filter with 15 ml of normal saline.
3) When 2 to 3 ml of saline remains in the filter flask reservoir, add a cell suspension of the lavage fluid for a sufficient volume to contain 200000 cells as determined by hemacytometer count.
4) When the cell suspension has nearly run through the filter but *not* come to dryness, add 10 ml of absolute ethanol to fix the cells on the filter.

5) When 1 ml of absolute ethanol remains in the flask reservoir, remove the filter and place it in 95% ethanol to await Papanicolaou staining. It is crucial that the filter not be allowed to dry in any of these steps or cell morphology will be lost.

## Cytocentrifuge preparations [26]

Cytocentrifugation preparations may be made using a Cytospin (Shandon Instruments, Pittsburgh, PA) or comparable instrument.

*Procedure:*
1) Add a cell suspension containing 100 000 cells, but limited in volume to less than 0.5 ml, to the funnel of the microscope slide holder.
2) The cells are centrifuged ($8.1 \times g$, 300 rpm, 10 min).
3) The slides may be air-dried (e.g., for Grocott methenamine silver stain), immediately fixed with a spray fixative (e.g., for Papanicolaou stain) or fixed in acetone (e.g., for immunohistochemical stains).

## Romanovsky stain [26]

The Diff-Quik stain is suitable for air-dried cytocentrifuge slides. This is a differential stain that may be used in place of the modified Wright-Giemsa stain, although the granules of eosinophils are not visualized as well. Staining is rapid and easily done, with the total staining procedure taking less than 30 s.

*Reagent (as one example out of several possibilities):*
1) Diff-Quik: Haeko Diff-Quik (catalog no. SP B4132-1, American Scientific Products, McGaw Park, IL.)

*Procedure*
1) Dip five times in fixative solution I (triarylmethane dye in methyl alcohol).
2) Dip five times in solution II (eosin Y),
3) Dip three times in solution III (buffered thiazine dyes).
4) Rinse in distilled water.

5) After staining, allow slide to dry and coverslip with a permanent mounting medium.

## Papanicolaou stain [26]

Although slight variations exist between laboratories, the Papanicolaou staining procedure is used in virtually all cytology laboratories. The procedure outlined below is used in many laboratories and provides excellent results on membrane filter or cytocentrifuge preparations of BAL fluid.

### Filters

1) Cellulose membrane filters.

*Reagents:* The following reagents are available from SurgiPath Industries, Northbrook, IL (of course comparable compounds provided by other manufacturers can be used depending on the local suppliers)

1) Papanicolaou stain: Harris hematoxylin (catalog no. HX400)
2) Orange G (catalog no. EX400)
3) EA-65 (catalog no. EX300)

*Procedure*: All stains and hydrating alcohols are filtered daily. The acid water and lithium solutions are prepared each day. In consecutive staining dishes:

1) Immerse 2 min in 95% ethanol.
2) Dip 10 times in 70% ethanol.
3) Dip 10 times in distilled water.
4) Immerse 1 min in Harris hematoxylin.
5) Dip once in acid water.
6) Dip 10 times in tap water.
7) Dip five times in lithium water.
8) Dip 10 times in tap water.
9) Dip 10 times in 70% ethanol.
10) Dip 10 times in 95% ethanol.
11) Immerse 1 min in OG-6.
12) Dip 10 times in 95% ethanol.
13) Dip 10 times in 95% ethanol (fresh solution).

14) Dip 10 times in 95% ethanol (fresh solution).
15) Immerse 3 min in EA-65.
16) Dip 10 times in 95% ethanol.
17) Dip 10 times in 95% ethanol (fresh solution).
18) Dip 10 times in 95% ethanol (fresh solution).
19) Dip 20 times in 100% ethanol (fresh solution).
20) Dip 10 times in xylene.
21) Dip 10 times in xylene (fresh fluid).
22) Coverslip slides with a permanent mounting medium.

### Grocott methenamine silver stain-microwave method [26]

The demonstration of fungi and *Pneumocystis carinii* is a major objective of BAL. A variety of stains are suitable for the identification of these organisms. Some are well suited for *P. carinii*, such as toluidine blue O and Gram-Weigert. Others, such as Calciflor white, are limited to fungal hyphae. Some authors favor the use of Grocott methenamine silver (GMS) [27, 28] stain in BAL specimens; other variations, such as Gomori methenamine silver stain, also work well. Silver stains demonstrate budding yeasts, yeast forms, fungal hyphae, and the cysts of *P. carinii*.

### Gram stain [26]

Bacteria may be demonstrated on cytocentrifuge or smear preparations of BAL fluid, using a standard Gram stain [26].

*Reagents:*

The following may be obtained from Fisher Scientific, Springfield, NJ (of course comparable compounds from other suppliers may also work well)
1) Crystal violet (certified) (catalog no. C581-10)
2) Ammonium oxalate (catalog no. A 679-500)
3) Potassium iodide (catalog no. P410-100)
4) Iodine (catalog no. 1137-100)
5) Safranin O (certified) (catalog no. 5670-25)

*Prepared reagents:*
1) Modified Hucker crystal violet

    a) Solution A: Dissolve 2 gm of crystal violet (certified) in 20 ml of 95% ethanol alcohol.

    b) Solution B: Dissolve 0.8 gm of ammonium oxalate in 80 ml of distilled water.

    c) Combine solutions A and B and store for 24 h. Filter prior to use.

2) Gram iodine: Grind 1 gm of iodine and 2 mg of potassium iodide in a mortar with a few milliliters of distilled water. When solubilized, transfer to an amber glass bottle and add distilled water to bring the total volume to 300 ml.

3) Acetone-alcohol: Combine 100 ml of 95% ethyl alcohol with 100 ml of acetone.

4) Safranin O

    a) Stock solution: Dissolve 2.5 gm of safranin O (certified) with 100 ml of 95% ethyl alcohol.

    b) Working solution: Combine 10 ml of stock solution with 90 ml of distilled water.

## Iron stain

The demonstration of iron within macrophages is useful in the evaluation of pulmonary hemorrhage, which may occur in a variety of disorders [26]. Thus the Mallory iron staining method seems appropriate.

*Procedure:*

Use this stain on dried and heat-fixed cytocentrifuge slides or smears.

In consecutive staining dishes:
Flood smear with crystal violet for 1 min.

2) Rinse in tap water.
3) Flood smear with Gram iodine for 1 min.
4) Rinse in tap water.
5) Decolorize with acetone-alcohol.
6) Rinse in tap water.
7) Immerse in safranin O for 10 s.
8) Rinse in tap water.
9) Dry, coverslip, and examine for organisms.

## In situ *DNA hybridization*

The rapid diagnosis of viral pathogens in organ transplant patients has become increasingly important as new antiviral drugs, such as Gancyclovir, have become available [26]. Several methods, such as fluorescent antibody study of viral cell culture, enzyme immunoassay, shell vial assay, and *in situ* DNA hybridization, facilitate the rapid diagnosis of viral infection. Of these, *in situ* DNA hybridization is particularly well suited to the direct microscopic study of alveolar macrophages, bronchial epithelial cells, or other cells recovered by BAL. Viral genome may be demonstrated within these cells through the use of an appropriately labeled viral DNA probe. Both radioisotopes and colorimetric reagents have been used to label DNA probes. Labeling with colorimetric reagents offers several advantages: the procedure is rapid, it does not require the handling of radioisotopes, and it employs many standard techniques familiar to immunohistochemistry laboratories [29]. Suitable DNA probes are available for many viruses that infect immunosupressed hosts. Brigati et al. [30], have applied this technique to adenovirus infected lung, and Myerson and others [31, 32] have demonstrated the value of DNA hybridization in the diagnosis of cytomegalovirus (CMV) pneumonia. Of particular importance has been the observation that many more cells are infected by CMV than actually have nuclear cytoplasmic inclusions. Because the cytologic diagnosis of CMV infection requires the identification of such inclusions, the sensitivity of cytology for detecting CMV is lower than that of conventional viral culture. For example, in the study by Hilborne et al. [33] the sensitivity of cytology for the detection of CMV infection was only 22% that viral culture.

*In situ* DNA hybridization is suitable for the rapid detection of CMV in BAL material. With tissue culture as a standard, direct *in situ* DNA hybridization utilizing a diaminobenzidine chromagen has reported sensitivity of up to 93%. Some authors have found *in situ* DNA hybridization useful in cases where CMV pneumonia was suspected but the pathognomonic inclusion bodies were not found on Papanicolaou-stained slides.

If *in situ* DNA studies are desired, it is worthwhile preparing additional cytocentrifuge slides on poly-D-lysine-coated glass slides. This coating allows better adherence of cells during the hybridization procedure.

## Immunocytochemical stains

Immunohistochemical stains have greatly aided the routine light microscopic examination of tissues in surgical pathology. A variety of monoclonal antibodies that recognize infectious agents and markers of cell differentiation are available. These techniques are readily applied to diagnostic cytopathology. Cell smears, cytocentrifuge slides, and membrane filters are all suitable for study. Particularly useful is the ability to decolorize Papanicolaou-stained slides, or to perform immunocytochemical stains directly over Papanicolaou-stained material [26]. Thus, special immunofluorescent (IF) and immunocytochemical techniques can be applied to better characterize the nature of some of the cells recovered from BAL, especially lymphocytes. These methods rely on the use of monoclonal antibodies directed against antigens present on the cell surface of lymphocytes and/or monocytes/macrophages. Monoclonal antibodies are basically used as a research tool in order to investigate the phenotypes of BAL cells. In addition, they can contribute to the diagnosis and clinical management of various interstitial lung disorders [3].

For IF technique the current method is staining and observation of viable cells in suspension. The cells are incubated either with a fluorochrome-labelled monoclonal antibody directly (direct IF technique) or with an unlabelled primary antibody first and then with a secondary labelled antibody directed against the primary antibody (indirect IF technique). Indirect techniques are more sensitive than direct techniques.

Peroxidase methods are most commonly used for immunocytochemical techniques. Newer methods are streptavidin-biotin-techniques or the use of alkaline phosphatase instead of peroxidase for labelling. A highly sensitive technique is the peroxidase antiperoxidase (PAP) technique, also called unlabelled antibody enzyme technique, where a PAP-immunocomplex is linked by a bridging antibody to the primary antibody. Advantages of immunocytochemical techniques are: Use of conventional light microscope, permanent recording of the reaction, excellent morphology, and a higher sensitivity than IF. A disadvantage of this immunocytochemical technique is: Double labelling, although possible, is very time consuming. In routine diagnostic monoclonals are for example used to demonstrate the predominance of T-suppressor cells (CD8) over T-helper cells (CD4) in hypersensitivity pneumonitis.

### Procedure (as one example out of a variety of techniques)

Cytocentrifuge slides of BAL cells should be fixed with an appropriate reagent [26]. The slides should not be permitted to dry, as this distorts cellular morphology and impairs immunoreactivity. Acetone or a modified Delaunay's fixative has been advocated for cell smears; either appears superior to ethanol and spray fixatives. In many instances it is also possible to perform immunohistochemical staining of previously stained materials, after removing the coverslip with xylene and decolorizing with acid alcohol. A typical avidin-biotin procedure is as follows:

1) Wash slides in 0.1 M phosphate-buffered saline (PBS), pH 7.6, for 5 min.
2) Incubate slides for 20 min in diluted normal serum prepared from the species in which the secondary antibody was made.
3) Blot excess serum from slide. Apply the primary antiserum and incubate for 30 min.
4) Wash slides for 3 min in PBS. Repeat.
5) Incubate sections for 30 min with biotinylated secondary antibody, directed against the primary antibody used in step 3.
6) Wash slides for 3 min in PBS. Repeat.
7) Incubate with avidin-biotin complex reagent.
8) Wash for 3 min in PBS. Repeat.
9) Incubate slides with diaminobenzidine solution. Check slides with a microscope during development to optimize ratio of staining to background.
10) Wash well in tap water.
11) Counterstain with hematoxylin.
12) Dehydrate with increasing grades of ethanol.
13) Clear in xylene and mount.

## Flow cytometry to quantify lymphocyte subsets

In order to electronically count lavage cells the flow cytometric method can be recommended if the technique is critically used and plausibility is tested by light microscopic controls. Flow cytometers provide one of the most advanced systems for detecting and quantifying surface and intracellular markers on cells in suspension [34–37].

### Principle of flow cytometry

In brief, operation of a flow cytometer with fluorescence activated cell analysis and sorting capabilities involves injecting cell suspensions, under pressure, into the centre of a stream of sheath fluid in a flow chamber establishing a co-axial flow which constrains the cells to the centre of the stream so that they flow in a single line. After emerging from the nozzle of the flow chamber, the narrow stream passes through a laser beam focused on the centre of the stream and intersecting it at right angles. As cells pass through the laser beam they scatter the laser light and also emit fluorescent light if they have been labelled with fluorochromes (e.g. labelled monoclonal antibodies).

Light scattered in the forward direction over a narrow angle (approximately 2° or 3° on either side of the beam) is collected by a forward angle scatter detector and converted to electronic signals which give an indication of the size of the cell. Light scattered at right angles (90° scattered light) is also detected and gives an indication of the internal characteristics of the cell such as granularity. Fluorescent light emissions are collected by a "collecting lens" and wavelengths of different colours (related to different fluorochromes) can then be directed to separate detectors (photomultiplier tubes) by means of a dichromic reflector. The signals are processed by an electronics console, amplified, and then digitized and passed to a computer for storage and analysis. If cell sorting is required, the computer can be used to define the population required (by setting a "sorting window" or "gate"), then the nozzle assembly is vibrated by a piezoelectric transducer to break the stream into drops. Drops containing a cell required can be positively or negatively charged and then deflected to the right or left as they pass two charged deflection plates. The deflected drops can then be collected into suitable sample tubes. Many different types of flow cytometer are available but the minimum requirement for most current applications is that the machine must be fitted with both forward angle and 90° scatter detectors and a minimum of two, or preferably three fluorescence detectors. For application with bronchoalveolar lavage (BAL) samples it is also important that the machine should have the capacity for logarithmic, as well as linear, acquisition of data and for non-rectangular "gating". Argon ion lasers may be tuned to produce beams of suitable wavelength to excite most commonly used fluorochromes, including fluorescein isothiocyanate (FITC) and phytoerythrin (PE), which are frequently employed in studies using monoclonal antibodies.

In general, flow cytometry should be used to count leukocytes and to quantify lymphocyte subpopulations in clinical routine, although there is a wide range of possibilities in detection of numerous cell markers for scientific purposes. Thus, for routine diagnostic use in man antibodies against lymphocyte surface anitgens are used as for example antibodies against T-cell associated protein (CD3), lymphocyte-MHC II-receptor (CD4), lymphocyte-MHC I receptor (CD8). For scientific use, however, there is a huge panel of antibodies available to identify special cell features, a problem that is beyond the scope of this chapter. Comparative studies have shown that flow cytometry yields equal or even better results than the conventional peroxidase-anti-peroidase (PAP) method for light microscopic assessment of lymphocyte subpopulations.

A major advantage of the former is providing a time sparing method by double labelling to study the parallel expression of two different surface markers on a single cell. Thus antibodies are usually conjugated with different fluorescence dyes (e.g. FITC [fluorescein-isothiocyanate, *green*], PE [phytoerythrin, *red*]). Disadvantages of IF techniques are: No permanent recording, no morphological details and interference with autofluorescence of macrophages. As a minimal panel for routine diagnostic it is recommended to use the following combinations of antibodies: CD45(FITC)/CD14(PE) (anti-human) to identify lymphocytes in general; antimouse $IgG_1$(FITC)/antimouse $IgG_2$ (PE) to detect the amount of unspecific label. CD3(FITC)/CD4 (PE) for determination of T-helper-cells; CD3(FITC)/CD8 (PE) for detection of T-suppressor cells; CD3(FITC)/CD19(PE) or CD20(PE) or CD22(PE) to discriminate B-cells (which normally are nearly absent in BAL); CD3(FITC)/CD57(PE) or CD16+56(PE) for detection of natural killer (NK-) cells; CD3(FITC)/ HLA-DR (PE) to assess the amount of activated T-cells.

## Preparation of samples

The cells recovered from the bronchoalveolar lavage are washed three times with Hank's solution, resuspended in cell culture medium (e.g. RPMI-1640) and then counted in order to prepare a cellular suspension at the concentration of $10 \times 10^6$ cells/ml. The viability of the cells is checked using the Trypan blue exclusion test. The percentage of dead cells must be less than 5%. Provided highly specific monoclonal antibodies are available, it is usually not necessary to separate different cellular components before testing samples. However, a morphological control must always be performed during the final microscopic count since, for instance, CD4-related monoclonal antibodies may stain with surface antigens belonging to the macrophagic lineage and thus may alter the final cell counts [38].

## Analysis by immunofluorescence

100 μl of the cell suspensions ($1 \times 10^6$ cells) are incubated for 30 min at 4 °C with the optimal amount of purified (indirect method) or conjugated (direct method) monoclonal antibody. The most widely used reagents are FITC and PE -conjugated monoclonal antibodies [39]. The amount of antibody to be used for each determination depends on its original concentration; in general, 5–20 μl represent the right amount.

Following the incubation, 2 ml of cold Hank's solution is added to the pellet and washed at 300 g for 10 min at 4 °C three times. If the indirect method had been used, a fluorescent anti-mouse immunoglobulin is then added. As a control, to demonstrate nonspecific immunofluorescence, the same quantity of anti-mouse immunoglobulin is added to a sample of cell suspensions that had not been previously incubated with monoclonal antibodies. Following a 30 min incubation at 4 °C, the sample is again centrifuged at 4 °C at 300 g three times. If the direct method is used, the control is represented by monoclonal antibodies without specificity for cells under study belonging to the same isotype as those utilized in the test and directly stained with fluorochrome. The pellet is then resuspended and the percentage of positive cells counted by flow cytometry. It must be taken into account that macrophages may show autofluorescence particularly in smokers.

Using the double fluorescence technique [40] it is possible to identify two different determinants simultaneously expressed on the membrane of the same cell. This concept deals with the use of two different fluorochromes (usually FITC and PE). Both these fluorochromes are excited by UV radiation but they display a different spectrum of light emission (green for FITC and red for PE). With the simultaneous use of an FITC-conjugated monoclonal antibody and a PE-conjugated monoclonal antibody, and changing the filter during evaluation with the fluorescent microscope, it is possible to identify cell subpopulations. To rule out the possibility that cells under study bind MoAbs via Fc-receptors, cell suspensions must be evaluated following incubation with gamma-globulin Cohn-fraction II and further washing.

Because of the modifications of the methods between different laboratories there are still insufficient data to recommend precise standardization of procedure. BAL cells are usually stained for flow cytometric analysis without the need for any prior separation of lymphocytes or other cell types. For satisfactory analysis of stained BAL samples by flow cytometry, it is essential to filter the stained samples (using a noncellular adherent material such as nylon gauze), immediately prior to running them through the instrument, to remove all clumps of cells and any residual mucus which can interfere with accurate cell analysis and risks clogging of the nozzle of the machine. It is also most important that there is minimal contamination of the sample with erythrocytes since they overlap and interfere with accurate analysis of the lymphocyte population due to their similar light scattering properties. When evaluating the results of flow cytometric measurements of BAL samples it is essential to selectively "gate" different cell populations for separate analysis because different types of cells in BAL have different amounts of background autofluorescence. Autofluorescence of lymphocytes is low and relatively constant, but autofluorescence of alveolar macrophages is much higher, especially in smokers, and can mask specific fluorescence on lymphocytes if the entire cell population is analysed.

## Electron microscopy

Electron microscopy aids the diagnosis of selected pulmonary diseases by BAL. One such disease is pulmonary alveolar proteinosis, a rare disease in which the alveolar spaces are filled with proteinaceous material, macrophages, and type II alveolar lining cells. Because the clinical features of slowly progressive pulmonary infiltrates, dyspnea, and fever are nonspecific, lung biopsy is usually required for diagnosis. However, BAL has been shown to be effective in the diagnosis of this disorder. Electron microscopic evaluation of cells obtained by lavage show concentric myelinoid figures within the cytoplasm of cells [41, 42].

Electron microscopy may also be used in the identification of eosinophilic granuloma or other disorders of the histiocytosis X triad. These conditions are characterized by the proliferation of Langerhans cells, which contain intracytoplasmic Bierbeck granules. The identification of these granules by electron microscopy is useful in the confirmation of this disorder [43].

## Differential cell counts

A differential cell count is usually performed on the BAL specimen because the relative proportions of inflammatory cells and lymphocytes may indicate which disease process or category of disease is present in the lung. Well-recognized examples include the elevated numbers of lymphocytes in sarcoidosis and hypersensitivity pneumonitis, neutrophils in idiopathic pulmonary fibrosis, and eosinophils in asthma. Information derived from the differential cell count may be used clinically to help predict response to therapy or to judge the effectiveness of therapy.

Given the potential significance of the differential cell count, one would expect it to be reliable and reproducible. However, this is not the case. If mucus is present in large airways and is not removed by filtration, inflammatory cells in the mucus will mix with alveolar fluid and distort the true picture of alveolar "inflammation". During the processing of lavage fluid, cells are variably lost in the centrifugation and washing procedures. Finally, the manner of slide preparation – cytocentrifugation *versus* membrane filtration – influences the relative numbers of inflammatory cells. Cytocentrifugation, the most common method of preparing cells for differential cell counts, causes an average lymphocyte loss of 20%. Worse still, the loss of lymphocytes is quite variable, ranging from none to over 50% [44]. By comparison, membrane filter preparations preserve lymphocyte numbers but cause a loss of neutrophils, as these cells are sheared by the filter [45].

Many laboratories (including our own) prefer to prepare both cytocentrifuge slides and membrane filters on all lavage specimens. The equipment required for preparing each is available in most laboratories. The preparation and staining of membrane filters requires approximately 2 h but yields excellent morphologic detail, which aids the identification of malignant cells in the lavage preparation.

In many laboratories a 500-cell differential cell count is done to express the relative number of macrophages, neutrophils, lymphocytes, eosinophils, airway epithelial cells, and squamous cells. It is crucial to recognize that the differential count of "normal individuals" is affected by the lavage technique and by cigarette smoking. Because of these factors, and the effect of specimen processing on the differential cell count, it is not possible to quote global "normal" values. Compared to nonsmokers,

*Table 13.1. Differential cell counts in BAL fluid [26]*

|  | Smoker without chronic bronchitis | | Nonsmoker | |
|---|---|---|---|---|
|  | Bronchial | Alveolar | Bronchial | Alveolar |
| Total cells (millions) | 3.6±0.6 | 104.3±9.4 | 4.1±0.6 | 28.0±3.5 |
| Macrophages | 56±4 | 89±2 | 63±3 | 79±3 |
| Neutrophils | 21±3 | 6±1 | 10±1 | 3±1 |
| Eosinophils | <1 | <1 | <1 | <1 |
| Lymphocytes | <1 | 2±1 | 3±1 | 13±2 |
| Ciliated cells | 17±3 | 2±1 | 19±2 | 4±1 |
| Squamous cells | 5±3 | 1 | 5±3 | <1 |

*Cell counts determined in cytocentrifuge preparations of fractionated BAL fluid. Values are means ± SEM.*

cigarette smokers have increased cell counts, with proportionately more macrophages and neutrophils.

The differential cell profile of unfractionated lavage specimens will differ from fractionated specimens. Until there is greater standardization of the methods used in lavage and specimen processing, careful attention must be given to the manner in which data are reported (Tab. 13.1).

## Cultures from BAL

### Microbial culture

Microbial culture of lavage fluid is an important part of specimen analysis, particularly if infection is suspected. Culture results may assist diagnosis in several ways.

First, although direct microscopic examination of the lavage specimen is effective in the identification of many infections, organisms may sometimes not be apparent. The direct identification of cytomegalovirus-infected cells is particularly troublesome, with some reports suggesting that only 22% of cases can be found by examination of Papanicolaou-stained material. Viral culture is capable of detecting virus-infected cells that do not manifest overt features of infection. Thus, the optimum diagnosis of infection requires both microbial culture and direct microscopic examination of BAL fluid.

Second, the specificity of diagnosis is enhanced through culture of the lavage specimen. In cases with only rare hyphal fragments, fungal culture is valuable for distinguishing *Aspergillus, Mucor,* and other organisms. Some fungi, such as *Aspergillus* and *Fusarium,* have identical cytomorphology and can only be distinguished by culture. Although cytomegalovirus and herpes simplex have well-defined cytomorphology, other viral respiratory pathogens do not. Viral culture may clarify otherwise nonspecific inflammation and epithelial alterations due to respiratory syncytial virus, echovirus, parainfluenza virus, adenovirus, or other pathogens.

Finally, the absence of growth in bacterial, viral, or fungal cultures of the lavage specimen is important negative information that may direct the diagnostic workup away from pulmonary infection and toward other disease processes such as malignancy or interstitial lung disease.

## Routine culture

The routine bacterial culture of BAL fluid is complicated by the presence of orally derived bacteria in virtually all specimens. Thus, α-hemolytic streptococci, *Neisseria* spp, coagulase-negative staphylococci, and other oral normal flora have been recovered in nearly 90% of the lavage specimens received in some laboratories. Because of this high prevalence of oral contamination, the practical problem becomes one of identifying pulmonary-based infection. Organisms typically recognized as normal oral flora may in some instances cause pneumonia, and well-recognized pulmonary pathogens (e.g., *H. influenzae, S. pneumoniae, S. aureus*) may be present in the oropharynx but not in the lungs.

Quantitative cultures may be practical for discriminating orally derived bacteria from those residing in the lung and causing pneumonia. When fewer than 1% squamous epithelial cells and more than $10^5$ colony-forming bacteria per milliliter are present in the lavage fluid, bacterial infection has been present in every case. The squamous epithelial cells serve as a marker for oropharyngeal contamination. In fact, bacteria are commonly seen coating these epithelial cells. When 1% or more squamous epithelial cells are present, the bacteria may be solely related to oropharyngeal contamination. Clinical correlation is required when fewer than $10^5$ colony-forming bacteria per milliliter are present, even when there are negligible numbers of squamous epithelial cells, because this finding may also reflect contamination.

The Gram stain may be of assistance in identifying cases of bacterial pneumonia. Neutrophils may be found that harbor Gram-positive or Gram-negative bacteria. The presence of intracellular bacteria, combined with a high colony count of a bacterial pathogen, is excellent evidence of pneumonia.

## Fungal culture

*Candida, Aspergillus, Cryptococcus, Histoplasma,* and members of the order Phycomycetes are the fungal organisms most frequently isolated from BAL fluid. In some laboratories, centrifuged sediment of lavage fluid is simultaneously cultured on Sabouraud's agar with chloramphenicol and gentamicin, and on Mycosel agar. The former inhibits the growth of nonpathogenic molds; the latter permits growth of virtually all fungi.

The significance of fungi in lavage fluid depends on which organism is isolated. The identification of *Aspergillus* and *Mucor* indicates a grave situation because of the propensity of these organisms to invade blood vessels and disseminate widely throughout the body. In a study, BAL was found to be a valuable first procedure to establish the diagnosis of invasive pulmonary aspergillosis. The greatest sensitivity and specificity are found with a combination of both cytologic examination and fungal culture.

It is extremely common to isolate *Candida* from BAL fluid. In a study [46], nearly 20% of specimens yielded *Candida* on fungal culture. However, only 7% of the specimens had more than three colonies; and 90% of patients from whom yeasts were cultured did not have clinical features of *Candida* pneumonia. This suggests that many of the yeasts identified by cytology or fungal culture are introduced into the lavage specimen through subclinical aspiration of oral materials, or by contamination of the bronchoscope during its passage through the oropharynx.

It is of interest to compare fungal culture and silver stains for the identification of *Candida* in lavage fluid. In approximately 14% of cases, both fungal culture and cytology detected yeasts in the lavage specimen. When many budding yeasts and hyphae (> 10/ slide) were present on cytologic preparation, numerous colonies were present on the fungal culture. Conversely, when few yeasts were detected on cytology (<3/slide), few colonies grew in culture. In only 6% of cases was fungal cultures positive for *Candida* without morphologic identification of yeasts. However, in 31% of cases yeasts were found on cytologic preparations without organisms being recovered on the fungal cultures. Typically, only a few nonbudding yeasts were found in the cytologic preparations in these cases. Again, these likely represent contaminants, rather than *Candida* pneumonia. Their frequent occurrence, however, indicates that the predictive value of rare yeasts in cytologic preparations for *Candida* pneumonia is low. Even among patients with *Candida* pneumonia, it is difficult to interpret fungal cultures. Each laboratory must develop its own philosophy on this question.

## Mycobacterial culture

Mycobacterial organisms in BAL fluid may be identified through the staining of smears or through mycobacterial culture. In some laboratories, the sediment smear from BAL fluid is routinely screened with a fluorescent auramine O technique. If fluorescent organisms are identified, a Ziehl-Neelsen carbolfuchsin stain is done on the same slide without decolorization. The auramine O stain is extremely practical, for screening may be accomplished in less than 1 min, compared to the 20 min required for the Ziehl-Neelsen stain. However, some mycobacteria, such as *Mycobacterium fortuitum,* do not fluoresce with auramine O. Some authors believe that a Ziehl-Neelsen stain is required to confirm a "positive" auramine O reaction, because pulmonary macrophages frequently contain substances that exhibit nonspecific fluorescence. Some authors emphasize that mycobacterial culture is extremely important in the identification of infections, since acid-fast or auramine O staining of lavage preparations have rarely yielded positive results [47].

## Viral culture

Viral culture of BAL fluid can only be recommended if there are clinical signs or there is justified suspicion of viral infection, especially in immuncompromised patients. And if these questions cannot be answered by assessment of viral antibody-titres or imunnocytochemically with antibodies to detect expression of viral antigens on the infected cells.

## Analysis of soluble components of the epithelial lining fluid

BAL samples not only the cellular components but also the soluble components of the epithelial fluid lining the lower respiratory tract [26]. The opportunity to sample the lower respiratory tract opens a wide field of research into the pathophysiology and biochemistry of the lower respiratory tract. As a result, many investigators have developed methods to assay a large number of components of the epithelial lining fluid of the lower respiratory tract. In this area of active research, the number of species detected in the lower respiratory tract continues to increase. Although the clinical application of this technology remains uncertain at present, several types of analysis have been undertaken. Major problems, however, emerge with all efforts undertaken to quantify intraalveolar compounds.

The majority of proteins present in blood plasma were also found in BAL fluid. The concentration of protein in lavage fluid varies for different proteins and also from study to study. The saline used for the lavage significantly dilutes the epithelial lining fluid that is sampled. Differences in BAL technique probably result in varying degrees of dilution, thus accounting for much of the variation among studies and individual investigators. Thus, some investigators "normalize" measurements to albumin, assuming that the albumin present in the epithelial lining fluid is diluted to the same degree as any species of interest. This method of expressing results was supposed to permit comparisons to be made among study groups and among investigators assuming that the albumin concentration in epithelial lining fluid is also comparable between groups. Up to now any attempt to calculate the "dilution factor" during the lavage, which would allow the epithelial lining fluid concentration to be calculated from the lavage fluid concentration has proven to be completely unsatisfactory. This spectrum of methods also includes assessment of lavage fluid urea concentration.

A variety of approaches have been used to measure the components of epithelial lining fluid sampled by BAL, including chemical assays, immunoassays, bioassays, and functional enzyme assays. Because of the dilution involved, the concentration of many species is quite low in BAL fluid. As a result, several methods have been employed to concentrate BAL fluids. Lyophylization, pressure filtration, and chemical extraction have all been used. Each has advantages and disadvantages for specific applications. Lyophylization tends to give efficient recovery but concentrates the salts present in the lavage, often necessitating a dialysis step. Aggregation of certain protein species can also be a problem in lyophylization. Pressure filtration is convenient and widely used, but is only applicable to species of relatively large molecular mass. The problem of quantifying soluble BAL constituents is considered in detail in the next chapter. Table 13.2 provides an overview on the concentrations assessed by a variety of non-comparable methods and thus should be seen from the point of view referred in the next chapter.

*Table 13.2. Analysis of soluble substances in BAL fluid [3, 26]*

| Solute | Approximate concentration* |
|---|---|
| Total protein | 70 µg/mL |
| Albumin | 20 µg/mL |
| Immunoglobulins | |
| IgG | 2.5–10 µg/mL |
| IgGI | 1.6 µg/mL |
| IgG2 | 0.8 µg/mL |
| IgG3 | 0.06 µg/mL |
| IgG4 | 0.18 µg/mL |
| IgA | 2.5–6 µg/mL |
| Free secretory piece | 700 ng/mL |
| IgM | 100 ng/mL |
| IgE | 0.06–0.3 ng/mL |
| $\alpha_1$-Antiprotease | 1–2 µg/mL |
| $\alpha_2$-Macroglobulin | 0.04 µg/mL |
| Low molecular weight bronchial inhibitor | + |
| Carcinoembryonic antigen | 0.8 ng/mL |
| Transferrin | 4 µg/mL |
| Fibronectin | 30–150 ng/mL |
| Leukocyte elastase | + |
| Collagenase | + |
| Angiotensin-converting enzyme | + |
| Lipid polar | 78 µg/mL |
| Lipid nonpolar | 45 µg/mL |
| Prostaglandin E | 200–2000 pg/mL |
| 6-keto-$F_{1\alpha}$ | 20–400 pg/mL |
| Thromboxane B | 25–85 pg/mL |
| Prostaglandin $F_{2\alpha}$ | 30 pg/mL |

*Solute concentrations are estimated for unconcentrated BAL fluid. The data are derived from variously reported concentrations and represent approximations. + = detected.

339

## Attempt to quantify lavage material

There have been made several attempts to calculate the amount of in-traalveolar fluid in order to assess the concentrations of soluble com-pounds in BAL with the intension to establish "normal values" for the latter in healthy individuals. This would create a powerful diagnostic tool for the detection of a variety of experimentally induced deviations in ani-mal studies as well as the diagnosis of lung diseases in humans compar-able to the broad use of serum parameters in clinical chemistry. The pri-mary basis for this would be to reliably estimate the amount of alveolar fluid harvested by the lavage method.

There have been attempts to solve the problem by comparing the con-centration of endogenous substrates in serum and lavage. Albumin [48] or urea [49] have been used. Also the "dilution" of exogenous markers such as methylene blue has been calculated [50]. The use of albumin has the disadvantage that the permeability of peripheral lung tissue changes in disease and is unknown in a given individual case. Urea is sensitive to osmotic transfer across the alveolar wall, and methylene blue yields sur-prisingly high values when compared with figures from morphologic calculations [51].

Of all the different approaches, no single one is completely satisfac-tory. Using these procedures noncritically, many misleading results have been obtained. The main problem is the determination of the very small amount of fluid that is present in the terminal airspaces and that must be seen as the basis for further quantitative analysis of BAL.

To address this problem, von Wichert et al. [52] carried out a compar-ative study with five markers: $^{99m}$Tc-DTPA, $^{51}$CR-EDTA, inulin, urea, and methylene blue in animal experiments as well as in patients who had agreed with informed consent to a BAL (The investigation was approved by the Ethical Committee of the Medical Faculty of the Philipps Univer-sity, Marburg, Germany). The marker substances were added to the lav-age fluid, and the "dilution" of the markers, i.e., the alveolar fluid, was calculated. The results showed that in animals with healthy lungs the tra-cer methods are able to calculate amounts of intraalveolar fluid that are comparable to morphologic findings. In animals as well as in humans, methylene blue and inulin were shown to be useless in determining alveolar fluid volume compared with the tracer methods. In humans, the calculations with the urea method and with TC-DTPA were in the same magnitude, but there was no individual correlation.

Thus, any "dilution" calculations are incorrect because the system is open or quasi-open. There is no way, at present, to solve the problem of the changing permeability of the alveolar wall, particularly in diseased states. The authors demonstrated that, at present, the methods to quantitate alveolar fluid volume lack precision and add nothing to a deeper understanding of alveolar biology. It should be a future task to develop a truly nondiffusible marker suitable for use in patients.

## Complications of lavage

One of the reasons why BAL is enjoying such general acceptance among scientists and clinicians is because of its noninvasiveness. This makes bronchoalveolar lavage possible to perform in virtually all patients except a few exceptions. Bronchoalveolar lavage is a very safe procedure, its side-effects are more or less comparable with those of routine fibreoptic bronchoscopy under topical anaesthesia. They include a reversible decrease of arterial oxygen saturation [53, 54], transient alterations of pulmonary mechanics [55], as well as potential alterations in cardiovascular functions [56, 57]. These alterations are nearly always reversible and usually are only of concern when dealing with critically ill patients [58]. Serious complications like significant bleeding, bronchial perforation, mediastinal emphysema, pneumothorax, and cardiac arrest are extremely rare [59].

As long as no other invasive techniques such as transbronchial lung biopsy or extensive bronchial brushing are performed the technique of bronchoalveolar lavage does not change the favourable side-effect profile as encountered with single fibreoptic bronchoscopy. The overall complication rate with bronchoalveolar lavage is reported between 0–2.3%; it rises to 7% if transbronchial lung biopsy is performed. The overall complication rate of open lung biopsy is reported to be 13%. So far no lethal complication directly attributable to BAL has been reported.

In comparison, the lethality for transbronchial lung biopsy is reported to be 0.2% and for open lung biopsy 1.8% [60].

Side-effects encountered with bronchoalveolar lavage are closely related to its procedures and technique [3]. Appropriate premedication is a prerequisite to successful bronchoalveolar lavage: local anaesthesia to avoid coughing and reflexes and sedatives to ensure cooperation of patients. Recommendations have been developed by the European BAL Task Group [3]. Pirozinsky et al. [61] reported the beneficial effect of pretreatment with ipratropium bromide which resulted in a higher BAL fluid return and lower oxygen desaturation, lower heart rate increase during the BAL procedure and minimized changes of pulmonary function. Special caution and possible pretreatment should be given to patients with bronchial hyperreactivity or patients with asthma. Side-effects of bronchoalveolar lavage can be minimized by not exceeding a lavage volume of 250 ml [3], by using BAL fluid at body temperature and physiological pH [9, 10].

Alveolar infiltration within 24 h after BAL has been repeatedly reported [9, 62, 63]. In a prospective study Gurney et al. [64] evaluated the radiographic manifestation of bronchoalveolar lavage. They reported increased consolidation of dependent lavaged lobes in 90% of cases when radiography was performed 30 min after lavage. Resolution of these opacities was gradual, 50% of them cleared after 6 h and after 24 h all opacities had cleared. The presence of these opacities correlated with the amount of the retained saline solution, was limited to the area lavaged and was not associated with clinical complications [64]. Other studies report similar observations where alveolar infiltration subsided within 24 or 48 h. The risk of alveolar infiltration increases with the size of instilled lavage fluid volume and numbers of lavaged segments. Significant abnormalities in the ventilation/perfusion ratio of lavaged segments could be observed when introducing significantly more than 300 ml of lavage fluid [10].

Fever some hours after BAL can be observed in about 10–30% of patients [9, 10, 62]. This can usually be treated sucessfully with antipyretics. The cause of fever so far is unclear; a bacterial origin seems unlikely. A recent case report suggests that fever after BAL is mediated by the release of excessive amounts of tumour necrosis factor (TNF) from mononuclear phagocytes [65]. If a total lavage fluid volume below 150 ml is used the percentage of occurrence of fever after BAL will not exceed 3% [63]. When lavage fluid up to 500 ml is used fever has been reported to occur in about 20% of patients [62]. If extensive volumes of lavage fluid are used and several lobes are lavaged at the same time fever may occur in nearly 50% of lavage patients [9].

Crackles within 24 h after lavage can be observed over dependent areas of the lung and are correlated to the volume of the instilled lavage volume [21, 66].

Wheezing and bronchospasm can be observed in hyperreactive patients up to 1 or 2 weeks after bronchoalveolar lavage. These findings are usually not observed in patients with normal bronchial reactivity. This clinical finding is usually correlated to some degree with transient deterioration of lung function [66].

Bleeding has only been anecdotally reported [63], even patients with thrombocytopenia have been successfully lavaged without major bleeding complications.

However, lavage should not be performed in patients with apparent clotting abnormalities (prothrombin time lower than 50%) or with significant thrombocytopenia (platelets lower than 20000 per ml).

BAL usually causes a transient deterioration of lung function parameters (forced expiratory volume in one second ($FEV_1$), vital capacity, peak expiratory flow and oxygen saturation) similar to that observed with routine fibreoptic bronchoscopy. However, the extent and duration of these lung function changes are strongly correlated to the amount of lavage fluid used, to the number of lavaged lobes [67] and in particular to the underlying bronchial status of the patients. Deteriorations of lung function are expressed more in patients with a history of asthma or chronic obstructive pulmonary disorders, as well as in patients with a relevant increase of bronchial hyperreactivity. Therefore, lung function prior to bronchoalveolar lavage has to be assessed and special care and monitoring has to be applied to patients with an underlying deterioration of their pulmonary function.

Although the safety of BAL performed in patients with mild asthma has been established special attention should be given to each patient with a history of a chronic bronchial disorder. Criteria and guidelines for specific selection of patients with chronic obstructive pulmonary disorders have been outlined by a consensus conference of the National Heart and Blood Institute [68]. Since bronchoalveolar lavage has so far no established clinical role in diagnosis and management of patients with chronic obstructive pulmonary disorders or asthma these guidelines are mainly applicable for research protocols.

## Preparation techniques in animals

Two methods of pulmonary lavage are usually used [69]. Living animals are lavaged under general inhalation anesthesia according to the method of Mauderly [70] or injection anesthesia. The second method is to kill the animal and lavage the excised lung. Wash volumes are based on the experience of the laboratories and thus are to some extent arbitrarily chosen. In one of these techniques prior to lavage the change in lung volume produced by applying 20 cm $H_2O$ airway pressure is determined [70]. Prior to lavage, in any case, the trachea should be cannulated to faciliate lavage fluid application and recovery. Each lavage, whether done *in vivo* or in the excised lung, consists of two consecutive washes with volumes equal to 80% of the estimated lung volume change at 20 cm $H_2O$ pressure and is performed with a 0.15 M NaCl solution.

The animals can be killed either just prior to lavage of the excised lung or just after lavage of the lung *in vivo*. Animals are brought to a deep plane of anesthesia with halothane and killed by a cervical dislocator (Cervical Dislocators, Inc., Wausau, WI).

Processing of the lavage fluid may be done as described in the above chapters. Briefly, the cellular fraction of the lavage fluid is removed by centrifugation at $300 \times g$ for 10 min. The cellular pellet is used for total cell counts and a differential nucleated cell count using for example Diff-Quik as the staining method. The lavage fluid supernatant may be used for all biochemical analyses.

To determine how variable is the content of lavage fluid from different species, bronchoalveolar lavage fluids from normal individuals of four species (hamster, rat, guinea pig, and rabbit) were compared for enzymatic and cellular content as well as total protein and sialic acid [69].

In addition, lavage fluid from young adult rats and hamsters was compared to that from older animals. Finally, the effect of the method of lavage on lavage fluid content was evaluated by comparing lavage fluid obtained from an excised lung with that from a lavage performed *in vivo*. In general, lavage fluids from the four species were similar. However, lavage fluid from guinea pigs had higher numbers of granulocytes and higher mean β-glucuronidase activities than fluids from other species. Rats had greater mean alkaline phosphatase activities, reflecting higher serum values of this enzyme. Older hamsters had more protein in their lavage fluid than younger animals, and older rats had lower elastase inhibitory activity than young rats. Performing lavage *in vivo*, as compared to *in vitro*, did not greatly alter the lavage fluid except for a trend toward a higher level of sialic acid in fluid taken from the living animal. Results yielded from animal models, however, have to be critically considered before they can be taken as tools to unravel the diseased state in humans.

# References

1 Crystal RG, Reynolds HY and Kalica AR (1986) *Chest* **90**: 122

2 Reynolds HY (1987) *Am. Rev. Respir. Dis.* **135**: 250

3 Klech H and Pohl W (eds) (1989) Technical Recommendations and Guidelines for Bronchoalveolar Lavage (BAL) *Eur. Respir. J.* **2**: 561

4 American Thoracic Society (1990) Clinical Role of Bronchoalveolar Lavage in Adults with Pulmonary Disease. Official ATS-statement. *Am. Rev. Respir. Dis.* **142**: 481

5 Pirozynski M, Silwinski P, Polubiez M, Zielinski J and Radwan L (1988) *Eur. Respir. J.* **1** (Suppl. 2): 312

6 Klech H, Haslam, P, Turner-Warwick M and 62 other contributors (1986) *Sarcoidosis* **3**: 113

7 Garcia JGN, Wolven RG, Garcia PL and Keogh BA (1986) *Am. Rev. Respir. Dis.* **133**: 444

8 Peterson MW, Nugent KM, Jolles H, Monick M and Hunninghake W (1988) *Am. Rev. Respir. Dis.* **137**: 79

9 Pingleton AK, Harrison GF, Stechschulte DJ, Wesselius I.J, Kerby GR and Ruth WE (1983) *Am. Rev. Respir. Dis.* **128**: 1035

10 Burns DM, Shure D, Francoz R, Kalafer M, Harrell J, Witztum K and Moser KM (1983) *Am. Rev. Respir. Dis.* **127**: 695

11 Reynolds HY, Fulmer JD, Kazmierowsky JA, Roberts WC, Frank MM and Crystal RG (1977) *J. Clin. Invest.* **59**: 165

12 Venet A, Clavel F. Israel-Biet D, Rouzioux C, Dennewald G, Stem MV, Vittecoq D, Regnier B, Cayrol E and Chretien J (1985) *Bull Eur. Physiopathol. Respir.* **21**: 535

13 Hunninghake, GW, Gadek JE, Kawanami O, Ferrans VJ and Crystal RG (1979) *Am. J. Pathol.* **97**: 149

14 Daniele RP, Elias JA, Epstein PE and Ross-man MD (1985) *Ann. Intern. Med.* **102**: 93

15 Davis, GS, Giancola MS, Costanza MC and Low RB (1982) *Am. Rev. Respir. Dis.* **126**: 611

16 Lam S, Leriche JC, Kijek K and Phillips E (1985) *Chest* **88**: 856

17 Dohn MN and Baughman RP (1985) *Am. Rev. Respir. Dis.* **132**: 390

18 Martin TR, Raghu G, Maunder RJ and Springmeyer SC (1985) *Am. Rev. Respir. Dis.* **132**: 254

19 Ettensohn DB, Jankowski MS, Duncan PG and Lalor PA (1988) *Chest* **94**: 275

20 Dhillon DP. Haslam PL, Townsend PJ, Primett Z, Collins J-V and Tumer-Warwick M (1986) *Eur J Respir Dis* **68**: 342

21 Reynolds HJ and Newball HH (1974) *J. Lab. Clin. Med.* **84**: 559

22 Davis WG, Rennard SI, Bittermann P and Crystal RG (1983) *N. Engl. J. Med.* **309**: 878

23 Costabel, U (1994) *Atlas der bronchoalveo-lären Lavage*, Thieme Verlag Stuttgart-New York

24 Costabel U (1988) *Prax. Klin. Pneumol.* **42**: 119

25 Haslam P, Turton C, Heard B et al. (1980) *Thorax* **35**: 9

26 Thompson, A and Ghafouri, M (1988) Processing and Analysis of Broncholaveolar Lavage Specimens. In: *Bronchoalveolar lavage*, J Linder and S Rennard (eds), p. 17, ASCP Press Chicago

27 Grocott RC (1955) *Am. J. Clin. Pathol.* **25**: 975

28 Brinn NT (1983) *I. Microtechnol.* **6**: 125

29 Unger ER, Budgeon LE, Myerson D et al. (1986) *Am. J. Surg. Pathol.* **10**: 1

30 Brigati DJ, Myerson D, Leary JJ et al. (1983) *Virology* **126**: 32

31 Myerson D, Hackman RC and Meyers JD (1984) *J. Infect. Dis.* **150**: 272

32 Myerson D, Hackman RC, Nelson JA et al. (1984) *Hum. Pathol.* **15**: 430

33 Hilborne L, Neiberg R, Cheng L et al. (1986) *Lab. Invest.* 26A

34 Parks DR and Herzenberg LA (1984) Fluorescence Activated Cell Sorting: Theory, Experimental Optimization and Application in Lymphoid Cell Biology. In: *Methods in Enzymology*, Kaplan NO and Colowick SP (eds) Academic Press New York

35 Pacheco Y, Cordier G, Perrin-Fayolle M and Revillard JP (1983) *Am. J. Med.* **73**: 82

36 Mornex JF, Cordier G, Pages J and Revillard JP (1983) *Monogr. Allergy* **18**: 178

37 Mornex JF, Cordier G, Pages J, Vergnon JM, Lefebvre R, Brune J and Revillard JP (1984) *J. Allergy Clin. Immunol.* **74**: 719

38 Steward SJ, Fujiinoto J and Levy R (1986) *J. Immunol.* **136**: 3773

39 Beuttner EH, Nisengard RJ and Albini B (1983) *Ann. NY Acad. Sci.* 420

40 Pizzolo G and Chilosi M (1984) *Am. J. Clin. Pathol.* **82**: 44

41 Costello JF, Moriarity DC, Branthwaite MA et al. (1975) *Thorax* **30**: 121

42 Martin RJ, Coalson JJ, Rogers RM et al. (1980) *Am. Rev. Respir. Dis.* **121**: 819

43 Basset F, Soler P, Jaurand MC et al. (1977) *Thorax* **32**: 303

44 Saltini C, Hance AJ, Ferrans VJ et al. (1984) *Am. Rev. Respir. Dis.* **130**: 650

45 Thompson A, Ghafouri M, Linder J et al. (1986) *Am. Rev. Respir. Dis.* **133**: A82

46 Linder J, Vaughan WP, Armitage JO et al. (1987) *Am. J. Clin. Pathol.* **88**: 421

47 Johnston WW, Frable WJ (eds) (1979) *Diagnostic Respiratory Cytopathology.* Masson Publishing New York

48 Low RB, Davis GS and Giancola MS (1978) *Am. Rev. Respir. Dis.* **118**: 863

49 Rennard SI, Basset G, Lecossier D et al. (1986) *J. Appl. Physiol.* **60**: 532

50 Baughman RP, Bosken CH, Loudon RG, Hurtubise P and Wesseler T (1983) *Am. Rev. Respir. Dis.* **128**: 266

51 Gehr P, Bachofen M and Weibel ER (1978)

*Respir. Physiol.* **32**: 121

52 von Wichert P, Joseph K, Müller B and Franck WM (1993) *Am. Rev. Respir. Dis.* **147**: 148

53 Kleinholz EJ and Fussel J (1973) *Am. Rev. Respir. Dis.* **108**: 1014

54 Dubrawsky C, Awe RJ and Jenkins DE (1975) *Chest* **67**: 137

55 Matsushima Y, Jones L, King E, Moysa G and Alton JD (1984) *Chest* **86**: 184

56 Shrader DL and Lakshiminarayan S (1978) *Chest* **73**: 821

57 Brach BB, Escano GE, Harrell JH and Moser KM (1976) *Chest* **69**: 335

58 Lindholm CE, Ollman B, Snyder JV, Miller EG and Grenvik A (1978) *Chest* **74**: 362

59 Pereira W, Kovnat DM, Anees Kahn M, Iacovino JR, Spivack ML and Snider GL (1975) *Am. Rev. Respir. Dis.* **112**: 59

60 Petro W, Linder O and Kaspar P (1989) *Atemw. Lungenkrkh.* **15**: 614

61 Pirozinsky M, Zaleska J, Radwan L and Zych D (1991) *Eur. Respir. Rev.* **1** (Suppl): 17s

62 Cole P, Turton C, Lanyon H and Collins J (1980) *Br. J. Dis. Chest.* **74**: 273

63 Strumpf IJ, Feld MK, Cornelius MJ, Keogh BA and Crystal RG (1981) *Chest* **80**: 268

64 Gurney JW, Harrison WC, Sears K, Robbins RA, Dobvy CA and Rennard SI (1987) *Radiology* **163**: 71

65 Standiford TJ, Kunkel SL and Strieter RM (1991) *Chest* **99**: 1529

66 Rankin JA, Synder PE, Schacter EN and Matthay RA (1984) *Chest* **85**: 723

67 Tilles TS, Goldenheim PD, Ginns LC and Hales CA (1986) *Chest* **89**: 244

68 Summary and Recommendations of a Workshop on the Investigative Use of Fiberoptic Bronchoscopy and Bronchoalveolar Lavage in Asthmatics (1985) *Am. Rev. Respir. Dis.* **132**: 180

69 Henderson RF, Mauderly JL, Pickrell JA, Hahn FF, Muhle H and Rebar AH (1987) *Exp. Lung Res.* **13**: 329

70 Mauderly J (1977) *Lab. Anim. Sci.* **27**: 255

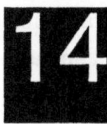

# Assessment of surfactant function

*B. Robertson and*
*S. Schürch*

The film of surface active material ("surfactant") that coats the terminal air-spaces and conducting airways is of vital physiological importance. It prevents end-expiratory alveolar collapse by reducing the contractile force of surface tension at low lung volumes, and furthermore constitutes a barrier involved in the pulmonary defence system. Lung surfactant has a crucial role in the process of neonatal adaptation by lowering the alveolar opening pressure. It also stabilizes the newly aerated alveoli during the first ventilatory cycles, allowing effective gas exchange soon after birth. Inadequate supply of surfactant material in the lungs of a premature newborn baby is characteristically associated with a type of respiratory failure known as respiratory distress syndrome (RDS), a major cause of neonatal morbidity and mortality [1].

Lung surfactant is secreted from alveolar type II cells as multilamellar packages of lipids and proteins. These "lamellar bodies" seem to contain all components required to generate the surface film at the air-liquid interfaces of the lung, including dipalmitoylphosphatidylcholine (DPPC), unsaturated phosphatidylcholine and phosphatidylglycerol, the hydrophilic surfactant-associated protein SP-A, and the hydrophobic proteins SP-B and SP-C. These proteins are instrumental in the transformation of secreted lamellar bodies to tubular myelin and for the subsequent adsorption of the surfactant lipids at the surface of the alveolar lining layer.

At least three physical properties of the surfactant system are essential for normal lung function, especially in the neonatal period. These are 1) rapid adsorption from the hypophase, 2) low film compressibility with a fall in surface tension to very low values during surface compression, and 3) effective replenishment of squeezed-out film constituents during surface expansion, probably achieved by the establishment of a surface-associated surfactant reservoir as will be explained in some detail below.

In this chapter, we will discuss different assay systems for *in vitro* evaluation of surfactant function. We will also review methods for determination of surface tension *in situ*, and the use of pressure-volume recordings for assessment of lung distensibility and stability as influenced by surfactant. Subsequent sections will deal with animal models of surfactant dysfunction, currently used for evaluating the potential of surfactant replacement therapy, and with problems related to surfactant inactivation – an important mechanism involved in the pathophysiology of many forms of lung disease including RDS.

## *In vitro* methods for assessment of surfactant function

A variety of systems have been used for determining the surface activity of surfactant materials derived from the lung. Among these are film balances, representing modifications of a Langmuir-type trough in combination with Wilhelmy plates, and a number of bubble methods, bubbles on a tube, captive and rotating bubbles [2]. In addition, the surface activity of pulmonary surfactant extracts can be assessed by foam stability tests using Newton black films [3] or the size distribution of microbubbles related to surfactant inhibition. In the following we will discuss the Langmuir-Wilhelmy balance, pulsating and captive bubble surfactometers and the assessment of microbubble stability.

### The Langmuir-Wilhelmy balance

In Langmuir's original balance [4], the surfactant film is confined on one side by a rigid, adjustable barrier and with a floating one on the other side. The force acting on the floating barrier was then measured directly to give the film pressure $\pi$, where $\pi = \gamma - \gamma_0$. $\gamma$ is the film surface tension and $\gamma_0$ is the surface tension of the substrate behind the barrier without the film. This technique, developed by Langmuir, had its origin in the work of Agnes Pockels [5] who showed that films could be confined by means of barriers (for the historical background, *see* [6]).

Today, Langmuir-Wilhelmy balances usually consist of a modified Langmuir trough of metal coated with Teflon or of solid Teflon, with a tightly fitting Teflon barrier (Fig. 14.1). Surface tension of the surfactant film is measured with a Wilhelmy dipping plate of platinum or other materials as described below (*see* [6] for a modern version). In addition to measuring a lowest achievable surface tension, this apparatus can also record surface-tension-area isotherm plots of material in the air-liquid interface.

The Langmuir-Wilhelmy method was introduced to study surfactant films by Clements in his pioneering studies on lung surfactant extracts [7]. The Langmuir-Wilhelmy method is easy to understand and provides an immediate analogue output of surface tension and film area. However, trough systems require large volumes (e.g. > 100 ml), and the barrier cannot be cycled easily at frequencies approaching normal breathing frequencies (e.g., 20 cycles per minute) as this creates waves. Cycling speeds for a full compression-expansion cycle of approximately 0.1 – 12 cycles/min and film area compressions of 50–90% relative to the fully expanded film have been used.

A wide range of trough sizes have also been employed with maximum areas of the film confined between the barrier and walls from about 50 cm$^2$ to more than 300 cm$^2$. If cycling speeds are to be compared, the film area change per unit time, e.g. in cm$^2$/min, has to be taken into account. Temperatures are usually stabilized at room temperature, ~ 22 °C, or at 37 °C. The trough may be filled to the required level with natural surfactant extract. In this case, relatively low concentrations, typically 50 µg/ml of phospholipid, are used because of the large

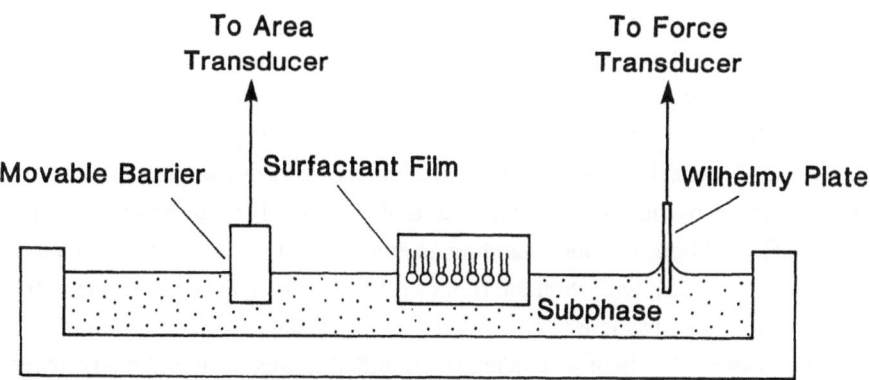

**Figure 14.1. The Langmuir-Wilhelmy surface balance**
A surfactant film is formed at the air-liquid interface either by adsorption of surfactant from the aqueous subphase or by spreading of surfactant material at the liquid surface. The subphase is contained in a Teflon Langmuir trough. The surface tension is monitored by a Wilhelmy plate. The surfactant film is compressed or expanded by the movable Teflon barrier.

volumes needed. Standard times of 5 min or more are observed for the surfactant film formation by adsorption before cycling is started.

Alternatively, the surfactant suspensions, typically at concentrations of 2 mg/ml of phospholipid, are applied carefully dropwise with a micro syringe onto a subphase of a salt solution, e.g. 0.9 % NaCl, 1.5 mM $CaCl_2$ buffered with HEPES to pH 6.9–7.2. Single drops of the suspension are formed at the tip of the syringe needle and the drop is placed by lowering the tip until the drop touches the aqueous subphase. Several drops are distributed over the surface while the resulting surface tension is monitored with the Wilhelmy plate. Surfactant suspensions may also be layered onto the subphase by letting single drops run down onto the surface along a clean glass rod that penetrates the air-liquid interface from the air phase. Again, a standard waiting period for the film formation is observed. Depending on the amount of surfactant placed onto the surface and on a particular waiting period, initial surface tensions of more than 50 mN/m to 22–25 mN/m (equilibrium) are observed. For further information on the Langmuir-Wilhelmy technique, we refer to [7–12].

Surfactant lipids may also be applied to the surface of the aqueous subphase from solutions of the lipids in a solvent system which contains chloroform. An example of a good solvent system for DPPC is chloroform:propanol:n-hexane (1:1:8, by volume). Propanol promotes spreading and n-hexane tends to keep the solution floating on the surface until the chloroform and the hexane have evaporated. (For problems with spreading solutions, *see* [13]).

An almost insoluble problem with trough systems is their tendency to "leak"; that is, they allow surface components to creep along constraining walls, and between the walls and the barrier. Leakage can be reduced by using tightly fitting barriers and by checking leakage along the barrier by measuring the surface tension behind the barrier during compression of the film [14]. Furthermore, continuous Teflon ribbons or bands standing on edge were used in the 1960s in a rectangular trough [15], with rhombic frames [16] or, more recently, a frame in the shape of a rounded triangle [17].

In contrast to the rhombic barrier, the rounded triangle offers the advantage of a linear displacement-surface area relation. However, even these Teflon ribbon balances have to be primed to better contain surfactant films. Leakage past the barrier can be eliminated by using continuous ribbons, but in order to prevent the film from occupying more interfacial area than that of the air-water interface, the thermodynamic driving force for surfactant spreading at the wall-water or barrier-water interfaces has to be reduced. This can be accomplished by reducing the interfacial free energy of these interfaces (about 50 mJ/m$^2$ for Teflon-water), by a priming process which makes the Teflon walls hydrophilic below the water line. Qiu and MacDonald [17] used sodium-naphthalene-tetrahydrofuran to make the Teflon surface below the water level hydrophilic. Goerke and Gonzales primed the Teflon walls and barrier of their surface balance with long chain di-saturated phosphatidylcholine and a solution of lanthanum chloride [18]. We have reduced surfactant creep along the Teflon ribbon of our rhombic balance by compressing spread films of dipalmitoyl or distearoyl phosphatidylcholine from the equilibrium surface tension of about 25 mN/m to near zero minimum surface tension by reducing the film area by 80–90% (overcompression), and by cleaning the surface area at minimum by aspiration. This process may be repeated several times to produce a hydrophilic surface below the water level. The principle is to build up a film of phospholipid at the Teflon-water interface with the polar heads of the phospholipids oriented toward the water and the fatty acid chains oriented toward the Teflon.

Another problem with the Langmuir-Wilhelmy balance is the contact angle at the three-phase line on the Wilhelmy dipping plate, usually a zero contact angle is assumed, that is the plate is completely wetted. As the surface tension falls upon film compression, the height of the meniscus decreases, often leaving behind a film of lipid material on the plate-air surface. Upon re-expansion of the film, the liquid meniscus must respread and advance upward on the Wilhelmy plate to increase the force transmitted to the recorder. Frequently, the contact angle upon re-expansion of the film is substantially higher than zero (contact angle hysteresis) causing erroneous results.

To reduce contact angle problems, careful cleaning, including chemical cleaning and/or flaming of the Wilhelmy plate, is necessary. In addition, the platinum Wilhelmy plates have to be roughened with fine sand paper or sandblasting is recommended (e.g. [19]). Gaines described the use of a strip of filter paper to measure the surface tension of insoluble monolayers [9]. Contact angle problems with pulmonary surfactant films can be nearly eliminated by using plates of filter paper [20].

In summary, minimum surface tension and film stability at tensions below equilibrium, typically 22–25 mN/m for pulmonary surfactant, depend on the careful preparation of the surface balance as films that produce low and stable minimum surface tensions in a carefully primed system show instability and much higher minimum tensions in a balance with untreated walls, especially at 37 °C, regardless of the geometry or arrangement of the moveable barrier. In addition, the potential problem related to the wetting properties of the Wilhelmy plate (non-zero contact angle) needs special attention.

### Bubbles on a tube: The pulsating bubble surfactometer according to Enhorning

In an attempt to overcome the difficulties with the Langmuir-Wilhelmy balance, some investigators have been using small air bubbles formed on subsurface tubes in cuvettes. Slama et al. [21, 22] described an oscillating bubble method for pulmonary surfactant studies.

Enhorning published his version of an oscillating bubble on a tube [23] (Fig. 14.2). This apparatus, known as the pulsating bubble surfactometer, has been widely used and has yielded a considerable amount of insight into dynamically compressed and expanded films from natural surfactant or compounds related to pulmonary surfactant (for review see [24]). The most common form of this apparatus is commercially available (Electronetics Corporation, Buffalo, New York). It consists of a bubble drawn from the atmosphere into a disposable plastic chamber at 37 °C containing as little as 20 μl of a suspension of the material to be tested. The bubble is oscillated between a maximum radius of 0.55 mm and a minimum radius of 0.40 mm which produces a surface area reduction of approximately 50%. The cycling frequency is usually about 20 cycles/min, but frequencies of 10 to 80 cycles/min. have also been used. The pressure across the bubble is continuously monitored with a pressure transducer. The surface tension is calculated by using the Laplace equation for a spherical interface. The bubble shape remains spherical, except when the surface tension falls to values below about 1 mN/m, where the bubble begins to flatten due to bouyancy, similarly to the larger bubbles in the captive bubble system described below. However, the lack of accuracy in the determination of surface tensions below about 1 mN/m because of the deviation from spherical shape at these tensions may not be important, since the minimum tension will be 1 mN/m or less, and whether the tension is, say, 0.5 or 0.8 mN/m does not usually concern the investigator interested in practical applications.

As in the Langmuir-Wilhelmy balance, there are still problems with surface leaks. They occur up the inner surface of the tube at the plastic-air interface as well as at the outer surface of the tube at the plastic-fluid interface by surfactant

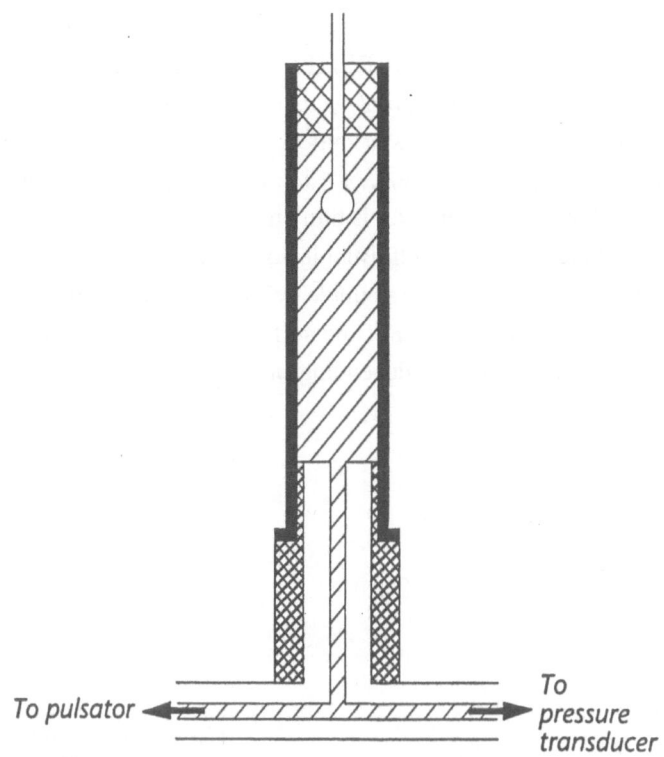

**Figure 14.2. The pulsating bubble surfactometer (PBS) according to Enhorning**

*A surfactant suspension is loaded into the bubble chamber. An air bubble is formed on the bottom of a plastic capillary open to the atmosphere. The bubble is periodically compressed and expanded by a pressure pulsator. The pressure across the bubble interface is monitored and the surface tension is calculated by the Laplace equation for a sphere.*

spreading, similarly to that in the surface balance at the Teflon-water interface. Leakage at the inner surface of the tube can be reduced by keeping the tube dry [25]. The method is not suitable to investigate the film stability at minimum surface tension (surface tension *vs.* time) at minimum bubble volume in the non-pulsating mode. The pulsating bubble is very convenient for examining the surface activity, now commonly named "biophysical activity" of samples under dynamic compression, as leakage is less of a problem if relatively high cycling frequencies are chosen.

## Captive bubbles

The captive bubble surfactometer (CBS) (Fig. 14.3) introduced by Schürch and co-workers [26, 27] offers a leak-proof system because the surface film is not interrupted by plastic walls, barriers or outlets. In this apparatus, the air bubble floats against a hydrophilic roof, e.g. of a 1% agarose gel, by buoyancy. At the air-agarose interface, the water layer is thin but sufficiently thick to prevent adhesion of the bubble to the gel itself. Bubble volume is controlled by varying the pressure in the sample chamber. As bubble volume is reduced, the surface area is reduced and the surface tension of the surfactant film at the bubble surface falls. The bubble shape changes depending on the surface tension, from more

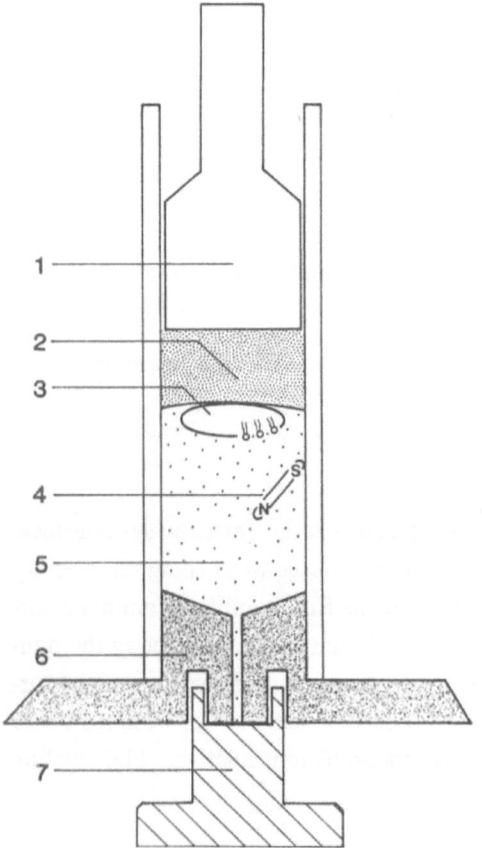

**Figure 14.3. The captive bubble surfactometer (CBS)**

1) Pressure tight piston; 2) 1% agarose gel; 3) air bubble with surfactant on its air-liquid interface; 4) stir bar; 5) surfactant suspension in chamber; 6) stainless steel base with inlet; 7) pressure tight plug. A bubble of atmospheric air 2–7 mm in diameter is drawn into the sample chamber to assume its resting position below the agarose gel. Bubble volume and, thus, bubble surface area is compressed or expanded by the changing pressure produced by the relative movement of piston and chamber. In the design of Putz and associates [28] the pressure changes are not driven directly with a piston, the bubble volume is regulated by an external pressure reservoir. Both approaches give equivalent results.

spherical to an oval shape. For bubbles larger than about 5 mm in initial diameter, the bubble shape assumes a thin disk as the surface tension falls towards zero. For surface tensions less than 1 mN/m up to about 30 mN/m, bubbles as small as 4 µl in volume (2 mm diameter) may be used in a sample volume of about 40 µl. However, usually bubbles of about 200 µl in volume (~ 7 mm diameter) are used in a sample volume of about 0.5 to 1.0 ml. Surfactant concentrations, usually expressed in total phospholipid per volume (mg/ml), can be used from as little as 50 µg/ml or less to a maximum of 1–2 mg/ml for the large chamber, 10 mm in diameter, while for the small chamber, 5 mm in diameter, a maximum concentration of 3 mg/ml may be used.

Surface tension, area and volume are calculated from bubble height and diameter, from video images [29]. For precision and accuracy of the method, *see* [26, 29]. If more elaborate imaging processing is available, then the axisymmetric drop shape analysis (ADSA-P) by Neumann and associates, originally published by Rotenberg et al. [30], can be used. ADSA-P is exceptionally accurate and very general, but one limitation is that it requires the measurement of at least 20 points defining the bubble perimeter for input into a complex iterative computation (for more information, *see* [29]). The CBS system can be used to construct quasi-static isotherms similar to those obtained in the Langmuir-Wilhelmy balance. Cycling frequencies from extremely slow to more than 60 cycles/min can be chosen.

There are several ways to evaluate film stability at near zero minimum surface tension.

*Bubble clicking:* Captive bubbles at low surface tension tend to spontaneously and rapidly revert to higher surface tensions if the surfactant is not sufficiently purified or if it has been degraded due to a variety of influencing factors (e.g. [31]). The phenomenon of spontaneous and rapid increase in surface tension accompanied by a reduction in surface area (rounding of the bubble) is referred to as "bubble clicking" [29]. Bubble clicking was first observed and extensively described by Pattle in several publications (e.g. [32, 33]). Pattle deduced from the clicking surfactant bubbles that the surfactant film reaches near zero surface tension. There is no contradiction between Pattle's conclusions and our interpretation of bubble clicking. He observed clicking on small bubbles, about 50 µm in diameter under a microscope glass slide. Such small bubbles tend to be spherical unless their surface tension is very low, less than 1 mN/m, where they tend to flatten due to buoyancy. He correctly concluded that these tiny bubbles did reach near zero surface tension because only then could he clearly see the spontaneous and rapid change of the bubble diameter corresponding to the change of the bubble shape from flat to round due to film instability. However in Pattle's case, it was not the imposed pressure which caused the reduction of the bubble volume, it was gas diffusion out of the bubbles which caused the film compression by the shrinking bubble area. In the CBS clicking is frequently observed on much larger bubbles which tend to be relatively flat at higher surface tensions. Bubble clicking upon bubble compression in the CBS means film instability at surface tensions from about 1 to 15 mN/m [26, 27].

*Surface tension* vs. *time:* Film stability can be assessed by holding the captive bubble at minimum volume (minimum surface tension) and by recording the bubble shape during a particular time period, e.g. 10 min. Surface tension *vs.* time plots can then be constructed. Films from natural pulmonary surfactant extract which contain SP-A and cholesterol as well as films from lipid extract surfactant (e.g. Curosurf, Chiesi Farmaceutici, Parma, Italy; or bLES, Biochemicals Inc., London, Ontario, Canada) demonstrate extraordinary stability at near zero surface tension, as surface tensions below 1 mN/m are observed for more than 10 min at 37 °C, after only about two compressions.

## Microbubble stability

The assessment of the surfactant quality by investigating microbubble stability is based on Pattle's observation of the extraordinary stability of microbubbles (about 40 μm in diameter) derived from the lung's lining layer [32]. These bubbles remained unchanged in size for long periods (60 min), and Pattle concluded the surface tension of the lung bubbles to be "zero". Later he called substances capable of reducing the air-water surface tension to 0.1 mN/m or less "fully surpellic" [34].

In 1979, Pattle and his coworkers developed the stable microbubble test for amniotic fluid to assess the quality of pulmonary surfactant. This test is based on the capacity of pulmonary surfactant to generate microbubbles which are less than 15 μm in diameter. The method to generate such bubbles in a particular suspension is described in [35, 36]. Briefly, an aliquot (about 40 μl) of amniotic fluid or gastric aspirate placed onto a microscopic slide is sucked into and expelled from a Pasteur pipette 20 times in 6 s to generate microbubbles. The aliquot with the bubbles is then placed onto a hollow slide which is inverted so that a hanging drop is formed. The slide is then examined under a microscope. The number (n) of microbubbles $< 15\,\mu m$ in diameter that are found in a 1 mm$^2$ field are counted. According to Pattle, if $n > 20$, RDS will not occur, while $n = 2$ to 10 and especially $n = <2$ suggest a high risk of RDS [35].

Chida [38] described refinements of the test based on his work and that of his Japanese colleagues [37–39]). For example, bubble counting could be reduced to 2 min and the test can give results in 10 min. The diagnostic accuracy of the test on amniotic fluid appears to compare favourably with that of biochemical and immunological tests. However, the test relies on counting the absolute number of bubbles below a certain size, and this number depends on the way the bubbles are produced. Standardisation among various clinical settings might be difficult.

Berggren et al. [40, 41] have modified the microbubble stability test by evaluating the size distribution of microbubbles using computer-aided image analysis to determine the median bubble diameter as a measure for the central tendency. In this approach, the bubbles are generated by vortexing the suspensions to be tested. Examples for test results are: the median bubble diameter of amniotic fluid from immature rabbit fetuses (27 days gestation) was 135 $\mu m$, whereas that from animals of 29 days gestation was 76 $\mu m$.

Surfactant (Curosurf, diluted to 5 mg/ml) was suspended in normal saline with 3 mM CaCl$_2$ and mixed with different concentrations of albumin and fibrinogen. Bubbles in the original surfactant suspension (control) had an average diameter of 27 $\mu m$ after 2 min. The diameter of bubbles generated in the presence of albumin (4 or 40 mg/ml) or fibrinogen (4 mg/ml) was four to five times larger than in the control study. It has been suggested that the method offers a rapid assessment of the influence of inhibitory agents on the surface activity of pulmonary surfactants.

The stability of gas bubbles in a liquid is dependent on the diffusion rate of the gas out of the bubble. The diffusion rate for a gas bubble in the liquid is a function of the gradient of the gas concentration across the bubble-liquid interface. In small bubbles, the pressure due to surface tension can be greatly elevated because the pressure difference across the bubble interface is inversely proportional to the radius of the spherical bubble as stated by the Laplace equation. For example, if the surface tension is 35 mN/m and the bubble radius is 1 $\mu m$, the total pressure inside the bubble is about 75 % above the normal atmospheric pressure, so outward diffusion is substantially enhanced. The lifetime of a gas bubble with a radius of a few micrometers in diameter was calculated to be only a few seconds, unless the pressure gradient becomes negligible due to a very low surface tension [42].

Therefore, the following explanation for the extended lifetime (stability) of small bubbles lined with surfactant is reasonable: microbubbles are generated by vortexing or by any other means. The size of a bubble just after its generation depends on properties important for fluid dynamic transport mechanisms and also on the rate of adsorption of surfactant molecules at the air-liquid interface. Relatively large bubbles at low surface tension will deform more easily in a shear field than bubbles at higher surface tensions [6] and will be ripped apart to form an array of smaller bubbles. These bubbles will then start to shrink in size by gas diffusion and, as a consequence, the surfactant molecules will be tightly packed for normal surfactant and close to zero surface tensions will be reached which, in turn, reduce the pressure gradient to very low values. Thus, diffusion is greatly reduced and is likely further reduced by the formation of a surface reservoir not only by *de novo* adsorption, but also by film overcompression at near zero surface tension [43, 44]. On the other hand, bubbles formed in abnormal, slowly absorbing surfactant will be larger on the average than those formed in normal surfactant suspensions, and relatively small bubbles will not survive because low surface tensions cannot be reached and diffusion will destroy these bubbles. Therefore in abnormal surfactant, there will be no bubbles in the range of a few micrometres in diameter, and the size of the surviving bubbles will be substantially larger than in normal surfactant [45].

## Adsorption

The concepts of adsorption and spreading are employed to describe the formation of a surfactant film at an interface, the boundary between two bulk phases. Adsorption means the accumulation of material at an interface. An exact definition of surface or interfacial adsorption requires a mathematical description of the interface and a specification of its location (e.g. [6, 46]). A decrease in surface tension with an increase in the concentration of a particular solute means that the solute is positively adsorbed at the interface. Any substance leading to this surface tension decrease is said to be "surface active" [46]. Adsorption is usually assessed by measuring the decrease in surface tension, but adsorption might also be investigated by employing the Gibbs adsorption equation which gives the number of surfactant molecules per unit area adsorbed at the surface if the relation between the bulk surfactant concentration and the resulting surface tension by adsorption is known (for review *see* [47]).

## The rate of adsorption

The adsorption and desorption processes depend on transport of solute to and from the interface. There are four major transport mechanisms: 1) diffusion, 2) thermal convection, 3) flow (convective transport) and 4) convective-diffusion processes (coupled transport).

The adsorption from turbulent or stirred solutions incorporates coupled transport of solutes by a combination of convection and diffusion [48]. All fluid interfaces contain an undisturbed layer of solution adjacent to the interface. Mass transport in this boundary layer occurs only by diffusion. The thickness of the boundary layer depends on temperature, stirring and the composition of the interface. It is up to 1 mm thick in unstirred systems and approaches 0.01 mm in well-stirred systems [48, 49].

If the bulk solution is kept stirred to within a distance $\Delta x$ of the surface, diffusion to the surface may be stationary. This will be possible if new solute is continuously being brought to the lower limit of the layer $\Delta x$ by convection and if back diffusion and depletion of the bulk solution can be neglected [49]. The rate of adsorption into the interface is then inversely proportional to the thickness of the boundary layer, i.e. the rate of adsorption is increased by reducing $\Delta x$ by stirring.

Experiments on the adsorption of molecular amphiphiles may show a decrease in the rate of adsorption due to an energy barrier, related to the energy needed to clear an area $\Delta A$ against the surface pressure $\pi$. On the other hand, the addition of surfactant-specific proteins, especially SP-C but also SP-B and SP-A in combination with SP-B, and SP-C, to surfactant lipids in solution, dramatically increases the rate of surfactant film formation by adsorption [31, 50–53]. It appears that the favourable free energy change in the adsorption process of lipid-protein aggregates more than compensates the energy barrier due to the surface pressure [54].

Graham and Phillips [55] and Birdi [56] have discussed the dramatic increase in the adsorption of proteins due to their unfolding at the air-liquid interface. Birdi [56] related the degree of unfolding to the polar:apolar ratio of the residues of a particular protein. These studies suggest that particular associations of the specific surfactant proteins (SP-A, -B, -C) with the phospholipids in surfactant aggregates promote adsorption by a configurational change at the air-liquid interface.

### Adsorption characteristics of pulmonary surfactants

Weibel and his associates demonstrated by electron microscopy the existence of an extracellular duplex lining layer of lung alveoli [57, 58]. They observed that parts of the surface film appeared as a lamellar superficial layer with repeating distances of 3.8 to 5.1 nm adsorbed to the surface film [57]. Recent studies have shown that the surfactant extracellular layer present in rabbit lungs *in vivo* is too thick to be a monolayer [59]. High power magnification of the film showed a polymorphous structure. At some sites multilayers covered the hypophase, at other sites the film appeared amorphous. These observations, together with *in vitro* depletion experiments [44], have led to the concept that the surfactant surface phase may be composed of more than a single monolayer and that the surplus material might act as a surface-associated reservoir for the formation of a surface active film [44]. Others found the surfactant film to be multilamellar [60, 61].

Film formation of lipid extract surfactants that contain SP-B and SP-C occurs in a cooperative movement of large collective units of surfactant molecules. This has been demonstrated recently in the captive bubble system by using porcine lipid extract surfactant (Curosurf) [43]. During these adsorption studies to the equilibrium tension, the surface tension tended to decrease in sudden, quick steps of 5–10 mN/m (adsorption clicks), corresponding to the adsorption of aggregates of $\sim 10^{14}$ phospholipid molecules ($\sim 120$ ng). Without exception, films formed in this manner appear already highly enriched in DPPC as seen by the extremely low compressibility close to that of DPPC. In contrast, films formed by gradual adsorption during several seconds to minutes may or may not show the same low compressibility as those formed by adsorption clicks. These latter films may then be purified by squeezing-out mechanisms previously described (e.g. [62]). Thus, both mechanisms of selective enrichment in DPPC are not mutually exclusive.

In addition, lipid extract films formed by rapid gradual adsorption within 1 to 2 s, or by adsorption clicks, to the equilibrium surface tension of 23–25 mN/m, tend to have film material in the surface associated surfactant reservoir in excess of three monolayers, and this excess material appears to be enriched in DPPC.

## Spreading

Spreading of one liquid, e.g. liquid 1, on another, e.g. liquid 2, occurs spontaneously if the spreading coefficient, S, is positive [6, 49, 63]. The spreading coefficient is defined as:

$$S = \gamma_2 - (\gamma_1 + \gamma_{12})$$

where
$\gamma_1$ = surface tension of liquid 1

$\gamma_2$ = surface tension of liquid 2 and

$\gamma_{12}$ = interfacial tension between the two liquids.

If the mutual solubility of the two liquids is negligible, and $S < 0$, spreading will not occur and a droplet of liquid 1 will form a lens. Mutual dissolution of the two liquids can substantially alter the surface and interfacial tensions, so that one must distinguish between the initial and final spreading coefficients. For liquids completely soluble in water, the interfacial tension $\gamma_{12}$ is assumed to be zero.

Exogenous surfactants for replacement therapy are aqueous suspensions of lipid aggregates. If a drop or bolus of such a suspension comes into contact with a liquid substrate of a relatively high surface tension, say 50 mN/m, the relatively large positive value of the spreading coefficient, $S = [50 - (25 + 0)]$ mN/m = 25 mN/m, causes the surfactant to spread rapidly before dissolution into the aqueous substrate occurs. Spreading is achieved through the development, ahead of the bulk of the drop, of a thin surfactant film on the substrate, along which the jump in surface tension occurs [64]. For this spreading process, accompanied with an increasing surface area of the spreading suspension, rapid adsorption and formation of a surfactant film of an equilibrium surface tension of 23–25 mN/m is important for maintaining the positive spreading coefficient. Thus, rapid adsorption is important for rapid spreading of surfactant.

The surface tension gradient along the air-liquid interface induces a flow (Marangoni flow [6]) that carries the surfactant along the interface and spreads the surfactant to regions of relatively low surfactant concentration (high surface tension) [64, 65]. The presence of an endogenous surfactant film reduces the spreading rate of exogenous surfactant. Furthermore, the endogenous surfactant, which is ahead of the advancing exogenous surfactant, undergoes a concentration increase due to area compression of the surface film at the air-liquid interface due to the spreading exogenous surfactant. So, the spreading exogenous surfactant can raise surfactant concentration in regions distal to its own location. This mechanism [65] might be important for the generation of low surface tensions at desired target sites, if the surfactant is delivered by aerosol.

In summary, exogenous surfactants that adsorb fast at the air-liquid interface to generate equilibrium surface tensions of 23–25 mN/m, will spread rapidly through the relatively large positive spreading coefficient, provided the surface tension of the endogenous surfactant is above that of the exogenous surfactant or the substrate. Lipid extract surfactants, among them Curosurf and bLES, adsorb within seconds to form films of an equilibrium surface tension of 23–25 mN/m and so are expected to also spread rapidly to regions of higher surface tensions.

## The measurements of adsorption and spreading

### Adsorption

Adsorption is usually measured by the rate of surface tension reduction (surface tension *vs.* time). If the relation between the amount (mass) of the accumulated surfactant in the surface (mass/unit area) and the surface tension is known, then adsorption can be expressed in $(\mu g \cdot cm^{-2} \cdot s^{-1})$.

*Method of King and Clements:* The apparatus of King and Clements consists of a stirred subphase in a Teflon beaker with surface tension being monitored by a Wilhelmy dipping plate [66]. As pointed out above, stirring reduces the thickness of the boundary layer and so reduces the complications associated with time-dependent diffusion processes. The subphase of the Teflon beaker is usually relatively large ($\geq$ 5 ml) but smaller beakers of any inert material, such as glass, might be employed.

*The pulsating bubble surfactometer:* The pulsating bubble surfactometer can be used in the pulsating mode where the small volume of the subphase is agitated by the oscillating bubble, but the system is probably not as well stirred as in the King and Clements method. In the non-pulsating mode, the bubble is held at maximum radius and the pressure drop across the bubble is monitored during adsorption. The rate of adsorption is likely influenced by the non-stirring condition.

*The captive bubble surfactometer:* As in the method of King and Clements, the subphase is well stirred with a magnetic stir bar. Two methods of bubble formation have been used for the adsorption measurements: in the first method, a relatively small bubble is introduced into the subphase. The bubble is then expanded within a small fraction of a second about tenfold in area by a sudden decrease in pressure. The initial amount of surfactant on the bubble surface before expansion is taken into account for the adsorption measurements [67].

In the second approach, a bubble of a given volume, usually about 7 mm in diameter depending on the chamber diameter, is formed within 0.10–0.13 s, the time of 3–4 frames on the TV monitor [43]. Again, the amount of surfactant during bubble formation has to be determined for an exact analysis of the adsorption rate.

## Spreading
*Spreading rates (distance/time) monitored by measuring surface tension with two Wilhelmy plates:* Joos and van Hunsel measured spreading kinetics of aqueous surfactant solutions on an oil phase [68]. A glass tube, 1 m long, with an inside diameter of 4 cm was cut along its axis and the resulting hemicylinder was filled with an oil phase. At one end the surface tension was monitored with a Wilhelmy plate. A second Wilhelmy plate was mounted at a distance X from the first plate. Distance X (direction parallel to longitudinal axis of the cylinder) could be changed by shifting the position of the second plate.

A drop of an aqueous surfactant solution was placed near the first plate. The surface tension measured with the first plate suddenly decreased. After time t, the surface tension at the second plate (distance X) suddenly decreased. The spreading rate at a particular point $X_i$ could be obtained from the plot of distance X *vs* time t. This method may be modified for studying spreading of pulmonary surfactants by using a long rectangular trough constructed of a material completely wettable by water (glass or stainless steel). The wettable surface allows the formation of a thin aqueous substrate to mimic the situation in the lung.

*Spreading rates (distance/time) monitored by recording the onset of motion using flow markers:* The fundamental theoretical work in fluid mechanics and transport phenomena related to spreading of pulmonary surfactant has been an active research area of Grotberg and his associates [65, 69–71]. Experimental approaches to surfactant spreading phenomena can be found in [69].

Time-dependent flows induced by a localised surfactant on a thin film were investigated. Glycerol layers of thickness, Ho, 2 mm and 0.7 mm were established in a 13.8 cm diameter Petri dish. A removable restraining collar of radius Ro was placed in the centre of the Petri dish, physically isolating the film of surfactant (oleic acid) inside the collar from the surface outside of the collar which was also modified with a surfactant film of a desired surface tension. The restraining collar permitted delivery of the oleic acid in a dilute solution of hexane, which was allowed to evaporate before the experiment commenced. Surface flows were visualised by dyed-glycerol markers placed on the surface at differing radial distances. Talc particles, cleaned by heating them to high temperatures [63] might also be used as markers, but they tend to interfere more with the surface flow than dye markers. The spreading experiments were recorded with a video camera and recorder. Slow motion play back of the experiments allowed accurate measurement of the onset of motion of the dye markers, which is a measure of the onset time for convective flow. More recent experimental work by Grotberg's group related to spreading of exogenous surfactants and problems of drug delivery using these surfactants will appear in the near future.

## Measurement of surface tension *in situ*

Alveolar surface tension can be determined *in situ* by placing droplets of test fluids with known surface tensions onto the alveolar surface and monitoring the shape of the droplets during various phases of the ventilatory cycle performed in quasi-static fashion. The method is based on the fact that a droplet of an inert oil with negligible solubility in water, when placed onto a surfactant film, changes its shape according to the film surface tension.

### Choosing a test fluid

As we have seen earlier, a droplet of a liquid 1 placed onto another liquid, 2 (for two liquids with negligible mutual solubility) will form a lens if the spreading coefficient, S, is negative, where $S = \gamma_2 - (\gamma_1 + \gamma_{12})$ (*see* Section on *Spreading*).

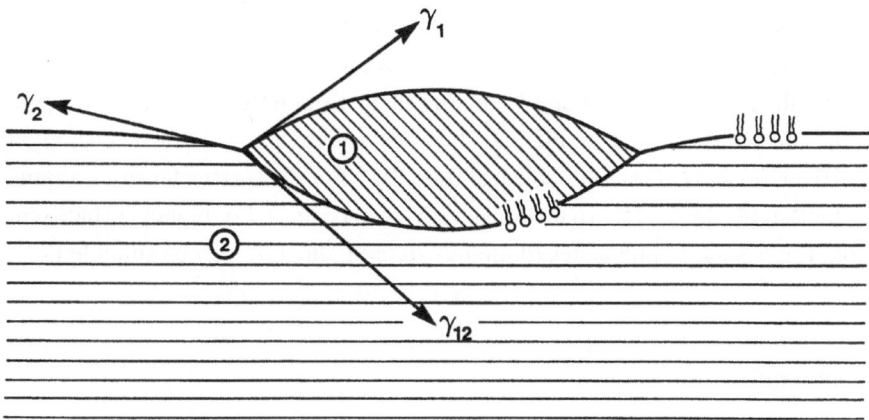

**Figure 14.4. Test fluid lens floating at the air-liquid interface modified by a surfactant film**
*The shape of the lens (diameter and angles) is given by the Neumann triangle relation which states that the vector sum of the surface tension forces per unit length at a point of the three-phase line is equal to zero.*

In this case, the droplet will assume an equilibrium shape which is character-ized by the three surface tension forces shown in the Neumann triangle relation [6].

$$\vec{\gamma_1} + \vec{\gamma_2} + \vec{\gamma_{12}} = 0$$

i.e. for equilibrium to be possible, the sum of the values of two of the tensions has to be greater than the value of the third, e.g.

$$\gamma_1 + \gamma_{12} > \gamma_2$$

If fluid 1 is to be used as a test fluid to estimate the surface tension of a surfact-ant film, the surface tensions of the test fluid, the film and the interfacial tension between test fluid and film are relevant parameters.

For the *in vitro* calibration, $\gamma_1$ of the test fluid is known and $\gamma_2$ may be mea-sured by the Wilhelmy plate, while $\gamma_{12}$ may be estimated by Antonoff's rule [6], which states that the interfacial tension between two fluids is approximately equivalent to the absolute value of the difference between the surface tensions of the two fluids, or

$$\gamma_{12} = |\gamma_2 - \gamma_1|$$

However, there are many exceptions to the validity of Antonoff's rule [6], and it should be only used as a guideline to choose a test fluid suitable to estimate the surface tension of the surfactant film *in situ* for a particular range.

For the range between 1 and 15 mN/m, fluorocarbon fluids of the lowest possible surface tension, e.g. FC 72 (3 MCo) which has a surface tension of 9–10 mN/m at 37 °C is a suitable test fluid [72]. For the surface tensions around 20 mN/m, FC 43, $\gamma = 15–16$ mN/m at 37 °C, can be used. For higher surface tension, fluids such as phthalates (dimethyl, dibutyl, dioctyl) may be suitable [73].

### Calibration

When a test fluid droplet is placed onto a surfactant film on a fluid substrate in a Langmuir-Wilhelmy balance, the lens diameter increases with the increasing and decreases with decreasing film surface tension in a reversible fashion. The

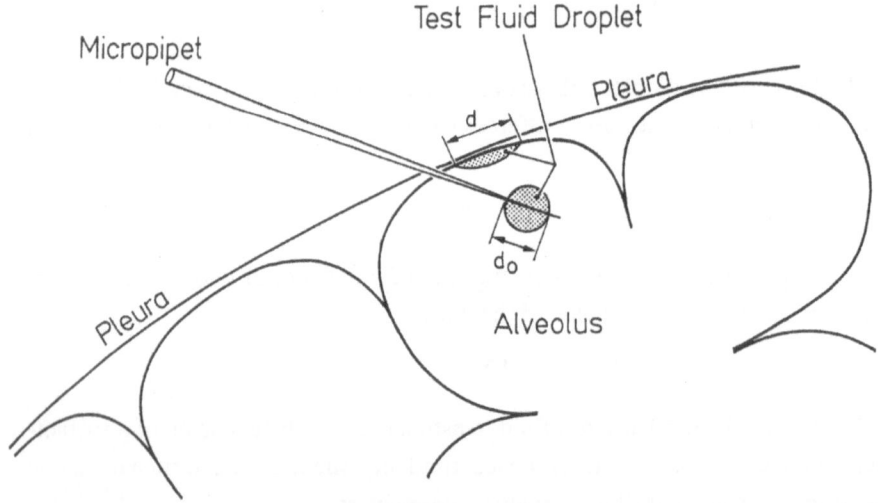

**Figure 14.5. Determination of alveolar surface tension in situ**
*A test fluid droplet (e.g. perfluorocarbon fluid) is formed at the tip of a micropipette inside an alveolus. The diameter of the drop before deposition is do. After deposition onto the alveolar surface, the drop spreads to a diameter d which is characteristic for the alveolar surface tension. This surface tension is determined from a calibration relation between lens diameter and film surface tension. The tip diameter of the micropipette is typically 1–2 µm, and $d_o$ is about 6–15 µm. The drop diameter inside an alveolus is determined with a microscope, using polarised light with transillumination if possible or epiillumination.*

diameter of the lens normalized to its spherical shape (relative diameter) is then plotted as a function of the film surface tension. On the other hand, if the relative diameter of the lens is known, the film surface tension can be determined by an inverse estimation procedure [74]. This is the basis for the direct determination of the *in situ* surface tension in the lung.

However, the model experiments have to be modified to simulate the morphology in the lung. In previous calibration experiments, the thickness of the subphase was reduced by supporting the surfactant film with a block of hydrated agar with its top surface slightly above that of the film on the fluid subphase. These experiments were conducted with a Langmuir-Wilhemly balance [72] or a captive bubble system [75, 76]. In contrast to a lens placed on top of a film on a liquid substrate, a lens placed onto a film on top of a thin layer of water, say 10 μm thick, has a larger relative diameter at the same film surface tension.

## *Alveolar micropuncture and surface tension* in situ

Droplets of inert test fluids as described above were placed onto alveolar surfaces of excised rat and cat lungs [72, 73, 75] (Fig. 14.5). Later experiments were conducted on continuously perfused rabbit lungs [76, 77]. The experiments confirmed that within the normal range of breathing, i.e. between 40 and 60% of total lung capacity (TLC), the surface tensions are between 1 and 10 mN/m, and further showed that the maximum surface tension at TLC is approximately 30 mN/m. Most importantly, further evidence could be provided that single alveoli are not individual units, but that some uniformity is ensured by both the tissue interdependence and the alveolar lining layer which forms a fluid continuum [78]. At a given volume, i.e. at a given total alveolar surface area, the surface tension was found to be the same in all alveoli regardless of their size [75].

## Influence of surfactant on static lung pressure-volume characteristics

The role of surface tension in lung mechanics was demonstrated already by von Neergard in 1929 [79], in his classical paper describing differences in pressure-volume properties between gas- and liquid-filled lungs. According to present understanding, surfactant material in the airspaces influences the static pressure-volume diagram of a lung inflated with air from a liquid-filled, collapsed, or actively degassed state in three important ways: first, it lowers the resistance to aeration that is due to capillarity in the finer conducting airways, reducing the opening pressure represented by the first inflection point of the inflation limb of the pressure-volume curve; second, it facilitates complete aeration of the lung, increasing maximal volume (or reducing the pressure required to establish maximal volume); and third, it stabilizes the lung during deflation, augmenting the amount of air retained in the lung at low transpulmonary pressure and preventing alveolar collapse at end-expiration.

Static pressure-volume diagrams are obtained by applying standardized stepwise increments and decrements of transpulmonary pressure (usually from 0 to 30 or 35 cm $H_2O$ and back to zero), and recording the resulting lung volume changes. Adequate time should be allowed for equilibration at each pressure level to make sure that truly static conditions are established, and volume calculations should be corrected for gas compression in the system. Alternatively, volume-pressure diagrams are generated by stepwise injection and withdrawal of known gas volumes into the lungs, while the resulting changes in airway pressure are recorded.

A simple system for pressure-volume recordings in multiple small experimental animals is illustrated in Figure 14.6 [80]. With this experimental design, the animals are tracheotomized and connected to a system of parallel narrow

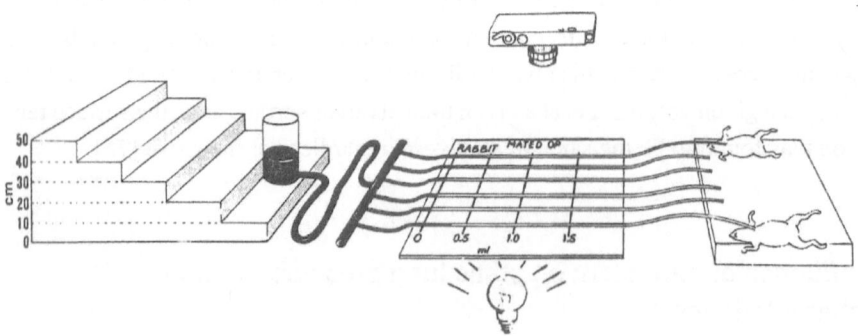

**Figure 14.6. Equipment for parallel recording of lung volumes in multiple experimental animals subjected to identical changes in intratracheal pressure**
A more detailed description is given in the text. From [80] with permission.

glass tubes, which at the other end contain columns of stained water. The fluid is continuous with that in a jar used for stepwise elevation of the insufflation pressure. Movements of stained water in the glass tubes, easily recorded photographically, represent volumes of air entering the lungs of individual animals. If fetal rabbits are examined and the animals are killed *in utero*, the lungs are liquid-filled and thus do not have to be degassed before the experiment.

Criteria for optimal performance of an exogenous surfactant in this experimental model have been outlined [81]. In surfactant-deficient immature rabbit fetuses (gestational age, 27 days), tracheal instillation of an effective surfactant substitute should improve lung stability during deflation to a mature level: static lung volumes above 40 ml/kg at 5 cm $H_2O$ deflation pressure indicate a satisfactory therapeutic response. Such volumes have been reported for immature rabbit fetuses treated with, for example Surfactant TA (Surfacten, Tokyo Tanabe, Tokyo, Japan), human surfactant isolated from amniotic fluid, and Curosurf, but not for animals treated with protein-free synthetic surfactants such as Exosurf (Burroughs Wellcome, Research Triangle Park, NC, USA) or a dry mixture of DPPC and unsaturated phosphatidylglycerol (for review, *see* [81]).

Surfactant-depleted lungs of adult experimental animals is an alternative system for testing the effects of exogenous surfactants on pulmonary pressure-volume characteristics. Bermel et al. [82] introduced a protocol for this purpose, in which excised, vacuum degassed rat lungs were lavaged 15 times via a tracheal cannula with a volume of normal saline corresponding to approximately 50% of TLC. During the subsequent volume-pressure measurements, the lungs were suspended by the tracheal cannula in a cylindrical Plexiglas chamber, heated to 37 °C. According to the original protocol, the lungs were inflated with a syringe pump at a rate of approximately 23 ml/min until transpulmonary pressure, measured with a low capacitance differential pressure transducer between the trachea and the chamber atmosphere, had reached a level of 30 cm $H_2O$. Following 15 min of stress relaxation, allowing additional inflation of air to maintain a transpulmonary pressure of 30 cm $H_2O$, deflation was begun at a rate of 2.3 ml/min and continued until a pressure of 0 cm $H_2O$ was reached (for further details of the experimental protocol, the reader is referred to the original description [82]). The repeated lavage procedure caused a significant shift of the deflation limb of the volume-pressure diagram to the right, indicating failure to stabilize the lungs at low transpulmonary pressures. In contrast to control animals, in which about 10% of TLC was retained in the lungs after deflation to a transpulmonary pressure of 0 cm $H_2O$, the corresponding figure for lavaged animals was only about 2%.

Hall et al. [83] used this model to characterize the physiological properties of various exogenous surfactants, currently used in clinical practice. They found that calf lung surfactant extract (CLSE; Rochester NY, USA) instilled via the airways of the lavaged lung, restored normal stability during deflation. With Exosurf, there was only a slight improvement of lung stability and with Survanta (Beractant, Abbott, North Chicago, IL, USA) an intermediate response. Interestingly, the physiological properties of Exosurf, as evaluated in this model as well as *in vitro* systems, could be improved by addition of hydrophobic proteins (SP-B, SP-C).

Static pressure-volume recordings provide important information on the physical properties of the alveolar surfactant film, especially during compression (deflation). However, a disturbance of lung mechanics secondary to moderately delayed surfactant adsorption may remain unrecognized, as long as time is allowed at each inspiration pressure level to equilibrate surface tension in peripheral airspaces [84]. A complete experimental evaluation of a surfactant substitute must therefore include studies on ventilated surfactant-deficient animals, as detailed in the following sections.

## Animal models for *in vivo* evaluation of exogenous surfactants

In the interest of space and consistency, the following sections will be restricted to *in vivo* models analogous to the "static" models described above, i.e. surfactant-deficient newborn animals and surfactant-depleted adult animals.

### Preterm newborn animals

RDS is a disease of prematurity and its characteristic pathophysiological features including low dynamic lung compliance, low functional residual capacity, poor oxygenation due to shunting of blood through collapsed portions of the lung, retention of $CO_2$, and increased leakage of plasma proteins into the airspaces, can be reproduced in various preterm newborn experimental animals (for review, *see* [85]). These animal models have also been used for testing the efficacy of surfactant replacement under *in vivo* conditions that to some extent simulate clinical routines in a neonatal intensive care unit. In the following paragraphs, experiments on preterm newborn rabbits will serve as a prototype for studies of neonatal lung function before and after surfactant treatment. Analogous experiments have been performed on larger experimental animals such as lambs and monkeys (for review, *see* [85]).

As indicated above, rabbit fetuses delivered at a gestational age of 26–27 days are nearly devoid of endogenous surfactant. Such immature animals are unable to generate the transpulmonary pressure required to expand the lungs at birth, and recordings of the first few breaths show that the small volume of air that enters the lungs with each inspiration is almost completely expelled during expiration. This implies a failure to establish adequate functional residual capacity (FRC). Survival of these animals depends on mechanical ventilation at birth, but lung function of the ventilated animal soon becomes further compromised by necrosis and desquamation of airway epithelium, and profuse leakage of plasma proteins into the alveolar spaces.

Ventilated immature newborn rabbits are suitable for *in vivo* evaluation of lung mechanics after surfactant replacement. One obvious advantage of this animal model is that the pregnant rabbit doe usually carries multiple fetuses, not infrequently as many as 10 or more in each litter. This facilitates parallel functional screening of different surfactant substitutes, with non-treated littermates serving as controls. On the other hand, the small size of these experimental animals (average body weight about 30 g at a gestational age of 27 days) precludes more invasive pathophysiological studies.

Several protocols for *in vivo* evaluation of surfactant substitutes in newborn rabbits have been described in recent years. In general, the fetuses are obtained by hysterotomy, anesthetized at birth with intraperitoneal sodium pentobarbital (suggested dose, 0.6 mg/kg), trachetotomized, kept in body plethysmographs at 37 °C, and paralyzed with intraperitoneal pancuronium bromide (suggested dose, 0.02 mg/kg). They are either ventilated individually [86] or connected in parallel to a common pressure-constant ventilator system. In the latter case, the litter may be subjected to a standardized sequence of insufflation pressures in order to obtain information on the approximate pressure level required to maintain adequate tidal volume [87, 88], or insufflation pressure can be individualized by means of water-locks [89] or valves at the outlet of the side limbs connecting the tracheal tube of each animal with the ventilator system. One simple way to individualize insufflation pressure in a common ventilator system of this type is illustrated in Figure 14.7 [90]. The ventilator is set at a working pressure of, for example, 50 cm $H_2O$, and by varying the length of the connecting tube for each animal, the resistance in the open side limb can be adjusted to provide the appropriate insufflation pressure, corresponding to the tidal volume defined by the protocol (usually about 10 ml/kg). Under these experimental conditions, treatment with surfactant increases dynamic compliance of an immature animal, delivered at a gestational age of 27.5 days, to a level corresponding to that of a mature newborn animal delivered 2 days later [90]. The level of positive end-expiratory pressure (PEEP) should be carefully standardized, especially in studies comparing various exogenous surfactants. The use of PEEP during mechanical ventilation influences several parameters of surfactant function, including dynamic lung compliance and

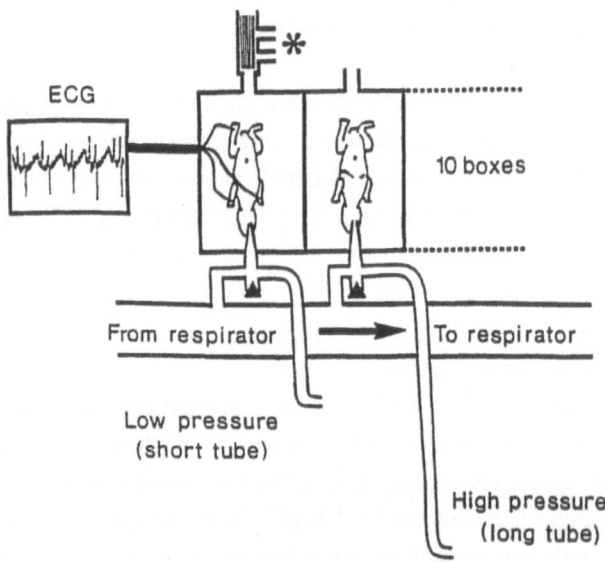

*Figure 14.7. Equipment for parallel ventilation of multiple experimental animals with standardized tidal volume, using a common ventilator and a multi-plethysmograph system*

From the common ventilator tube, narrow high-resistance tubes lead to each tracheal cannula, continuing as open outflow limbs. Tidal volumes are recorded with a Fleisch tube (*) connected to each plethysmograph box. The pressure delivered to each animal is kept at the level required to maintain the tidal volume defined by the protocol by adjusting the length of the open outflow limb, or by adjustable valves (not shown in the figure). (▲) pressure transducer. From [90] with permission.

lung permeability, and these effects may differ for different surfactants, in part depending on their content of surfactant proteins [91, 92].

Passive expiratory flow-volume recordings, generated from the paralysed, ventilated rabbit pups can be used for determination of the expiratory time constant, a parameter strongly influenced by surfactant function. Studies by Noack et al. [93] on immature newborn rabbits have shown that, after treatment with an appropriate dose of modified natural surfactant, this time constant is prolonged by approximately 100%, indicating stabilisation of the airways during expiration. The model can also be used for assessment of end-expiratory gas volume, an equivalent of FRC. If the animals are ventilated with nitrogen for a few minutes before termination of the experiments and the tracheal tube is clamped at end-expiration, then the difference between lung volume (in ml), determined by water displacement as described by Scherle [94], and lung weight (in g) is a good approximation of lung gas volume (in ml).

Lung permeability can be investigated in newborn rabbits (as well as in other experimental animals) by intravenous injection of for example radiolabelled albumin at a standardized time point, and quantification of the marker in lung lavage fluid and lung tissue at the end of the experiment [95]. For assessment of alveolar-to-vascular leakage, the marker is added to the liquid-filled airspaces at birth and quantified in blood sampled after a defined period of ventilation. In other studies, heterologous (human) albumin was used as intravenously injected marker, and the quantity of this protein in lung lavage fluid was assessed by immunodiffusion [96]. Regardless of the method employed, the data are concordant in showing that there is a substantial bidirectional leakage of protein in the ventilated immature lung and that this leakage is strongly influenced by treatment with surfactant. Lung permeability to macromolecules can therefore be regarded as an important, albeit non-specific, parameter of surfactant function.

A uniform pattern of well-aerated alveoli is another good indicator of normal surfactant function. Surfactant deficiency or dysfunction on the other hand is characterized by an irregular expansion pattern with overexpansion of preterminal airspaces during inspiration and wide-spread alveolar collapse at end-expiration (for reasons explained above). These features can be demonstrated in histological lung sections provided that the lungs are fixed under well standardized conditions. Before fixation, the lungs should be expanded with air at a transpulmonary pressure of 30 cm $H_2O$; this pressure should then be lowered to 10 cm $H_2O$, which is maintained while the lungs are perfused via the pulmonary arteries with, for example, a mixture of 3.5% formaldehyde and 1% glutaraldehyde. This method preserves the alveolar expansion pattern at a critical point of the pressure-volume curve, and the addition of glutaraldehyde to the fixative renders the specimen suitable for both light and electron microscopy. The volume density ($V_V$) of the alveolar spaces is easily assessed by conventional point counting, using total parenchyma as reference volume, and irregularity of the expansion pattern with a large field-to-field variability is reflected by a high coefficient of variation for the volume density measurements CV ($V_V$). These and other stereological parameters of alveolar expansion can also be determined by automated image analysis in binarized images of the histological lung sections [97].

In newborn animals, the alveolar $V_V$ determined by these methods is correlated with the compliance of the lungs. A surfactant deficient lung is thus characterized by low values for both $V_V$ and CV ($V_V$), whereas lungs with adequate lung surfactant function and good compliance have a high alveolar $V_V$ associated with low CV ($V_V$). The irregular expansion pattern of an immature lung treated with a suboptimal dose of surfactant is reflected by intermediate values for $V_V$ and high values for CV ($V_V$). Ventilation of a surfactant-deficient lung also results in disruption of airway epithelium, with formation hyaline membranes in bronchioles and alveoli. Treatment with an effective surfactant should prevent these lesions, and an optimal response to surfactant therapy in an immature lung is therefore characterized by a combination of well expanded alveoli and absence of epithelial lesions in the airways (for review, *see* [98]).

## In vivo *lung lavage*

As expected from the static pressure-data cited above, a deficiency of alveolar surfactant can be induced in live mature neonatal or adult experimental animals by repeated lung lavage [99]. This model has been used extensively to study the *in vivo* effects of surfactant replacement in, for example, newborn piglets, and adult guinea pigs and rabbits. As expected, such surfactant-depleted animals have reduced lung compliance and fails to stabilize their lungs at end-expiration. Following the lavage procedure, there is a significant fall in arterial $PO_2$ due to intrapulmonary shunting, but this can be restored to prelavage level by rapid treatment with an adequate dose of surfactant, and the animal can subsequently be weaned from the ventilator [100]. The therapeutic effect of surfactant in this model depends on ventilation with PEEP [101], and on the mode of surfactant administration. For example, a bolus of surfactant instilled in the trachea is distributed more uniformly, and is much more effective than the same material administered by slow infusion into the central airways (Fig. 14.8) [102]. Comparative evaluation of surfactant substitutes thus calls for a well standardized experimental procedure.

The original protocol, proposed by Lachmann et al. [99] for experiments on adult guinea pigs has been modified slightly by other investigators (e.g. [102]) but the basic principles remain unchanged. The lungs of the anesthetized, tracheotomised, and ventilated experimental animals are washed several times via the airways with normal saline (30–35 ml/kg). Between and after each lavage maneuver, the animals are subjected to constant pressure ventilation with 100% oxygen, a peak pressure of 26–30 cm $H_2O$, a frequency of 30/min and 33–50% inspiration time. Respiratory failure is defined as a fall in $PaO_2 < 7$ kPa [98].

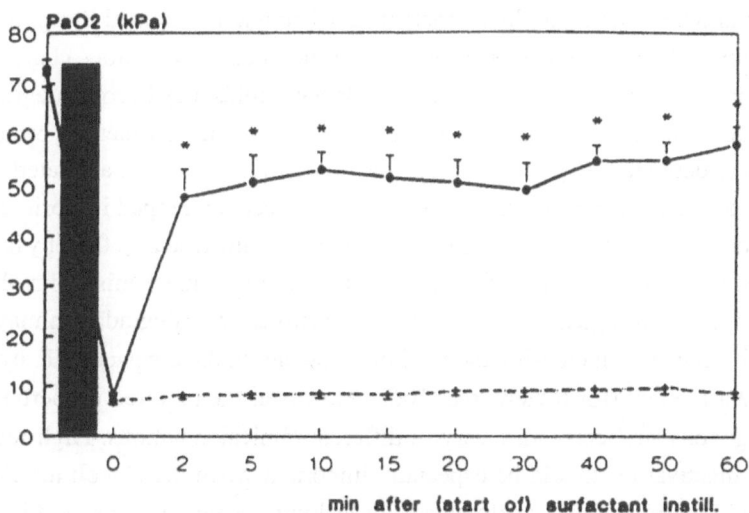

Figure 14.8. Arterial $PO_2$ (mean, SEM) in adult rats ventilated with 100% oxygen, before and after repeated lung lavage and subsequent treatment with Curosurf (200 mg/kg), administered via the airways either rapidly as a bolus (●—●) or by slow infusion over 45 min (+--+) The time axis is discontinuous. Shaded column represents saline lung lavages, time 0 onset of surfactant treatment. The differences between the groups are statistically significant (p < 0.01) during the time period 2–60 min. From [102] with permission.

Repeated *in vivo* lung lavage is a rather clean model of surfactant depletion, involving no other initial insult to the pulmonary parenchyma. However, prolonged ventilation of the surfactant-depleted lungs leads to airway epithelial disruption, intraalveolar edema, hyaline membranes, and recruitment of granulocytes [103]. These inflammatory changes may inactivate surfactant in the airspaces (*see* below), and the response to exogenous surfactant may therefore vary with the time interval between the lavage procedure and surfactant treatment. Satisfactory results, characterized by rapid restoration of pre-lavage levels for PaO$_2$, have been obtained with modified natural surfactants [100–103] as well as with artificial surfactants based on hydrophobic synthetic peptides [104, 105].

## Comments

Surfactant function may be disturbed in several forms of neonatal lung disease other than RDS. For example, surfactant may become inactivated by aspirated meconium or by leaking plasma proteins in inflammatory conditions characterized by increased alveolar permeability. Surfactant lipids may become degraded by phospholipases produced by invading bacteria, and surfactant proteins cleaved or deranged by proteases and free radicals released from activated granulocytes and macrophages. Surfactant may also become trapped in fibrin clots (this could happen both in RDS and in inflammatory lung disease), thereby being retracted from its normal site of action. Irrespective of the mechanisms involved in the pathophysiological events, surfactant inactivation or degradation may be counterbalanced by increasing the pool of surfactant in the airspaces, i.e. by replacement therapy (for review, *see* [106]). However, the required properties of the exogenous surfactant may vary in different clinical situations. High resistance to inactivation should be especially important when the alveoli are filled with aspirated meconium or flooded with leaking plasma proteins, and bacteriostatic effects are potentially important in case of infectious pneumonia. Both resistance to inactivation and mode of interaction with bacteria and viruses depend on the composition of the surfactant preparation, expecially its content of specific proteins [107, 108]. The hydrophilic surfactant protein SP-A (absent in all exogenous surfactants prepared by extraction with organic solvents) both increases resistance to inactivation by plasma proteins and stimulates phagocytosis and killing of bacteria by alveolar macrophages. SP-D (likewise absent in commercially available surfactants) has an even stronger, but otherwise similar effect on alveolar macrophages.

Within the near future, a new generation of surfactant substitutes, based on synthetic peptides mimicking the structure and function of the natural surfactant proteins, will probably compete on the market with currently available modified natural and protein-free synthetic surfactants. These preparations could perhaps be tailored to optimize resistance to inactivation or interaction with phagocytic cells. An interesting example, illustrating this concept, is the recently developed artificial surfactant peptide $KL_4$ (consisting of repeat sequences of lysine and leucine) [109]. An artificial, physiologically active surfactant made from the $KL_4$-peptide and synthetic lipids is significantly more resistant to inactivation by hypochlorous acid (a reactive oxidizing species released by activated granulocytes) than is Survanta [110].

The *in vitro* test systems described above (Wilhelmy balance, pulsating bubble surfactometer, and captive bubble) are suitable for testing resistance to surfactant inactivation. Various concentrations of surfactants can thus be exposed to different amounts of "inhibitor", either mixed with the surfactant preparation or added by means of a hypophase exchange system (available in modern versions of the pulsating bubble and captive bubble systems). Animal models of meconium aspiration syndrome, neonatal pneumonia, lung hypoplasia, and the "adult" form of acute respiratory distress syndrome (ARDS), allowing *in vivo* testing of various exogenous surfactants with particular reference to physiological and bacteriostatic effects, have been developed in recent years (for review, *see* [111, 112]). New surfactant substitutes should be carefully studied in these models, as well as in models of lung immaturity, before final evaluation in clinical trials.

# Acknowledgements

This work was supported by Swedish Medical Research Council (Project No. 3351), Konung Oscar II:s Jubileumsfond, the Medical Research Council of Canada and the Alberta Heritage Foundation for Medical Research.

# References

1 Walther FJ and Taeusch HW (1992) Patho-physiology of Neonatal Surfactant Insuffi-ciency: Clinical Aspects. In: *Pulmonary Surfactant. From Molecular Biology to Clinical Practice,* Robertson B, van Golde LMG and Batenburg JJ (eds), p. 485, Elsevier Amsterdam

2 Chung JB, Shanks PC, Hanneman RE and Frances EI (1990) *Colloids Surfaces* **43**: 223

3 Exerowa D, Lalchev Z, Marinow B and Orgnyanov K (1986) *Langmuir* **2**: 664

4 Langmuir I (1917) *J. Am. Chem. Soc.* **39**: 1848

5 Pockels A (1891) *Nature* **43**: 437

6 Adamson AW (1990) *Physical Chemistry of Surfaces* (Fifth Edition). John Wiley and Sons New York

7 Clements JA (1957) *Proc Soc. Exp. Biol. Med.* **95**: 170

8 Adam NK (1968) *The Physics and Chemistry of Surfaces.* Dover Publications, New York

9 Gaines GL (1972) *J. Colloid Interface Sci.* **60**: 210

10 Scarpelli EM (1968) *The Surfactant System of the Lung.* Lea and Febiger, Philadelphia

11 Hildebran JN, Goerke J and Clements JA (1979) *J. Appl. Physiol.* **47**: 604

12 Notter RH (1984) Surface Chemistry of Pulmonary Surfactant: The Role of Individual Components. In: *Pulmonary Surfactant,* Robertson B, Van Golde LMG and Batenburg JJ (eds), p. 17, Elsevier Amsterdam

13 Munden JW and Swarbrick J (1973) *J. Colloid Interface Sci.* **42**: 657

14 Boonman A, Machiels FHJ, Suik AFM and Egberts J (1987) *J. Colloid Interface Sci.* **120**: 452

15 Clements JA, Hustead RF, Johnson RP and Gribetz I (1961) *J. Appl. Physiol.* **16**: 444

16 Schoedel W, Slama H and Hansen E (1971) *Pfluegers Arch.* **322**: 336

17 Qiu R and MacDonald RC (1994) *Rev. Sci. Instr.* **62**: 500

18 Goerke J and Gonzales J (1971) *J. Appl. Physiol.* **51**: 1108

19 Notter RH and Morrow PE (1975) *Annals Biomed. Engin.* **3**: 119

20 Schürch FS (1975) Thesis, The University of Western Ontario

21 Slama H, Schoedel W and Hansen E (1971) *Pfluegers Arch.* **322**: 355

22 Slama H, Schoedel W and Hansen E (1973) *Respir. Physiol.* **19**: 233

23 Enhorning G (1977) *J. Appl. Physiol.* **43**: 198

24 Possmayer F (1991) Biophysical Activity of Pulmonary Surfactant. In: *Fetal and Neona-tal Physiology,* Polin RA and Fox WW (eds), p. 459, WB Saunders Philadelphia

25 Putz G, Goerke J, Taeusch HW and Clements JA (1994) *J. Appl. Physiol.* **76**: 1425

26 Schürch S, Bachofen H, Goerke J and Possmayer F (1989) *J. Appl. Physiol.* **67**: 2389

27 Schürch S, Bachofen H, Goerke J and Green F (1992) *Biochim. Biophys. Acta* **1103**: 127

28 Putz G, Schürch S, Goerke J and Clements JA (1994) *J. Appl. Physiol.* **76**: 2389

29 Schoel WM, Schürch S and Goerke J (1994) *Biochim. Biophys. Acta* **1200**: 286

30 Rotenberg YL, Boruvka L and Neumann AW (1983) *J. Colloid Interface Sci.* **93**: 169

31 Schürch S, Possmayer F, Cheng S and Cockshutt AM (1992) *Am. J. Physiol.* **263**: L210

32 Pattle RE (1955) *Nature* **175**: 1125

33 Pattle RE (1958) *Proc. Roy. Soc. B* **148**: 217

34 Pattle RE (1976) The Lung Surfactant in the Evolutionary Tree. In: *Respiration of Amphibious Vertebrates,* Hughes GM (ed.),

p. 234, Academic Press New York

35  Pattle RE, Kratzing CC, Parkinson CE et al. (1979) *Br. J. Obstet. Gynaecol.* **86**: 615

36  Chida S (1995) A Stable Microbubble Test for Antenatal and Early Neonatal Diagnosis of Surfactant Deficiency. In: *Surfactant Therapy for Lung Disease*, Robertson B and Tauesch HW (eds), p. 107, Marcel Dekker New York

37  Chida S, Fujiwara T, Takahashi A, Kanehama S and Kaneko J (1991) *Acta Paediatr. Jpn.* **33**: 15

38  Chida S and Fujiwara T (1993) *Eur. J. Pediatr.* **152**: 148

39  Chida S, Fujiwara T, Konishi M, Takahashi H and Sasaki M (1993) *Eur. J. Pediatr.* **152**: 148

40  Berggren P, Eklind J, Linderholm B and Robertson B (1992) *Biol. Neonate* **61**(suppl 1): 15

41  Berggren P and Linderholm B (1996) *Biol. Neonate* **69**: 133

42  Epstein PS and Plesset MS (1950) *J. Chem. Phys.* **18**: 1505

43  Schürch S, Schürch D, Curstedt T and Robertson B (1994) *J. Appl. Physiol.* **77**: 974

44  Schürch S, Qanbar R, Bachofen H and Possmayer F (1995) *Biol. Neonate* **67**(suppl 1): 61

45  Schürch S, Wallace JA, Wilkinson MH and McIver DJL (1989) Protein Adsorption at Air Water Interfaces Stabilised by Phospholipids Related to Pulmonary Surfactant: Microbubbles as an Ultrasonic Contrast Agent. In: *Surfactants in Solution*, Mittal KL (ed.), Plenum Press New York

46  Overbeek JTG (1971) *Colloid and Surface Chemistry Study Guide* (third printing, 1981), Lectures, Massachusetts Institute of Technology, Center for Advanced Engineering Study, MIT

47  Chang C-H and Franses EI (1995) *Colloids Surfaces* **100**: 1

48  Andrade JD (1985) Principles of Protein Adsorption. In: *Surface and Interfacial Aspects of Biomedical Polymers*, Andrade JD (ed.), p. 1, Plenum Press New York

49  Davies JT and Rideal EK (1963) *Interfacial Phenomena*, Academic Press New York

50  Curstedt T, Jörnvall H, Robertson B, Bergman T and Berggren P (1987) *Eur. J. Biochem.* **168**: 255

51  Hawgood S, Benson BJ, Schilling J, Damm D and Clements JA (1987) *Proc. Natl. Acad. Sci. USA* **84**: 66

52  Yu S-H and Possmayer F (1990) *Biochim. Biophys. Acta* **1046**: 233

53  Qanbar R, Cheng S, Possmayer F and Schürch S (1996) *Am. J. Physiol.* **271**: L572

54  Damodaran S and Song KB (1989) Adsorption of Protein of the Air-Water Interface: Role of Protein Conformation. In: *Surfactants in Solution*, Mittal KL (ed.), p. 391, Plenum Press New York

55  Graham DE and Phillips MC (1979) *J. Colloid Interface Sci.* **70**: 415

56  Birdi KS (1973) *J. Colloid Interface Sci.* **43**: 545

57  Weibel ER and Gil J (1968) *Respir. Physiol.* **4**: 42

58  Gil J and Weibel ER (1969/70) *Respir. Physiol.* **8**: 13

59  Schürch S and Bachofen H (1995) Biophysical Aspects in the Design of a Therapeutic Surfactant. In: *Surfactant Therapy for Lung Disease*, Robertson B and Taeusch HW (eds), p. 3, Marcel Dekker New York

60  Grossmann G and Robertson B (1975) *Acta Paediatr. Scand.* **64**: 7

61  Ueda S, Izumi T, Ishii N, Matsumoto S, Hayashi K and Okayasu M (1982) *J. Jpn. Med. Soc. Biol. Interface* **13**: 26

62  Clements JA (1977) *Am. Rev. Respir. Dis.* **115**: 67

63  Gaines GL (1966) *Insoluble Monolayers at Liquid-Gas Interfaces*. Interscience Publishers, John Wiley and Sons New York

64  Grotberg JB (1994) *J. Fluid Mech.* **26**: 529

65 Grotberg JB, Halpern D and Jensen OE (1995) *J. Appl. Physiol.* **78**: 750

66 King RJ and Clements JA (1972) *Am. J. Physiol.* **223**: 715

67 Putz G, Goerke J and Clements JA (1994) *J. Appl. Physiol.* **77**: 597

68 Joos P and Van Hunsel J (1985) *J. Colloid Interface Sci.* **106**: 161

69 Gaver DP and Grotberg JB (1992) *J. Fluid Mech.* **235**: 399

70 Jensen OE and Grotberg JB (1992) *J. Fluid Mech.* **240**: 259

71 Jensen OE, Halpern D and Grotberg JB (1994) *Chem. Engin. Sci.* **49**: 1107

72 Schürch S, Goerke J and Clements JA (1976) *Proc. Natl. Acad. Sci. USA* **73**: 4698

73 Schürch S, Goerke J and Clements JA (1978) *Proc. Natl. Acad. Sci. USA* **75**: 3417

74 Williams EJ (1959) *Regression Analysis.* John Wiley and Sons New York

75 Schürch S (1982) *Respir. Physiol.* **48**: 339

76 Schürch S, Bachofen H and Weibel ER (1985) *Respir. Physiol.* **62**: 31

77 Bachofen H, Schürch S, Urbinelli M and Weibel ER (1987) *J. Appl. Physiol.* **62**: 1878

78 Bastacky J, Lee CYC, Goerke J, Koushafar H, Yager D, Kenega L, Speed TP, Chen Y and Clements JA (1995) *J. Appl. Physiol.* **79**: 1615

79 von Neergaard K (1929) *Z. Ges. Exp. Med.* **66**: 373

80 Enhörning G and Robertson B (1972) *Pediatrics* **50**: 58

81 Fujiwara T and Robertson B (1992) Pharmacology of Exogenous Surfactant. In: *Pulmonary Surfactant. From Molecular Biology to Clinical Practice,* Robertson B, van Golde LMG and Batenburg JJ (eds), p. 561, Elsevier Amsterdam

82 Bermel MS, McBride JT and Notter RH (1984) *Lung* **162**: 99

83 Hall SB, Venkitaraman AR, Whitsett JA, Holm BA and Notter RH (1992) *Am. Rev. Respir. Dis.* **145**: 24

84 Kobayashi T, Li W-Z, Tashiro K, Takahashi R, Waseda Y, Yamamoto K and Suzuki Y (1996) *J. Appl. Physiol.* **80**: 62

85 Robertson B (1992) Animal Models of Neonatal Surfactant Dysfunction. In: *Pulmonary Surfactant. From Molecular Biology to Clinical Practice,* Robertson B, van Golde LMG and Batenburg JJ (eds), p. 459, Elsevier Amsterdam

86 Yukitake K, Brown CL, Schlueter MA, Clements JA and Hawgood S (1995) *Pediatr. Res.* **37**: 21

87 Berggren P, Curstedt T, Grossmann G, Nilsson R and Robertson B (1985) *Exp. Lung Res.* **8**: 29

88 Kobayashi T, Nitta K, Ganzuka M, Inui S, Grossmann G and Robertson B (1991) *Pediatr. Res.* **29**: 353

89 Ikegami M, Berry D, Elkady T, Pettenazzo A, Seidner S and Jobe A (1987) *J. Clin. Invest.* **79**: 1371

90 Sun B, Kobayashi T, Curstedt T, Grossmann G and Robertson B (1991) *Eur. Respir. J.* **4**: 364

91 Rider ED, Jobe AH, Ikegami M and Sun B (1992) *J. Appl. Physiol.* **73**: 2089

92 Rider ED, Ikegami M, Whitsett JA, Hull W, Absolom D and Jobe AH (1993) *Am. Rev. Respir. Dis.* **147**: 669

93 Noack G, Curstedt T, Grossmann G, Nilsson R and Robertson B (1990) *Respiration* **57**: 1

94 Scherle W (1970) *Mikroskopie* **26**: 57

95 Robertson B, Berry D, Curstedt T, Grossmann G, Ikegami M, Jacobs H, Jobe A and Jones S (1985) *Respir. Physiol.* **61**: 265

96 Anceschi MM, Robertson B, Broccucci L. Barbati A, Grossmann G, Hedenborg L, Lundberg E, Petrelli A, Zaccardo G and Cosmi EV (1990) *Exp. Lung Res.* **16**: 593

97 Rigaut JP and Robertson B (1986) *Pediatr. Pathol.* **6**: 11

98 Robertson B and Lachmann B (1988) *Exp. Lung Res.* **14**: 279

99 Lachmann B, Robertson B and Vogel J (1980) *Acta Anaesthesiol. Scand.* **24**: 231

100 Bambang Oetomo S, Reijngoud D-J, Ennema JJ, Okken A and Wildevuur ChRH (1988) *Lung* **166**: 65

101 Kobayashi T, Kataoka H, Ueda T, Murakami S, Takada Y and Kokubo M (1984) *J. Appl. Physiol.* **57**: 995

102 Segerer H, van Gelder W, Angenent FWM, van Woerkens LJPM, Curstedt T, Obladen M and Lachmann B (1993) *Pediatr. Res.* **34**: 490

103 Berggren P, Lachmann B, Curstedt T, Grossmann G and Robertson B (1986) *Acta Anaesthesiol. Scand.* **30**: 321

104 Sood SL, Balaraman V, Finn KC, Britton B, Uyehara CFT and Easa D (1996) *Am. J. Respir. Crit. Care Med.* **153**: 820

105 Häfner D, Germann PG and Hauschke (1994) *Pulm. Pharmacol.* **7**: 319

106 Walther FJ (1995) Surfactant Therapy for Neonatal Lung Disorders Other than Respiratory Distress Syndrome. In: *Surfactant Therapy for Lung Disease*, Robertson B and Taeusch HW (eds), p. 461, Marcel Dekker New York

107 Günther A and Seeger W (1995) Resistance to Surfactant Inactivation. In: *Surfactant Therapy for Lung Disease*, Robertson B and Taeusch HW (eds), p. 269, Marcel Dekker New York

108 van Iwaarden F and van Golde LMG (1995) Pulmonary Surfactant and Lung Defense. Interactions of Surfactant Proteins with Phagocytic Cells and Pathogens. In: *Surfactant Therapy for Lung Disease*, Robertson B and Taeusch HW (eds), p. 75, Marcel Dekker New York

109 Cochrane CG and Revak SD (1991) *Science* **254**: 566

110 Merritt TA, Amirkhanian JD, Helbock H, Halliwell B and Cross CE (1993) *Biochem. J.* **295**: 19

111 Robertson B (1995) Experimental Models for Evaluation of Exogenous Surfactants. In: *Surfactant Therapy for Lung Disease*, Robertson B and Taeusch HW (eds), p. 239, Marcel Dekker New York

112 Robertson B (1996) *Arch. Dis. Child* **75**: F1

# Cell culture

Cell culture

# 15 Isolation of type II alveolar epithelial cells

*J.S. Lwebuga-Mukasa*

In this chapter we will briefly review the techniques available for isolation and culture of type II pneumocytes and describe in detail a technique for the rapid isolation of adult rat type II cells. The lung consists of 40 different cell types of which type II cells make up 15% [1]. Type II alveolar epithelial cells are important for normal lung function [2] and in regeneration of lung epithelium following injury [3, 4]. They synthesize and secrete surfactant phospholipids and proteins that are required for lowering surface tension at low lung volumes. Type II cells also participate in many other functions such as inflammatory and immune responses, oxidant metabolism, fluid transport, and electrolyte transport. To investigate how these functions are regulated, it is important to study pure type II cell populations. Many different methods have been developed to isolate type II cells for study *in vitro* (reviewed in [5]). *In vitro* studies are still limited by the rapid loss of differentiated functions of type II cells in culture [6]. Furthermore, the most commonly used isolation techniques require culturing type II cells for 1–2 days before they are available for study. Most techniques that permit isolation and immediate study of type II cells either have limited cell yields [5] or require specialized equipment not routinely available. In this chapter, we will discuss the techniques available for type II cell isolation and describe a method for isolation of adult rat type pneumocytes for immediate use.

## Why do we need to isolate cells for *in vitro* studies?

Because type II cell isolation requires investment of time and resources, it is important to first determine whether the question to be studied does indeed require the use of isolated cells. Next, we need to determine whether adequate numbers of the cells will be obtained for the planned studies. Consideration should be given to whether the expected cell purity will permit reasonable interpretation of the data. To address some specific questions, it may be reasonable to use a cell line and/or lung slices in combination with immunocytochemistry and/or *in situ* hybridization. The observations made on these systems can then be combined with selected experiments with primary isolated cells.

## Strategies for isolation of type II cells

We have not found a universally applicable type II cell isolation technique. Strategies for type II cell isolation vary depending on the developmental stage of the lung (i.e. embryonic, fetal, neonatal, or adult) and with species. Some procedures described for one species may not work as well with another species. Hence, the investigator needs to empirically optimize the isolation conditions for a given system. For example, as reviewed by Dobbs [5], type II cell size varies among and within species, state of lung growth and development, functional state and repair. Such variations need to be taken into account when choosing a type II cell isolation method. This may be especially challenging when human adult lung tissue is utilized and the investigator has no control over sample-to-sample variations. A number of reports have been published using human type II cells, e.g. [7–9].

The age of animals from which cells are to be isolated needs to be considered. This is important because cells isolated from lungs at different developmental stages may show different biosynthetic functions and other characteristics. Isolation of fetal type II cells presents special challenges because the cells at different developmental stages may not have all the functional features of mature type II cells. Investigators in this area have used an explant system or subcultured pre-type II cells on collagen sponges [10, 11]. Despite variations in details, type II cell isolation techniques from diverse systems share a number of common steps: removal of blood products from the lung, enzymatic digestion of the tissue; mechanical separation or loosening of the cells to free them from structural components, selective recovery of dissociated cells and finally, char-acterization of isolated cells. We will consider each of these steps separately.

# Methods

## Steps in type II cell isolation

### Removal of blood products and alveolar macrophages

Serum components contain inhibitors that block enzymatic digestion of tissues. It is therefore important to remove serum from the lungs to prevent protease inhibitors from interfering with enzymatic digestion of the tissue. In the rat, this is most easily accomplished by perfusion of the pulmonary vascular tree with a needle or catheter inserted in the right ventricle, until the lungs look white. Alveolar macrophages are a potential contaminating cell population. These cells are found in the airways and the alveolar spaces. Alveolar macrophages are removed by several installations of Ca-free saline buffer via the airway, and by allowing the fluid to drain out by gravity. The adequacy of the lavages in removing the macrophages needs to be assessed for the system being studied.

### Dissociating lung tissues with digestive enzymes

### Selecting the enzyme combinations

The next step is to dissociate type II cells from their tight epithelial connections and attachment to the alveolar basement membrane. This step requires enzymatic digestion. A number of enzymes, singly or in combinations, have been reported including pancreatic elastase, trypsin, clostridial collagenase, pronase, and dispase. These enzymes are either instilled in the airways, into the alveolar space, or incubated with minced lung tissue.

Most commonly, the enzyme solution is instilled in the airways and the tissue incubated at 37 °C for varying periods of time, which is empirically determined to provide maximum release of epithelial cells with minimum disruption of the interstitial layer. Alternatively, lungs may also be perfused with the digestive enzyme mix [12]. To release type II cells, the enzymes have to digest proteins involved in the formation of cell–cell interactions as well as those involved in cell–basement membrane interactions. Once the cells have been loosened from the tissue, mechanical disruption is usually required to obtain free cell suspensions. To minimize contamination with airway epithelial cells, large airways are dissected away from the alveolar tissue, prior to the mechanical disruption. Filtration through a coarse Nytex filter removes collagenous tissue and large cell clumps.

## Recovery of dissociated cells

### Strategies for selective isolation

The free cell suspensions contain mixtures of cells from which type II cells need to be isolated. For this reason, a number of approaches have been described for selective capture of type II cells. Earlier methods used density gradient centrifugation with albumin, Ficoll, or Metrizamide. This approach takes advantage of differences in buoyant densities of type II and other cells. The buoyant densities of type II cells depend on the phospholipid content of type II cells and the cell size in comparison to the other cell types. Positive selection techniques have been described in which cell surface marker protein or lectin binding characteristic has been used in combination with flow cytometry and more recently, with an antibody linked to magnetized beads. Cell separation using magnetic beads in combination with an antibody to a cell surface component has also been utilized in isolation of murine type II cells [13]. These investigators used intratracheal instillation of dispase and agarose followed by mechanical dissociation. The cell suspension was then subjected to negative selection with antibody. Alternatively, a negative selection approach has been taken in parallel studies in which the contaminating cells, usually alveolar macrophages, were removed by selective adhesion on the IgG of Fc-coated dishes. Studies involving isolation of subpopulations of type II cells use centrifugal elutriation [14].

The most frequently used method is that of selective cell adherence because of its relative ease and good cell yields [15]. Following elastase dissociation of lung cells, alveolar macrophages and leukocytes are removed by selective adhesion to tissue culture vessels coated with normal goat IgG or antibodies to common leukocyte antigen [15, 16]. Type II cells, which lack Fc receptors, remain in suspension but subsequently, adhere to culture vessels in presence of serum over 16–24 h. Lymphocytes and most other contaminating cells remain in suspension [5]. Using this approach, type II cell preparations that are greater than 90% pure can be obtained in good yields. A major drawback to this technique is the required prolonged incubation of type II cells (16–24 h) before they are available for study.

Type II cell isolation by centrifugal elutriation [17] requires expensive, specialized equipment. While the technique provides highly purified type II cells and subtypes of type II cells, it suffers from low cell yields and prolonged isolation times. Cell sorting techniques require surface labeling and considerable sorting times which may be complicated by problems with sterility and low cell yields [18, 19]. Another technique which uses lectin agglutination to remove macrophages has also been described [20]. However, this procedure requires adhesion of type II cells to separate them from other cells. A combination of natural fluorescence and orthogonal light scatter have been shown to discriminate between type II cells, macrophages and monocytes. However, this technique has not been widely applied since its description [21]. A technique that permits isolation of type II cells in good yields and purity for immediate assay would be especially useful.

Our laboratory has observed that 0.1 to 1 mM $Mn^{2+}$ promoted rapid adhesion of type II cells on fibronectin coated vessels and dishes coated with a genetically engineered 75 000 kDa polymer protein ProNectin-F (Protein Polymer Technologies, Inc., San Diego, CA) [22]. The protein contains repeating Arginine-Glycine-Aspartate (RGD) sequences interspersed with silk peptide segments [23, 24]. We used porcine pancreatic elastase, in combination with a low concentration of trypsin, to dissociate the lung cells. Macrophages were removed by 1 h adhesion on purified, normal goat IgG-coated Petri dishes. Non-adherent type II cells were then adhered on the ProNectin-F-coated dishes in presence of 0.5 mM $Mn^{2+}$. Adherent type II cells were then detached by a brief treatment with 0.025% trypsin in 2 mM EDTA in HEPES buffered saline pH 7.4. Isolated type II cells were immediately used for studies of cell adhesion and spreading on different extracellular matrix components in the presence of different divalent cations. This technique reduced the period between cell lung dissociation and time of study from the previous 16–24 h to 2–2.5 h following the cell dissociation step.

## Characterization of isolated type II cells

Once the cells have been isolated, it is important to assess the purity of the isolation. The ideal type II cell marker would be easily detected by a readily available assay that could be performed on a relatively small number of the cells, preferably non-destructively. The assay should be specific for type II cells. An increasing number of reagents [18, 25, 26] are becoming available which should in the future permit development of a panel of markers characterizing type II cells.

### *Morphology*

Transmission electron microscopy is "the gold standard" for the morphological characterization of type II cells. By this technique type II cells are recognized as cuboidal cells with numerous cytoplasmic lamellar bodies, the storage organelles of surfactant phospholipids. The apical surface contains microvilli. Lamellar bodies have been described in other cell types. Electron microscopy technique is time consuming, expensive, and requires specialized equipment.

The limitations of transmission electron microscopy technique have led to the development of alternative techniques for type II cell identification: a commonly used technique involves the use of tannic acid and osmium tetraoxide introduced in [27]. In this technique the lamellar bodies containing surfactant phospholipids are stained intense black with osmium tetraoxide in the presence of tannic acid. The cytoplasm can be counter-stained with eosin. The cells can be evaluated with an ordinary light microscope. The limitation of this technique is that non-epithelial cells, such as macrophages that have ingested lamellar bodies, may be mistaken for type II cells. However, in most cases, when this technique is combined with another characteristic, it can be used as an adequate identifying feature of type II cells. Papanicolau stain has been combined with alkaline phosphatase or phospholipid profile in the characterization of isolated type II cells [28].

## Surfactant phospholipid profile

Characterization of type II cells based on surfactant phospholipids is based on the recognition that adult type II cells have a phospholipid profile rich in phosphatidyl choline, at least 60% of which is disaturated; two to 8% of the phospholipids are phosphatidyl glycerol. However, characterization solely based on the phospholipid profile can be misleading since the characteristic pattern is rapidly lost in culture. Furthermore, cell characterization using this technique is laborious and in itself requires substantial numbers of cells that may not be available in some studies. Moreover, during some developmental states or during rapid remodeling, type II cells may not express the characteristic phospholipid profile.

## Immunochemical techniques

Antibodies to SP-A, -B and -C have been used for identification, during early fetal lung development, of type II cells. Among the three, SP-C is specific for type II cells in mature lungs. However, SP-C is expressed in other epithelial cells, but becomes restricted to distal airspaces as the lung matures. SP-A and SP-B are also expressed by Clara cells. Outside the lung, other cells in the gastrointestinal system have been reported to express combinations of the surfactant associated proteins. These markers share the limitation described for phospholipids in that they are rapidly lost in cells maintained in culture. Patterns of expression of the surfactant proteins depend on maturation stage and functional status. Furthermore, immunostaining for these proteins requires permeation of the cells. These limitations have stimulated a search for a cell surface marker for type II cells.

A number of such reagents have been reported [18, 25, 26]. Antibodies to pneumocin: antibodies to these cell surface glycoproteins can be used as surface markers of type II cells. Pneumocin is however also expressed on Clara cells. Its expression decreases when type II cells are maintained in culture on plastic. Alkaline phosphatase: alkaline phosphatase can be found in a number of epithelial cell types and is not a unique marker of type II cells [7]. However, when combined with other characteristics, alkaline phosphatase can be used as a functional marker of type II cells [7–9].

## Adhesion and culture on different substrata

Since type II cells rapidly lose their differentiated functions in culture, there is a major interest in developing systems that may permit maintenance of the differentiated state. A variety of systems have been developed for type II cell culture. Selection of a culture system depends on the question the investigator wishes to study. Most commonly, the investigator seeks to isolate and use type II cells within the first 24 to 48 h following cell isolation. This allows cell recovery from the isolation, and at the same time the type II cells retain some features of differentiated type II cells. However, isolated type II cells may express a wider repertoire of integrins and increase their synthesis of extracellular matrix components than they normally do in intact tissue.

### Selection of CO₂ atmospheric conditions

Type II cells are usually cultured in a $CO_2$ atmosphere of 10%. This is believed to more closely simulate the $CO_2$ environment in the lung. Interestingly, there has been very little information about the effect of $CO_2$ environment on type II cell functions.

### Selection of substrata for culture

Differentiation and function of alveolar type II cells can be regulated by culture of the cells on floating collagen gels. Collagen gels have been used in studies of type II cell differentiation in culture [29].

Matrigel is a laminin-rich reconstituted basement membrane fraction from EHS sarcoma. It has been used to culture type II cells. Cells cultured in Matrigel gel form alveolar structures and retain a number of differentiated features of type II cells. However, the presence of bound growth factors in Matrigel may complicate interpretation of some observations.

The contributions of soluble growth factors must be considered. A number of cytokines and growth factors have been shown to regulate type II epithelial differentiation and function. Of great interest is the keratinocyte growth factor which has been reported to promote type II cell growth *in vivo* [30], decrease hyperoxia-induced mortality in rats [31] and induce expression of differentiated function in cultured type II cells [32]. Soluble growth factors may become bound on culture substrata. At these locations, the factors may achieve much higher concentrations than would be expected in solution.

Selection of animal species: the rat is the most commonly used species because it is economical to maintain in the laboratory. As a result, there already exists a large body of information about isolation and culture techniques and developmental issues using rat cells. However, species differences must be taken into account when generalizing results. There is less information about type II isolation in murine systems which are most frequently needed for recombinant studies.

## Mn⁺⁺-enhanced technique for pneumocyte isolation (this procedure was adapted from [22])

*Reagents*

Dulbeccos's Modified Eagle's Medium (DMEM), penicillin and streptomycin, and trypsin 1:250 were purchased from Gibco (Grand Island, NY). Fetal calf serum (FCS) was purchased from Hyclone (Logan, UT). Type I collagen was purchased from Collagen Corporation (Palo Alto, CA). Mouse type IV collagen, human fibronectin, Matrigel and mouse laminin were obtained from Collaborative Research (Bedford, MA). Purified normal goat IgG was purchased from Cappel/Organon Teknika Corporation (Durham, NC). ProNectin-F was purchased from Protein Polymer Technologies (San Diego, CA). Porcine pancreatic elastase lot #887651 (specific activity 76.6 units/mg) was from Elastin Products Incorporated (Pacific, MO). All other reagents were of the purest grade available and were purchased from Sigma (St. Louis, MO). Nytex mesh was obtained from Tetko (Elmsford, NY).

## Type II Cell Isolation

Type II alveolar epithelial cells were isolated from four adult 150–200 g Sprague Dawley male or female rats from Harlan Sprague Dawley (Indianapolis, IN). Each animal was killed by a lethal injection with 4 g of Pentobarbital intraperitoneally and heparin 550 units in a total volume of 1 ml. The chest was opened and the pulmonary vascular bed perfused with 30 ml of N-2-Hydroxyethylpiperizine-N'-2-ethanesulfonic acid (HEPES)-buffered saline pH 7.4, containing: 140 mM NaCl, 5 mM KCl, 2.5 mM $Na_2HPO_4$, 5 mM glucose, and 10 mM HEPES (Solution I), through the right ventricle to remove blood. The lungs were lavaged with five 10 ml aliquots of solution I at 4 °C to remove free alveolar macrophages.

Cell dissociation was then accomplished by intratracheal instillation of two 10 ml aliquots of Solution II (140 mM NaCl, 5 mM KCl, 2.5 mM $Na_2HPO_4$, 5 mM glucose, 1.4 mM $CaCl_2$, 1.9 mM $MgCl_2$ and 10 mM HEPES pH 7.4), containing porcine pancreatic elastase 30 units/ml and trypsin 1:250 at 50 mg/ml. The lungs were incubated for 20 min in a water bath at 37 °C in a total volume of 160 ml. Following the incubation, the lungs were removed with a pair of sterile forceps from the enzyme solution. The enzyme digestion was stopped by instillation of two 10 ml aliquots of solution II containing 30% fetal calf serum (FCS) and DNAse type I at 5 mg/ml. The digested lungs were teased to a fine suspension with forceps to free the cells. The cell suspension was incubated at 37 °C for 10 min to allow DNAse to degrade the freed cell DNA. The cell suspension was then filtered sequentially through 110, 41 m Nytex filters (Tetko, Elmsford, NY). The cell pellet was obtained by centrifugation at 1400 rpm in a Centura 7R IEC centrifuge (International Equipment Company, Needham Heights, MA) for 10 min at 4 °C. The supernatant was centrifuged at the same rate for a second time and the two pellets were pooled. The cells were washed twice with 40 ml aliquots of solution II. The cells were then resuspended in 40 ml of DMEM, containing 10% FCS, Penicillin 100U units/ml and Streptomycin 100 mg/ml. Five ml aliquots were plated on 100-mm diameter Petri dishes (Falcon, Oxnard, CA), previously coated with purified normal goat IgG at 500 mg/ml. The plates were incubated at 37 °C in a humidified atmosphere of 10% $CO_2$ to remove macrophages as described by Dobbs et al. [15]. Following the incubation, non-adherent cells were removed and pelleted by centrifugation at 1400 rpm in the Centura 7R IEC centrifuge for 10 min at 4 °C. The cell pellet was washed once with 45 ml of HEPES-buffered saline pH 7.4, containing 1% radioimmunoassay (RIA) grade serum bovine albumin (BSA), 5 mM glucose and 5 mM KCl. The cells were then resuspended in 40 mls of the same buffer containing 0.5 mM $Mn^{2+}$. Five ml aliquots of the cell suspension were plated on 100-mm diameter Petri dishes coated with fibronectin, at 25 mg/ml or ProNectin-F at 10 mg/ml and prepared according to the supplier's instructions (Protein Polymer Technologies, San Diego, CA).

The cells were incubated for 45 min at 37 °C in a humidified atmosphere of 10% $CO_2$. Following the incubation, non-adherent cells were removed and replated on a fresh set of dishes coated with ProNectin-F for an additional 45 min. Adherent cells from the two incubations were washed three times with solution I containing 2 mM EDTA and detached with 0.025% trypsin in the presence of 2 mM EDTA, and HEPES-buffered saline pH 7.4. The cells were washed twice with HEPES-buffered saline pH 7.4, containing 1% RIA-grade BSA, 5 mM glucose and 5 mM KCl. Cell purity was assessed by the tannic acid stain technique [27] and by immunofluorescence staining with monoclonal antibody 4AmAb which recognizes pneumocin, a sialoglycoprotein apical membrane of type II pneumocytes [25, 26]. Cell viability was determined by Trypan Blue dye exclusion.

Greater than 90% of type II cells adhered to ProNectin-F coated plates within the first 45 min of incubation. An additional 10% adhered when the cell suspension from the first adhesion was incubated on fresh ProNectin-F coated Petri dishes. Ciliated cells formed small aggregates of 3–10 cells that remained in suspension. Few type II cells were observed when non-adherent cells from the second incubation were plated overnight in DMEM containing 10% fetal calf serum, overnight on tissue culture plastic.

Type II cells rapidly adherent to the artificial substrate in presence of $Mn^{2+}$ were harvested by trypsinization in the presence of 2 mM EDTA. The cells were obtained in good yields, had excellent viability, and were immediately available for functional studies. $Mn^{2+}$ enhances freshly isolated type II cell adhesion to fibronectin, type IV collagen and reconstituted basement membrane Matrigel. The majority of the $Mn^{2+}$-enhanced adhesion can be accounted for by an RGD dependent mechanism since it can be blocked by the (RGDS), but not the inactive (RGES) peptide. Freshly isolated type II cells adhered poorly to laminin and type I collagen, and there was no apparent enhancement of adhesion by $Mn^{2+}$.

Native fibronectin and ProNectin-F can be used in the isolation procedure. However, the use of ProNectin-F is attractive for several reasons. ProNectin-F is commercially available and cheaper than the intact fibronectin. Binding to a restricted domain of the ligand avoids potential problems arising from cell interactions with other domains of fibronectin. The uniform nature of the substrate provided by ProNectin-F provides a unique opportunity for study of cell interaction with this ligand on specific type II cell functions. In addition, the presence of multiple RGD sites on the recombinant molecule provide a much higher concentration of cell adhesion sites than is achievable by coating the substratum with intact fibronectin. Plates coated with the artificial substrate can be stored in dry form. The utility of this technique for isolation of type II cells from rat lungs of different ages and possibly different developmental stages remains to be investigated.

A potential limitation of this procedure is that it requires exposure of the cells to $Mn^{2+}$ and ProNectin-F for a brief period of time. We have shown that 0.5 mM $Mn^{2+}$ is effective in enhancing type II cell adhesion to both fibronectin and ProNectin-F. In another study using a rat type II cell derived cell line LM5, we have observed that $Mn^{2+}$ concentrations as low as 100 nM enhance cell attachment to fibronectin. However, the effect of the brief exposure to $Mn^{2+}$ and ProNectin-F on specific type II cell functions needs further study. Despite these potential limitations, the benefits obtained from having highly purified type II cells available in good yields for immediate study far outweigh the potential limitations. Furthermore, the use of a ProNectin-F-coated substratum in presence of $Mn^{2+}$ may offer a potential alternative to poly-lysine coated dishes as a means of adhering freshly isolated type II cells while their functions are under study.

Other divalent cations $Co^{2+}$ and $Ni^{2+}$ also promoted cell adhesion to fibronectin and ProNectin-F, but to a lesser magnitude than that observed for $Mn^{2+}$. $Ca^{2+}$ did not significantly enhance type II cell adhesion to fibronectin or ProNectin-F. $Zn^{2+}$ and Cadium were inhibitory. Differences in $Mn^{2+}$, $Co^{2+}$ and $Ni^{2+}$ enhancement of type II cell adhesion were less pronounced when cells were plated on fibronectin compared to ProNectin-F.

In this type II cell isolation protocol, fibroblast contamination was minimized by using elastase as opposed to collagenase, which was applied directly to the epithelial lining by instilling it in the airway, and by limiting the digestion to 20 min, which has been shown to leave the interstitium relatively intact [5].

Type II cells attach to fibronectin by a number of integrin receptors. It is believed that the $a_5b_1$ integrin is a specific receptor for fibronectin and interacts with the RGD cell binding site of integrin receptors [37]. The potential roles of the various receptors in adhesion of type II cells to fibronectin or ProNectin-F remain to be determined. In contrast to the rapid cell adhesion to fibronectin, primary isolated type II cells attach slowly to laminin, suggesting either a lower number of the laminin receptors, their apparent removal with cell dissociating enzymes or inactivation during the isolation process.

---

# Discussion

## Limitation of studies of isolated cells

The response of isolated cells may not completely reflect the behavior of parent cells *in situ*. In fact, none of the currently available techniques is suitable for cell isolation for all different studies. Cell isolation with enzymatic techniques may destroy spatial relationships that are critical to normal cellular functions and maintenance of the differentiated state.

Culture of cells on artificial substrata may result in either up- or downregulation of functions, such as integrin and ECM components, that are normally expressed at low levels *in situ*. Because of the above limitation it is necessary to relate the observations made on isolated cells to those of cells *in vivo* or *in situ*.

## Alternatives to cell isolation

Despite careful standardization of isolation procedures, primary isolated cells vary from one cell preparation to another, in purity, quantity and quality of cells. In addition, the biological characteristics of the cells change even during the first 48 h when most studies are performed. For some study questions it is desirable to initiate studies with a cell line and subsequently confirm or relate the observations on primary isolated cells and *in situ*. Several immortalized type II cell derived cell lines have been described [33–36].

Studies utilizing immunocytochemical techniques when combined with *in situ* hybridization may provide functional and biosynthetic information without need for cell isolation.

## Acknowledgments

Supported by Grants R01-HL-41854 and R01-HL-46735 to JLM from the United States Public Health Service.

## References

1 Crapo, JD, Barry BE, Gehr P, Bachofen M and Weibel ER (1982) *Am. J. Respir. Dis.* **126**: 332

2 Mason RJ, Dobbs LG, Greenleaf RD and Williams MC (1977) *Fed. Proc.* **36**: 2697

3 Adamson IYR and Bowden DJ (1974) *Lab. Invest.* **80**: 35

4 Evans MJ, Cabral LC, Stephens RJ and Freeman G (1974) *Chest* **65**: Suppl. 63

5 Dobbs LG (1990) *Am. J. Physiol.* **258**: L134-L147

6 Liley HG, Ertsy R, Gonzalez LW, Odom MW, Hawgood S, Dobbs LG and Ballard PL (1988) *Biochim. Biophy. Acta* **961**: 86

7 Edelson JD, Shannon JM and Mason RJ (1988) *Am. Rev. Respir. Dis.* **138**: 1268

8  Edelson JD, Shannon JM and Mason RJ (1989) *Am. Rev. Respir. Dis.* **140**: 1398

9  Mason RJ, Apostolou S, Power J and Robinson P (1990) *Am. J. Respir. Cell Mol. Biol.* **3**: 571

10  Post M, Barsoumian A and Smith BT (1986) *J. Biol. Chem.* **261**: 2179

11  Kresch MJ, Dynia DW and Gross I (1987) *Biochim. Biophys. Acta* **930**: 19

12  Bundschuh DS, Uhlig S, Leist M, Sauer A and Wendel A (1995) *In vitro* **31**: 684

13  Corti M, Brody AB and Harrison JH (1996) *Am. J. Respir. Cell Mol. Biol.* **14**: 309

14  Rami J, Sasic SM and Rooney SA (1991) *Am. J. Physiol.* **260**: L577-L585

15  Dobbs LG, Gonzalez R and Williams MC (1986) *Am. Rev. Respir. Dis.* **134**: 141

16  Weller NK and Karnovsky MJ (1986) *Am. J. Pathol.* **122**: 91

17  Greenleaf RD, Mason RJ and Williams MC (1979) *In vitro* **15**: 673

18  Funkhouser JD, Cheshire LB, Ferrara TB and Peterson RD (1987) *Dev. Biol.* **119**: 190

19  Wilson JS, Steinkamp JA and Lehnert BE (1986) *Cytochemistry* **7**: 157

20  Simon RH, McCoy JP, Chu AE, Dehart PD and Goldstein IJ (1986) *Biochim. Biophys. Acta* **885**: 34

21  Rochat TR, Casale JM and Hunninghake GW (1988) *J. Lab. Clin. Med.* **112**: 418

22  Lwebuga-Mukasa JS (1994) *Am. J. Respir. Cell Mol. Biol.* **10**: 347

23  Cappello J (1992) Genetic production of synthetic protein polymers. Materials Research Society Bull; XII (10): 48

24  Cappello J and Crissman J (1990) *Polymer Preprints Am. Chem. Soc.* **31**: 193

25  Lwebuga-Mukasa JS (1991) *Am. J. Respir. Cell. Mol. Biol.* **4**: 479

26  Lwebuga-Mukasa JS, (1991) *Am. J. Respir. Cell Mol. Biol.* **4**: 489

27  Mason RJ, Wallxer SR, Henson JE and Williams MC (1985) *Am. Rev. Respir. Dis.* **131**: 786

28  Kikkawa Y and Yoneda K (1974) *Lab. Invest.* **30**: 76

29  Sugihara H, Toda S, Miyabara S, Fujugana C and Yonemistsu N (1993) *Am. J. Pathol.* **142**: 783

30  Ulich TR, Yi ES, Longmuir K, Yin S, Biltz R, Morris CF, Housley RM and Pierce GF (1994) *J. Clin. Invest.* **93**: 1298

31  Panos RJ, Bak PM, Simonet WS, Rubin JS and Sith LJ (1995) *J. Clin. Invest.* **96**: 2026

32  Sugahara K, Rubin JS, Mason RJ, Aronsen EL and Shannon JM (1995) *Am. J. Physiol.* **269**: L344 -L350

33  Steele MP, Levine RA, Joyce-Brady M and Brody JS (1992) *Am. J. Respir. Cell Mol. Biol.* **6**: 50

34  Mallapalli RK, Floerchinger CS and Hunninghake GW (1992) *In vitro* **28**: 181

35  Wikenheiser KA, Vorbroker DK, Rice WR, Clark JC, Bachurski CJ, Gil HK and Whitsett JA (1994) *Proc. Natl. Acad. Sci. USA* **90**: 11029

36  Driscoll KE, Carter JM, Iype PT, Kimmero HL, Crosby LL, Aardema MJ, Isofort RJ, Cody D, Chestnut MH, Burns JL et al. (1995) *In vitro* **31**: 516

37  Pytela R, Pierschbacher MD and Ruoslahti E. (1985) *Proc. Natl. Acad. Sci. USA* **82**: 5766

# 16 Endothelial cells

T. Stevens, G.H. Brough, T.M. Moore,
P. Babal and W.J. Thompson

The lung was thought to be a metabolically inactive organ until 1925, when Starling and Verney suggested otherwise [1]. Endothelial cells have in common with the lung that historically these cells were thought to be metabolically inactive, serving only as a physical barrier to separate blood from tissue. Indeed, it is easy to understand how this early view of endothelium was conceived and that it was difficult to envision how endothelial cells could be metabolically active. These cells are only $\approx 0.2\,\mu M$ in diameter across their cytoplasmic regions and electron micrographs demonstrate few mitochondria, Golgi, and endoplasmic reticulum [2], especially when compared to metabolically active cells like hepatocytes and cardiomyocytes. Further, endothelial cells are non-excitable, e.g. lacking action potentials [3] and possessing a low reliance upon mitochondrial production of ATP to meet their metabolic demands [4].

The concept that endothelial cells are inert has passed. We now recognize that endothelial cells regulate a variety of functions including hemostasis, white blood cell trafficking, hormone metabolism, blood pressure, vascular growth, and permeability [2]. Endothelial cell functions in the lung are particularly important by virtue of the organ's large vascular surface area. Moreover, endothelial cell biology has been greatly advanced by investigators who studied predominantly the pulmonary circulation [2, 5–7]. Many of the advances in pulmonary endothelial cell biology and the view of endothelial cells as a metabolically active tissue arose from three seminal observations: (i) bradykinin is cleared from blood with a single pass through the lung [8], (ii) angiotensin II is not cleared from blood with a single pass through the lung [9], and (iii) angiotensin I is activated upon a single pass through the lung [10]. Ultimately, Dr. Una Ryan and colleagues would discover that endothelial cells possess an enzyme, angiotensin converting enzyme (ACE), which inactivates bradykinin and converts angiotensin I to angiotensin II [2], a potent vasoconstrictor that also promotes aldosterone production in the adrenal gland. These data were among the early studies that confirmed the lung and vascular endothelium are metabolically active.

Progress in endothelial cell biology was slowed initially because target cells were difficult to isolate and maintain in culture. It was possible to evaluate hormone clearance in the intact pulmonary circulation, for example, but was not possible to effectively determine the role of endothelial cells in this process. Thus, it was clear isolation of endothelia would be required to address the specific role of endothelial cells in such metabolic processes. In the 1960–70s a few laboratories reported methods for isolating endothelia from systemic vascular beds [11, 12]. The use of these cells in endothelial cell biology was generally fruitful. While not routine, it was clear that endothelia possessed phenotypic distinctions between vascular beds. Thus, direct application of data obtained from systemic endothelial cells to pulmonary endothelial cells was not well justified. To address this issue – and specifically issues regarding clearance of bradykinin from the lung and conversion of angiotensin I to angiotensin II within the lung – techniques were devised by Ryan and coworkers to culture endothelial cells from the pulmonary artery of large animals [13]. Comprehensive studies were conducted to demonstrate that both endothelial cells *in vivo* and in culture possessed similar markers, suggesting phenotypic similarity. For example, endothelia *in vivo* or *in vitro* possess in common: a characteristic cobblestone morphology (see Troubleshooting), factor VIII antigen, LDL receptors, extensive specialized membranous invaginations called caveolae and Weibel-Palade bodies (not necessarily characteristic of pulmonary endothelia, however) (Fig. 16.1) [2]. After verifying these morphological characteristics it was shown that endothelial cells cultured from pulmonary arteries inactivate bradykinin and convert angiotensin I to angiotensin II, due to expression of ACE. Thus, not only could primary and early passage endothelial cells be isolated and cultured, but the cells exhibited certain physiological processes in common with endothelial cells *in vivo*.

While these hallmark observations demonstrated endothelial cells could be isolated and cultured from large vessels, other studies showed ACE expression throughout the microcirculation [14]. Given the large microcirculatory surface area of the lung and immunolocalization of ACE to the microcirculation, investigators reasoned that most inactivation of bradykinin and conversion of angiotensin I to angiotensin II would occur within capillaries of the microcirculation [2]. Moreover, many studies in pulmonary physiology were/are conducted using

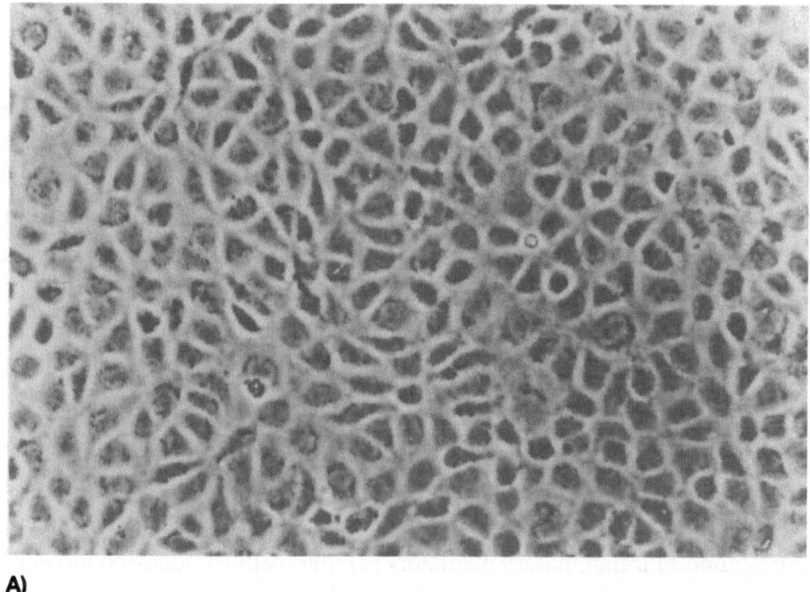

**A)**

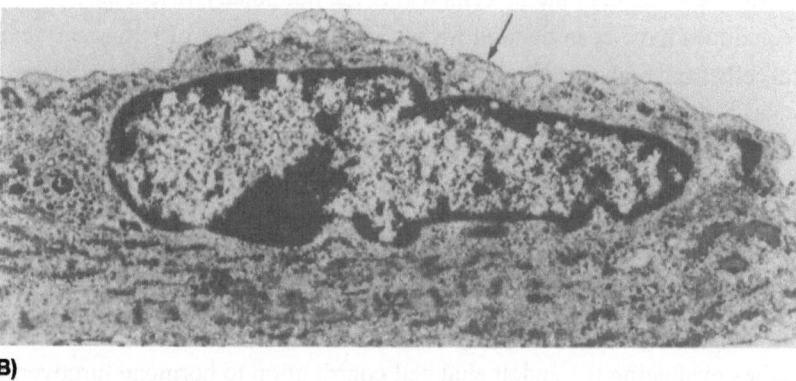

**B)**

*Figure 16.1. Pulmonary artery endothelial cells grow to confluence and exhibit a characteristic cobblestone morphology*

*The cells exhibit contact inhibition and under usual conditions do not overgrow. A) Phase contrast micrograph of 12th passage pulmonary artery endothelial cells (×250). B) TEM of cultured pulmonary artery endothelial cells showing extensive caveolae (arrow), Golgi apparatus (G) near the nucleas, fibrillar material below the nucleus (asterisk), and rough endoplasmic retuculum distributed throughout the cytoplasm (×20000). Photographs adapted from [6].*

small animals, and obtaining large numbers of endothelial cells from pulmonary arteries of small animals proved difficult. Hence, there existed a need to subculture pulmonary microvascular endothelia and study the metabolic activity of these cells. In accordance with the need to culture microvascular cells, Habliston and coworkers [5], and subsequently other investigators [15–17], isolated and characterized pulmonary microvascular endothelial cells from small animals. These cells retained many features of systemic and large vessel pulmonary endothelia, yet were quite clearly phenotypically distinct cells. In contrast, however, microvascular endothelial cells were thinner and possessed fewer actin-like filaments. Perhaps most strikingly, Chung-Welch et al. found that bovine pulmonary artery endothelial cells exhibited a smooth surface, whereas microvascular endothelial cells exhibited a remarkable array of projections when assessed by scanning electron microscropy (Fig. 16.2). Using preparations described below, we have also made similar observations comparing conduit *vs.* microvascular endothelial cells from rat lungs (Fig. 16.3). Functional data suggests that production of neuro-humoral inflammatory mediators [7], intercellular adhesion molecules [18], signal transduction pathways [19] and semi-selective barrier properties [17] differ between endothelial cells within the pulmonary vasculature.

Techniques have been devised for isolation and culture of pulmonary endothelial cells from both conduit vessels and the microcirculation of large and small animals. Since endothelial cells derived from different vascular sites exhibit marked heterogeneity, investigators seeking to study properties unique to a particular segment of the pulmonary circulation should be advised to utilize cells from that segment. As an example, arterial endothelial cells are pivotal in regulation of pulmonary artery pressure and also smooth muscle cell growth. Thus, endothelial cells derived from larger vascular segments are likely suitable to study production of vasoactive, pro-proliferative and anti-proliferative autocoids. In studies evaluating the endothelial cell contribution to hormone turnover, an-

*Figure 16.2. Macrovascular and microvascular pulmonary endothelial cells appear morphologically distinct*

*A) Cultured pulmonary artery endothelial cells possess a smooth surface when analyzed by SEM (×2000). B) Cultured pulmonary microvascular endothelial cells exhibit extensive projections when analyzed by SEM (×4500). C) Fingerlike projections are apparent on pulmonary microvascular endothelial cells when evaluated using low-power micrographs of surface replica. D) Projections are also apparent on microvascular endothelial cells when viewed by TEM (×12000). Photographs adapted from [2, 7].*

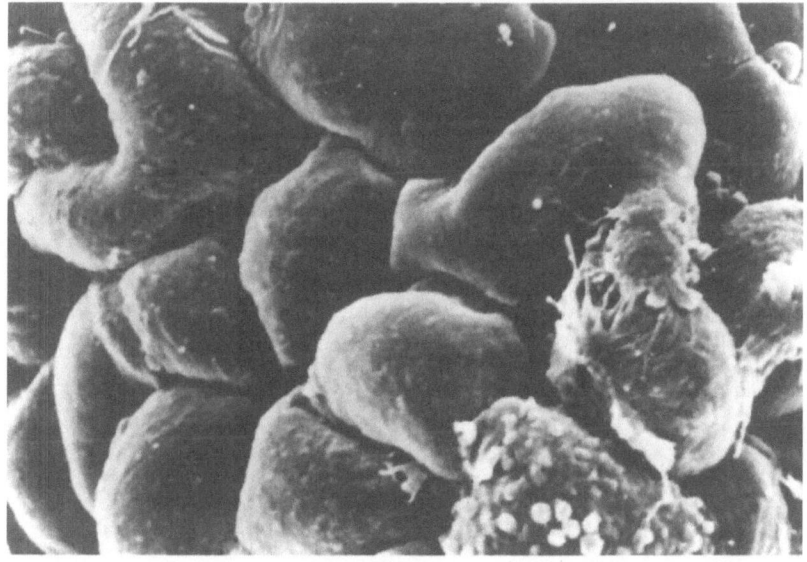

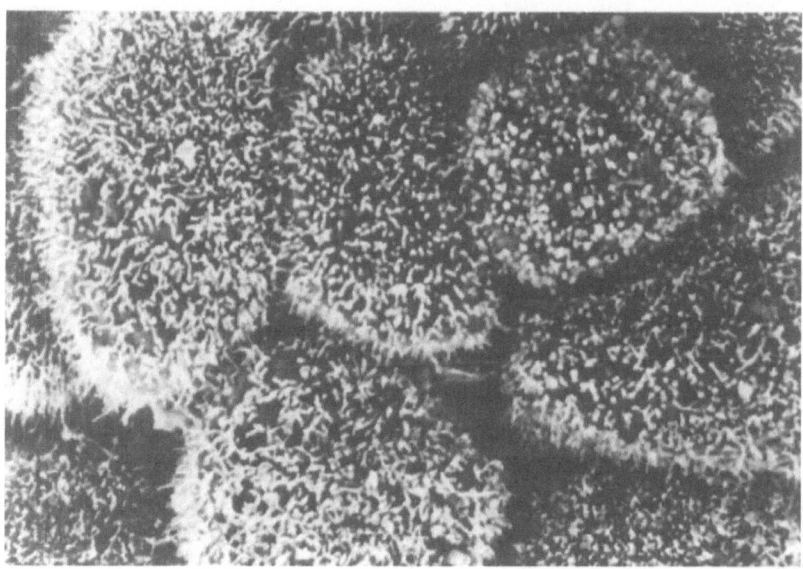

*Figure 16.2A, B*

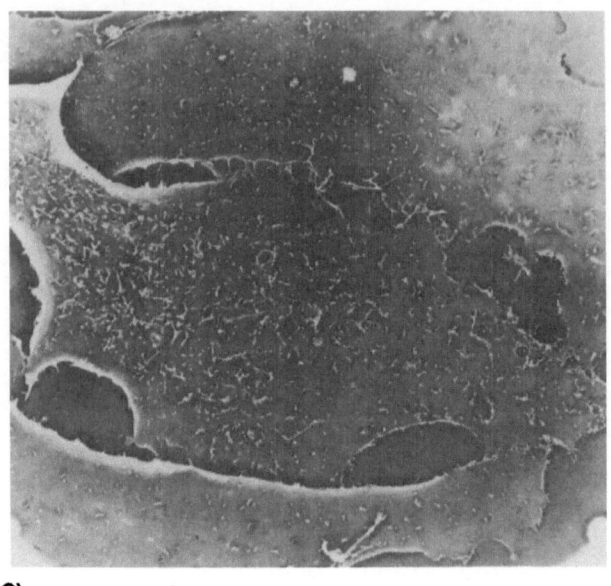

**C)**

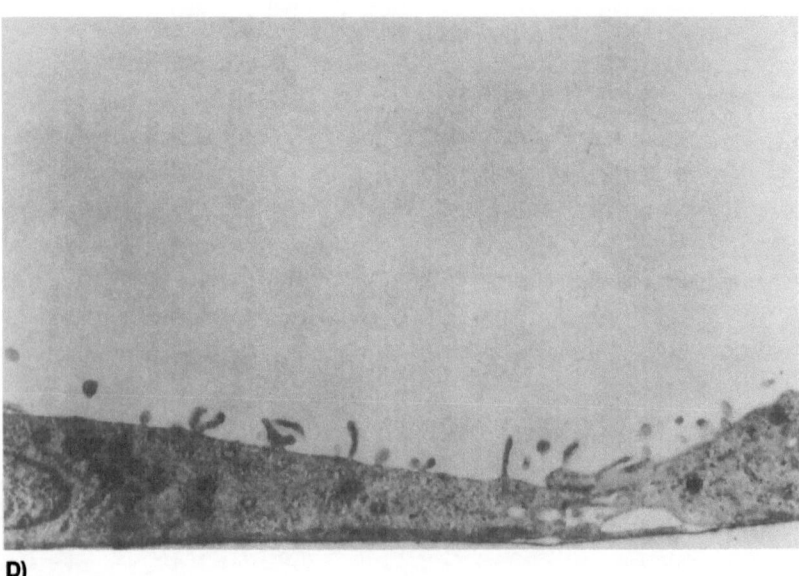

**D)**

*Figure 16.2C, D*
*(Legend see p. 406)*

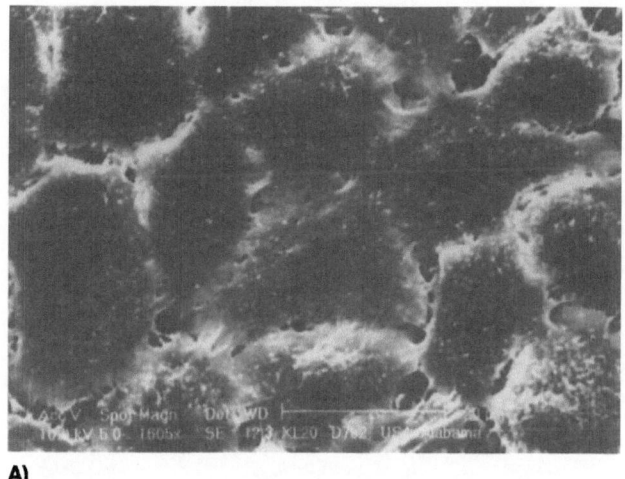

**A)**

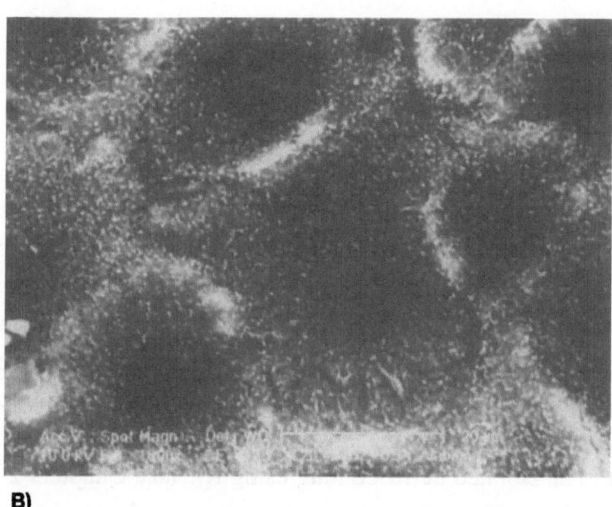

**B)**

*Figure 16.3. Rat macrovascular and microvascular endothelial cells as described by scraping and retroperfusion techniques, respectively*

*Cells were grown to confluence on glass, fixed using 3% glutaraldehyde, dried in $CO_2$ critical point, and analyzed by SEM and TEM ($\times$1600). A) Cultured pulmonary artery endothelial cells demonstrate some fingerlike projections and gaps between cells. B) Cultured pulmonary microvascular endothelial cells showing more extensive fingerlike projections, few gaps between cells, and a larger surface area compared with their main artery counterpart. C) Cultured microvascular endothelial cells possess close cell-cell apposition, as suggested by B).*

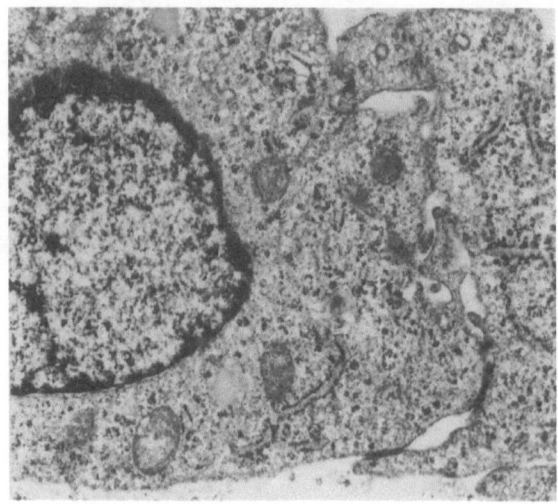

*Figure 16.3C (Legend see p. 409)*

giogenesis, white blood cell trafficking, or pulmonary edema, investigations should utilize microvascular endothelia. Historically, however, microvascular endothelial cells have been more difficult to isolate than cells from larger vessels.

Isolation and culture of endothelia from different lung segments have allowed progress in endothelial cell biology, especially when studies performed *in vitro* are vertically integrated with established models of intact pulmonary circulation. Examples include studies of endothelial cell permeability, where microvascular permeability is assessed *in vivo* and *in vitro* using tracer molecules (*see* Chapters 8 and 9), and in an isolated perfused lung using $K_{f,c}$ (*see* Chapters 2 and 8). All told, these studies provide a comprehensive way to investigate mechanistic questions regarding control of endothelial cell barrier properties. Beyond this though, *in vitro* experiments allow more comprehensive mechanistic studies to be performed that may not be presently possible in the setting of an intact organ. To cite an example again with respect to endothelial cell barrier properties, it is possible to evaluate mechanisms of endothelial cell-cell and cell-matrix tethering *in vitro* [20]. Future studies will be required to assess how cell-cell and cell-matrix tethering control events like acute barrier disruption and other endothelial cell functions like angiogenesis in the intact circulation.

*In vitro* assessments of endothelial cell function are not without problems. One difficulty is cultured endothelial cells may not retain their *in vivo* phenotype. Indeed, this problem has plagued investigators throughout the history of endothelial cell cultures, adding support to the idea that formulation of vertically integrated experiments is the preferred approach to addressing experimental problems. Investigators using cultured cells should demonstrate that in regard to the question under study, cultured cells do maintain their *in vivo* phenotype. Another problem is that while endothelial cells are easily identified from other contaminating cells, e.g. smooth muscle cells or fibroblasts, criteria clearly defining specific types of endothelial cells are still needed. Without question, the advances made by utilizing isolated cells far outweighs the problems and difficulties associated with their use.

To summarize, research has identified that endothelial cells are metabolically active cells involved in the regulation of hemostasis, white blood cell trafficking, hormone metabolism, blood pressure, vascular growth, and permeability. Isolation and culture of endothelial cells from different vascular segments of the lung can be achieved, both from large and small animals. Because of endothelial cell heterogeneity, isolates should be employed in accordance with the researcher's specific question, e.g. macrovascular *vs.* microvascular problem. Outlined below are published procedures available for procurement and culture of endothelial cells from various species and anatomic locations.

## Material and methods

### Tissue culture of pulmonary artery endothelial cells

The protocol described is for isolation of bovine pulmonary artery endothelial cells although it can be modified to accomodate other species, even small animals. Indeed, Figure 16.3 compares rat pulmonary artery endothelial cells obtained using a slight modification of the technique discussed below with pulmonary microvascular cells obtained using retroperfusion (*see* Section on *Tissue culture of pulmonary microvascular endothelial cells: Method* 2). It is noteworthy that whereas it is relatively easy to reproducibly generate pulmonary artery endothelial cell cultures from large animals, it is difficult to reproducibly generate pulmonary artery endothelial cell cultures from rat.

## Equipment/media and chemicals

- Sterile serological pipets (5, 10, 25 ml sizes).
- Rat tooth forceps, scissors (large and small).
- 100×20 mm plates (Falcon).
- 15 ml conical sterile (Falcon).
- 25, 75 cm [2] tissue flasks (Corning).
- Laminar flow hood, class II.
- Microscope, inverted phase contrast.
- 95–100% ethanol.
- Phosphate Buffered Saline (PBS; sterile).
- MEM D-val modification (Sigma).
- MEM (Sigma).
- Trypsin-EDTA solution (10×: 5 g porcine trypsin, 2 g EDTA·4Na per liter) (Sigma).
- 37 °C, 5% $CO_2$ humidified incubator for tissue culture.
- Antibiotic/antimycotic solution (100×: 10 000U penicillin, 10 mg streptomycin, 25 ug amphotericin B per ml: Sigma).
- Penicillin/streptomycin solution (100×: 10 000U penicillin, 10 mg streptomycin per ml: Sigma).
- Collagenase (Crude Type 1a: Sigma).
- Calf Bovine Serum.
- Non-Essential Amino Acids (100×: Sigma).

## Solutions/media preparation

- Media for tissue transport
  To 500 ml bottle of MEM add:
  1) 5 ml of antibiotic/antimycotic solution (100×).
  2) 5 ml of 200 mM L-glutamine (Sigma).

- Media for tissue processing (i.e., collagenase treatment)
  To 250 ml bottle MEM add:
  1) 2.5 ml of penicillin/streptomycin solution (100×).
  2) 1.25 ml of Non-Essential Amino Acids (NEAA).
  3) 0.05% (w/v) Collagenase.
- Full Growth Media (250 ml)
  1) Start with 200 ml of sterile-filtered MEM D-val modification pH 7.3–7.4 that is prepared according to the supplier's instructions.
  2) Add 50 ml of calf bovine serum (CBS), then add 2.5 ml of penicillin/streptomycin and 1.25 ml NEAA.
  3) Swirl gently to mix and store at 4 °C. Only warm volumes for use from this bottle.

### Macrovascular endothelial cell isolation procedure

- Obtain fresh heart and lungs with attached great vessels from an abattoir.
- Dissect main pulmonary artery (PA) free from pericardium and aorta with a scalpel (one 2-inch segment per primary flask of cells desired).
- Immediately place PA vessel segment into a sterile specimen cup or clean, sterile glass beaker (250 ml size) containing tissue transport media. Immediately upon return to the laboratory transfer PA to fresh tissue transport media.
- Perform all subsequent work under laminar flow biosafety cabinet on a sterile drape. Work on a flat surface – a styrofoam container top works well.
- Sterilize scissors by ethanol and flame, allow to cool, and remove bifurcation of vessel. Carefully remove any extraneous fatty and connective tissue from the outside of PA segment with rat tooth forceps and scissors.
- Submerge vessel segment into sterile PBS several times to remove blood, etc.
- Sterilize instruments, then cut the artery segment. Cut the segment into two pieces that are roughly equal in size.

- Place tissues sections, luminal surface down, into 3 ml of media containing collagenase type 1a (0.05% w/vol) (*see* Section on *Solutions/media preparation*) on a plastic 100 mm dish. Place in a 5% $CO_2$ incubator at 37 °C for 10 min.
- Wet a cell scraper with Full Growth Media. Gently scrape luminal surface of vessel withsingle strokes, covering each area only once. Do not push too hard to avoid collecting underlying fibroblasts or smooth muscle cells. *Note*: Avoid small arteriolar portals into aorta vessel, excise if possible or avoid the area because collagenase treatment may draw other (contaminating) cells into that area when you scrape off endothelial cell layer.
- Swirl scraper in 4 mls of Full Growth Media to shake off cells. Triturate and culture in a 25 $cm^2$ flask. Place the flask in a 37 °C, 5% $CO_2$ humidified incubator.

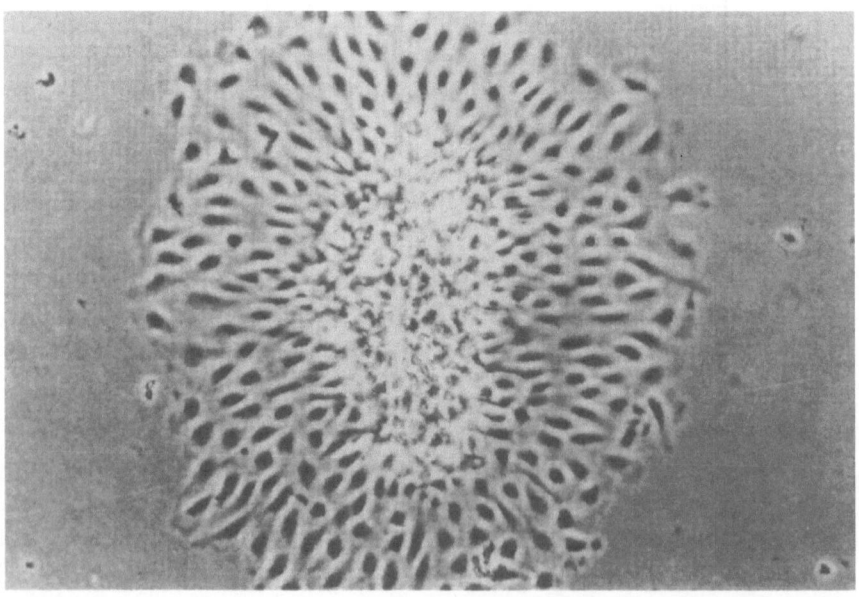

*Figure 16.4. Newly seeded primary cultures of endothelial cells obtained by scraping appear as small clumps or sheets (×200)*
*Photographs adapted from [6].*

- On the next day, observe flasks for adherent cells (small, discrete colonies should be observed, Fig. 16.4) and replace with fresh growth media. Replace growth media on cells roughly twice per week.
- At roughly 7 days, cells will be ready for subculture.

## Tissue culture of pulmonary microvascular endothelial cells: Method 1

This method takes advantage of the large number of microvessels found in the lung periphery. The technique was described by Del Vecchio et al., [15] using bovine tissue and Magee et al. [21] using rat tissue. The method described below by Stevens et al., [19] reports a modification of these techniques for bovine lung.

### Equipment/media and chemicals

- Media:
  1) RPMI-1640 (Whittaker Bioproducts)
  2) Dulbecco's phosphate buffered saline (Gibco)
  3) Hank's Balanced Salt Solution, $Ca^{2+}$ and $Mg^{2+}$- free (Irvine Sci.)
  4) Hank's Balanced Salt Solution (Irvine Sci.)
  5) $Ca^{2+}$ and $Mg^{2+}$-free phosphate buffered saline (cmf-PBS)
  6) Human umbilical vein endothelial cell (HUVEC) conditioned media – sterile filtered
- Collagenase (1000 U/ml: $\geq 125$ U/mg dry weight CLS2) (Worthington Biochemical Corp)
- ENDOGRO (bovine retinal derived growth factor VEC TEC Inc.)
- 160 micron NITEX nylon mesh (TETKO)
- 2% gelatin (Sigma)
- Fetal Bovine Serum
- Trypsin-EDTA solution (10×: 5 g porcine trypsin, 2 g EDTA·4Na per liter) (Sigma)
- 6 mm cloning cylinders (Bellco Glass Inc)
- 7.5% sodium bicarbonate solution

- Bovine Serum Albumin (Sigma #A5403, fraction V powder)
- 35 and 20×100 mm tissue culture dish (Falcon #3001, #3002)
- 96, 48, 24, and 12 well tissue culture plates
- 25, 75 and 150 cm$^2$ tissue flasks
- 15 and 50 ml sterile conical tubes
- Small, fine, curved forceps, large forceps with teeth, and sharp microscissors
- Sterile disposable drape or underpad
- Sterile silicon vacuum grease
- 70% ethanol

## Solutions/media preparation

- Plating media (incomplete) – mix and sterile filter
  1) RPMI-1640
  2) 20% FBS
  3) 70 µg/ml heparin
  4) 6.7 µg/ml (ENDOGRO)
  5) 1% penicillin/streptomycin/glutamine
- Plating media (complete) – mix and sterile filter
  1) 1 part HUVEC conditioned media (maintenance media with any HUVEC culture which can be obtained from the ATCC or alternatively by contacting authors)
  2) 3 parts incomplete media (*see* above)

## Microvascular endothelial cell isolation procedure

- Obtain bovine lung from an abattoir. Place whole lobe into plastic bag on ice and promptly return to laboratory.
- Rinse the outside of lobe with 70% ethanol, on sterile drape (also soaked with 70% ethanol).
- Separate pleural sheath from the periphery of the lung.
- Remove 10 segments of tissue roughly 2 cm in diameter. Limit tissue collection to the parenchymal portion of lung (do not cut too deep) and wash thoroughly with cmf-PBS.

- Place tissue fragments into a small beaker with cmf-PBS and mince finely with microscissors (to < 1×1 mm size).
- Use a spatula to transfer minced pieces into a 50 ml conical tube containing 10 ml of 1000 U/ml collagenase (CLS2) and 5% BSA in cmf-PBS. Wrap Parafilm around the tube cap and place on rocker for 30–45 min at 37 °C.
- Pour through the NITEX membrane (pre-wash mesh with cmf-PBS before filtering). Wash with approximately 30 ml cmf-PBS into a 50 ml conical tube.
- Centrifuge at 200×g for 10 min to obtain a cell pellet.
- Aspirate the supernatant and resuspend the pellet in plating media. Wash three times using HBSS, repeating 5 min spins.
- Resuspend cells in 10–20 ml of plating media and plate cells onto 5–10 gelatin coated 35 mm Petri dishes with 2 ml suspension per dish (dilute gelatin to 1% with sterile tissue grade water 1 day prior to the procedure: use 1.5 to 2 ml on each dish, place at 37 °C for 1 h, then remove residual gelatin and allow to dry). Place into 37 °C, 5% $CO_2$ incubator.
- On the next day, wash cells twice with HBSS and add fresh media. Observe cells daily for endothelial cell patches.

### Endothelial cell procurement

- While viewing cells under a phase microscope, select those areas that exhibit typical endothelial cell morphology.
- Select cell patches by removing the surrounding non-endothelial cells with a syringe and needle. After scraping, wash vigorously three times with cmf-PBS to remove detached cells.
- Isolate cell patches with a sterile glass cloning ring. Coat the bottom, outer edge of the cloning ring with sterile vacuum grease to obtain a good seal and place firmly over the cells of interest.
- Harvest the cells inside each ring with 1× trypsin. Inactivate trypsin with growth media and transfer cells to a 96-well gelatin coated plate. (Wash the plate with HBSS prior to seeding cells).

- Culture cells for 1–2 weeks and begin subculture to achieve cell homogeneity.
- Subculture cells from each "pure" culture into one well (gelatin coated) of a 24-well plate. Once confluent, subculture cells into six well plate (gelatin coated). Allow the cells to grow to confluency again. Repeat the cloning ring process if necessary.
- When you are certain that your cultures are pure, subculture cells into a gelatin-coated, 75 cm$^2$ flask.

## Tissue culture of pulmonary microvascular endothelial cells: Method 2

This method for isolating and culturing rat pulmonary microvascular endothelial cells was modified from that described previously by Ryan and White [22] in the laboratory of W.J.T. [17]. Equipment and supplies necessary for performing this experiment can be found in Chapter 3 regarding lung isolation and perfusion and above, regarding isolation of microvascular endothelial cells.

### Solutions/media preparation

- Initial lung perfusate: Krebs balanced salt solution can be prepared as per the supplier's instructions and supplemented with sodium bicarbonate (30 ml of a 7.5% solution/liter) and 4% bovine serum albumin (18 ml of a 30% solution/150 ml of buffer). The 30% albumin solution should be prepared a day in advance to allow for complete dissolution of the albumin in sterile water.
- Cell harvesting perfusate: To prepare 125 ml, add to Aim V serum-free media (Gibco) the following:
  1) 5 g bovine serum albumin (4% final) (Intergen Bovuminar standard powder)
  2) 50 mg hyaluronidase I (Sigma)
  3) $7.5 \times 10^5$ microbeads (Dupont, NEN 50 µm diameter). Beads are incubated with collagen IIII (1 µg/ml) for 1 h at room temperature and washed with PBS.

- Wash media: The media used for washing the cell-microbead suspension harvested from the isolated lung consists of the following:
    1) RPMI-1640 media (Sigma) containing 25% fetal bovine serum (Intergen)
- Plating media: The media used for plating the harvested endothelial cells consists of the following:
    1) One part endothelial cell-conditioned media (Endothelial cell conditioned-media can only be obtained from prior endothelial cultures; maintenance media with any endothelial cell culture which can be obtained from the ATCC or alternatively by contacting authors).
    2) Two parts RPMI-1640 containing 20% rat serum and 0.1% gentamicin. The pooled rat serum can be stockpiled in advance by using donor rats for collection.
- Maintenance media (feeding or growth media): One liter of the cell culture maintenance media consists of the following:
    1) DMEM
    2) 0.1% gentamicin (Gibco; 10 µg/ml)
    3) 0.05% amphotericin B (Sigma; 0.25 µg/ml)
    4) 1% penicillin/streptomycin solution (Sigma; 100 U/100 µg/ml)
    5) 3.7 g sodium bicarbonate
    6) 20% fetal bovine serum (After passage 10, the fetal bovine serum content can be switched to 10 %)

*Microvascular endothelial cell isolation procedure, lung isolation*

Detailed methodologies for isolating and perfusing animal lungs can be found in chapter 3 of this volume. A brief description of the rat lung isolation procedure follows here. It should be noted however that this method has been adapted for use in rabbit lungs and lobes of larger animals [5, 6].
- Anesthetize rats (CD strain; Charles River Breeding Laboratories; 250–350 g) with sodium pentobarbital (50 mg/kg i.p.).
- Perform a tracheostomy and establish positive pressure ventilation using room air [Harvard rodent respirator; $V_t = 10$ ml/kg; respiratory

rate = 55 breaths per min; positive end expiratory pressure (PEEP) = 2.5 cmH$_2$O].

- Perform a sternotomy and inject heparin (300U) into the left ventricle. After 5 min cannulate both the pulmonary artery (by way of the right ventricle) and left atrium (by way of the left ventricle). Establish an initial lung perfusion while the lungs are *in situ* with initial lung perfusate. Wash the pulmonary vasculature free of the majority of blood elements (use approximately 75 ml of non-recirculating perfusate). Establish a recirculating perfusion (50 ml) that is driven by a peristaltic pump (Gilson Minipuls). Perfusate flow rate should be constant and set at 0.03 ml/min/g rat body weight. Recirculating perfusion should be established for approximately 25 min.

## Endothelial cell procurement

- The lung perfusate should be switched to the cell-harvesting perfusate containing approximately 600 collagen-coated microbeads/ml perfusate.
- The direction of perfusate flow should be alternated from anterograde to retrograde and perfusate containing the endothelial cell-bound microbeads collected from both the arterial and venous cannulas. After the first 125 ml of harvesting perfusate has been collected, an additional 125 ml of harvesting perfusate, devoid of enzyme and microbeads, should be perfused into the lungs and collected. Perfusate collection should be performed on ice.

## Establishment of primary cultures

- The suspension of harvesting perfusate, beads, and cells should be centrifuged at 200× g (4 °C) for 5–10 min. The pellet is washed three times by suspension with 25 ml of prechilled wash media and centrifugation.
- The washed bead pellet is suspended in 36 ml of plating media and aliquoted (1.5 ml) to a 24-well plate. After 24 h of culture, approxi-

mately 0.7 ml of the suspended cells are removed and replated to a 24-well plate. The volume of media in all dishes is adjusted to 1.5 ml.

- After 3 days 0.3 ml of fresh rat serum is added to the cultures, and after 10 days refresh 1 ml of media.
- To selectively promote endothelial cell growth, the established primary cultures are supplemented with 100 µg/ml heparin (Calbiochem), 150 µg/ml Endothelial Cell Growth Factor (Collaborative Biomedical Research), and 10 µl of a 10 µg/ml rat epidermal growth factor solution (Biomedical Technologies Inc.). MEM D-val modification (*see* Section on *Tissue culture of pulmonary artery endothelial cells*) may also be used with supplements. After passage 3, cells maintained in maintenance media and after passage 10, FBS is reduced to 10%.

## Verification of endothelial cells

- Endothelial cells can be characterized by morphology. It may be difficult, however, to discern endothelial cells from other cell types before patches are formed. Indirect immunofluorescence is commonly utilized as an identifying criteria using Factor VIII antigen antibody binding, uptake of acetylated LDL, and *Ulex europaeus I* (UEA-I) lectin binding.
- Antibody and lectin labeling: Fix cells grown on coverslips with 100% methanol for 10 min. Add anti-human Von Willibrand's Factor antibody (Dako, Glostrup, Denmark), diluted 1:100 in phosphate buffered saline, to the fixed endothelial cells and allow to incubate for 60 min. Antibody labeling can then be detected with a labeled secondary antibody suitable for immunofluorescence.
- Acetylated LDL uptake: DiI-AC-LDL (20 µg/ml)(Biomedical Technologies, Stoughton, MA) can be incubated with endothelial cells for 4 h at 37 °C in a $CO_2$ incubator. Labeled cells are then fixed (10 min) with 3% formaldehyde in PBS and fluorescence analyzed.

# Discussion

Endothelial cells cultured and grown from either the pulmonary artery or microvasculature should exhibit a characteristic cobblestone pattern at confluence. Differences between macrovascular and microvascular cells can be seen at the subcellular level or utilizing lectin binding criteria, but are difficult to discern using phase contrast or bright field light microscopy. Each cell type should grow to confluence, exhibit contact inhibition, and not overgrow in culture. It is advisable to determine the growth rate of early passage cells to enable comparison with later passages.

Isolation of endothelia from large vessels by scraping is a widely appreciated method for obtaining cells. This method is currently used by multiple laboratories due largely to the ease at which pure cells can be isolated and the large numbers of cells (e.g. from large animals) that can be obtained. As discussed above, these may be the preferred cells for studies relating to control of blood pressure, but may not be the preferred cell type for studies relating to permeability. Morphological and functional data support the notion that macrovascular and microvascular endothelia express unique phenotypes. Therefore, it is advised to utilize cells from the site most relevant to your specific experimental question.

Two different techniques for isolating microvascular endothelial cells have been presented above. The fundamental question relating to microvascular endothelial cell isolation is, from which vascular site are the cells derived? Microvascular cells by definition may represent small arteries, capillaries and small veins. Thus, even within microvascular cells there may be mixed or heterogenous phenotypes of endothelia. Still, these cells are bound to be more similar than macrovascular *vs.* microvascular cells. It is unclear whether the cells obtained by cutting the external face of the lung differs from those obtained by retroperfusion, *per se*. We expect that similar populations of cells will be obtained although similarities and differences of cells obtained by these techniques has not been tested. It therefore seems reasonable from an experimental standpoint to use either technique, likely the one which can most easily be adapted to your laboratory setup. While technically demanding and perhaps easier to perform in laboratories familiar with perfused organ techniques, establishment of a lung perfusion set-up *per se* should not dictate the method chosen to obtain cells.

It is noteworthy that early passage endothelial cells from various organs including lung are now commercially available. Procuring cells through commercial vendors, while convenient, is not yet the preferred route by most investigators with the possible exception of use of human, organ-specific cells. Typically these cells and the media required for their culture are expensive, and the cells themselves are limited in the number of viable passages. It has been our experience that commercially available cells need to be fully characterized in the investigator's laboratory.

## Troubleshooting

*The cells obtained in primary culture are contaminated with cells staining negative for factor VIII antigen or LDL receptor. How can I select endothelial cells?* In primary cultures endothelial cells may be contaminated with other cell types, e.g. fibroblasts or smooth muscle cells. Over time, if contaminant cells grow faster than endothelial cells they may in fact overtake the culture. Techniques for insuring endothelial cell purity in primary cultures have therefore been developed. First, since endothelial cells grow effectively without L-valine whereas other cell populations do not, media complete with D-valine instead of L-valine is available for use in endothelial cell cultures. We commonly utilize MEM with the D-valine modification for this purpose. Use of D-valine MEM however does not guarantee that the culture will be free of contaminating cells. Thus, cells may be selected based upon their gross morphology using clonal rings. With clonal rings one may select a region with the culture which exhibits the morphology characteristic of endothelia, place the ring around that region, and scrape off the remaining cells. Subsequent clonal expansion will therefore reflect the cells selected by the ring. Alternatively, one may select cells using methods such as fluorescence activated cell sorting (FACS) or dilution cloning. It has been our experience that the dilution limit is two cells in the case of dilution cloning because single cells did not proliferate. We anticipate the next generation of endothelial cell selection methods will mimic the established fractionation procedures available in other cell types, e.g. lymphocytes.

*I am interested in microvascular and not macrovascular endothelial cells. How can I verify that my cell population is from the microcirculation?* As demonstrated in the preceding discussions, microvascular endothelial cells differ from macrovascular endothelial cells in both morphology and function. Thus, microvascular cells can be identified partly by their TEM and SEM morphologic characteristics. Upon analysis by TEM microvascular endothelial cells are thinner and possess fewer actin-like filaments. These cells also have a greater density of plasmalemmal vesicles and more extensive intercellular junctions. Upon analysis by SEM microvascular endothelial cells exhibit a remarkable array of projections (glycocalyx) that relates to glycoproteins differentially glycosylated. This heterogenous expression of glycosylation within pulmonary vascular segments can be used to identify microvascular endothelial cells [15, 18]. Binding of certain lectins to endothelial cells fulfills this criterion, where *Lycopersicum esculentum, Ulex europaeus I, Ricinus communis*, and *Arachis hypogaea* agglutinins interact with microvascular and less with macrovascular endothelial cells. In contrast, *Bandeiraea simplicifolia* and *Caragana arborescens* agglutinins interact with macrovascular endothelial cells and not microvascular endothelial cells. A caution for using lectins to define endothelial cell populations is that further work may be necessary to quantitate lectin binding, and cells from different species may demonstrate different patterns of lectin receptors.

*Cells lose their characteristic cobblestone pattern or any given functional response with successive passages. How can I prevent this de-differentiation?* Utilization of cells in culture provides a means of addressing mechanistic questions without many of the confounding variables present in the intact circulation. However, an important determinant is that endothelial cells do not differentiate with regard to their *in vivo* phenotype. While some change in endothelial behavior in culture is unavoidable, it is the investigator's responsibility to validate that the functional response *in vitro* is similar to the response observed in the intact circulation. Previous studies have determined that the longer cells are maintained in culture the more likely they are to de-differentiate. Furthermore, it is appreciated that trypsin, or exposure of cells to proteases, increases the rate at which cells de-differentiate. Thus, when passaging cells exposure to trypsin should be avoided. Cells can instead be scraped off the flask and then re-seeded. Since endothelial cells grow in sheets, scraping will generate sheets of cells that cannot be accurately counted. Precise cell counts are not necessary for routine passaging, however, and therefore this technique is acceptable for amplifying cell colonies. In contrast, the use of trypsin or Viokase is indicated when cells are transferred from large flasks to smaller plates for experiments in which good single cell dispersion and accurate cell counts are needed.

*My primary isolates commonly become contaminated. How can I prevent this contamination?* Tissue should be procured in media containing antibiotic and antimycotic, and subsequent tissue culture should be performed using sterile technique as described above. However, contamination at some point in your cell culture experience is almost unavoidable. The simple rule is that there is no substitute for sterile technique, and once a flask is infected throw it out and do not try to "rescue" the culture. Sufficient evidence is not available to determine whether previously infected cultures of cells behave in a manner similar to otherwise uninfected cultures. Given the time and money invested in the proposed experiments, it is simply not worth the risk.

It is noteworthy that endothelial cells may possess endogenous bacteria. As an example, the rat microvascular cells isolated using the retroperfusion technique described above have phagocytic activity. Endothelial intracellular vesicles can contain bacteria identical to endogenous species. Should endothelial cells burst, these bacteria do not replicate in culture media due to the penicillin, streptomycin, and gentamicin. These bacteria are also sensitive to third generation cephalosporins.

*What is the influence of substratum on endothelial cell morphology and function?* Endothelial cells are commonly allowed to lay down their own matrix when plated on plastic or glass. However, the morphology and function of cells grown on sufaces containing collagen and gelatin, matrigel and/or a variety of other matrices clearly differs. Furthermore, it is becoming clear that cell-matrix interactions greatly alter endothelial cell behavior. Since it is difficult to accurately reproduce the cell's *in vivo* substratum, to a large extent the surface on which cells are plated will depend upon your study questions. It is clearly important however to consider the potential influence of the matrix on your observed response.

*While the characteristic morphology of endothelial cells is cobblestone in nature, certain vascular segments in vivo possess endothelial cells that are elongated and aligned in the direction of blood flow. How do I address this issue in culture?* A cobblestone morphology has been generally utilized to identify healthy endothelia in culture. However, such a cobblestone morphology is only seen in low blood flow, low blood pressure vascular segments *in vivo*. In areas of high flow in particular endothelia are slightly elongated and aligned in the direction of flow. Thus, studies conducted on cells from high flow vascular segments may best represent the *in vivo* environment by recreating such an alignment *in vitro*. Interestingly, endothelial cells also align with flow *in vitro* and thus it is possible to mimick the *in vivo* environment.

# References

1 Mineau-Hanschke R, Wiles M, Morel N, Hechtman H and Shepro D (1990) *Microvasc. Res.* **39**: 140

2 Ryan U and Ryan J (1984) *Circulation* **70**: III-46

3 Adams D, Barakeh J, Laskey R and van Breeman C (1989) *FASEB J.* **3**: 2389

4 Dobrina A and Rossi F (1983) *Biochim. Biophys. Acta* **762**: 295

5 Habliston D, Whitaker C, Hart M, Ryan U and Ryan J (1979) *Am. Rev. Resp. Dis.* **119**: 853

6 Ryan U (1984) *Environmental Health Perspectives* **56**: 103

7 Chung-Welch N, Shepro D, Dunham B and Hechtman H (1988) *J. Cell Physiol.* **135**: 224

8 Ferreira S and Vane J (1967) **30**: 417

9 Hodge R, Ng K and Vane J (1967) *Nature* **215**: 138

10 Ng K and Vane J (1967) *Naure* **216**: 762

11 Lewis L, Hoak J, Maca R and Fry G (1973) *Science* **181**: 454

12 Gimbrone M, Cotran R and Folkman J (1974) *J. Cell Biol.* **60**: 673

13 Ryan U, Clements E, Habliston D and Ryan J (1978) *Tissue Cell* **10**: 535

14 Caldwell P, Seegal B, Hsu K, Das M and Soffer R (1976) *Science* **191**: 1050

15 Del Vecchio P, Siflinger-Birnboim A, Belloni P. Holleran L, Lum H and Malik A (1992) *In Vitro Cell Dev. Biol.* 28A:711

16 Hewett P and Murray J (1993) *Microvasc. Res.* **46**: 89

17 Diwan H, Thompson W, Lee A and Strada S (1994) *Biochem Biophys Res Comm* **202**: 728

18 Schnitzer J, Siflinger-Birnboim A, Del Vecchio P and Malik A (1994) *Biochem. Biophys. Res. Comm.* **199**: 11

19 Stevens T, Fouty B, Hepler L, Richardson D, Brough G, McMurtry I and Rodman D (1997) *Am. J. Physiol.* **272**: L1

20 Moy A, Van Engelenhoven J, Bodner J, Kaymath J, Keese C, Giaever I, Shasby S and Shasby D (1996) *J. Clin. Invest.* **97**: 1020

21 Magee J, Stone A, Oldham K and Guice K (1994) *Am. J. Physiol.* **267**: L433

22 Ryan U and White L (1986) *J. Tissue Cult. Meth.* **10**: 9

# Histology

# Studying lung ultrastructure

*H. Fehrenbach and*
*M. Ochs*

The study of ultrastructure comprises a wide field of techniques and instrumentations that are used to investigate the organisation of an organ, its tissues, and their cells at the subcellular level all the way down to molecules. The central theme is: How are these components organized in space, i.e. how do they look in three dimensions, and how are they arranged in 3-D with respect to one another?

In conventional electron microscopy, we have the choice of studying ultrastructure by means of scanning (SEM) or transmission (TEM) electron microscopes [1]. From SEM we may gain some information about the external aspects of an object as, for example, direct 3-D views of cells, their surface differentiations like cilia or microvilli, and their regional distribution. From TEM we may learn something about the internal aspects of cells and their organelles as, for example, the organisation of microtubules within a cilium, the arrangement and distribution of an organelle within a cell. While SEM is performed on the whole specimen, TEM requires that a skillful person (perhaps from the next EM unit) will cut ultrathin sections (50–100 nm) of the specimen. However, be aware of the fact that the 3-D object has been transformed into a two-dimensional section. To extract the information about the object's organization in space from the 2-D section, we have to do either 3-D reconstruction using serial ultrathin sections, which is very cumbersome, or use an appropriate sampling scheme to be able to apply stereological techniques.

This chapter is intended to give anyone without experience in ultrastructural research a basis to integrate a study of lung ultrastructure into an own experimental design. We will not go into theory and practice of running an EM lab, or of using highly sophisticated ultrastructural methods (for comprehensive information, *see* [2–4]). Rather, we will focus on the first steps of conventional procedures, i.e., fixation, sampling, and tissue processing that will allow to get a proper sample of the specimen, prepared in an appropriate way so that colleagues from the EM and stereology units will not criticize us for giving them a biased sample of cell mash for examination. For integrating an ultrastructural study into an own experimental design, rather than just trying to obtain a nice picture to illustrate a paper, we have to take into account some essentials.

The aim of fixation is to preserve the organization of tissues, cells, and organelles with as minimal alterations from the living state as possible, ideally at the molecular level. Further, fixation should protect the specimen against potential alterations caused by subsequent treatments as, for example, rinsing, dehydration, embedding, sectioning, vacuum and exposure to the electron beam. Since structural alteration starts with the removal of a specimen from the living organism, fixation should be performed *in situ* within the shortest time possible after death or at the end of an experiment. Further, all parts of the organ should be homogeneously well preserved. Since no fixation procedure is available that satisfies all the demands, the choice of a particular fixation procedure is always a compromise (for review, *see* [3–8]).

Quantification by means of stereology is essential for comparative ultrastructural studies. And whenever the intention is to measure or count anything from specimens, we have to take special care to use a proper sampling scheme (for review of recent assumption-free stereological methods (*see* e.g. [9–13]). In most instances, the aim of sampling will be to obtain a collection of tissue blocks, sections, and finally micrographs that are representative of the whole organ. Therefore, each site of the lung should have the same chance to be selected for the study. The most effective procedure to accomplish this is known as systematic random sampling, in which the first item in the sample is chosen randomly, but then determines the position of all other items (e.g. [12]). This principle is pertinent to all stages from slicing of the lung, excision of tissue blocks, recording of micrographs, and analyzing the structures of interest. At each stage of the selection process systematic random sampling has to be performed. If, at any stage, the chain is broken, this will result in a biased sample impairing the accuracy of the measurements (e.g. [13]). Very often, absolute values of stereologic parameters are needed to obtain an appropriate description of what has happened to the organ. Therefore, stereological data are at best related to the total volume of the lung, which can be determined either by fluid displacement or by application of the Cavalieri principle [14]. In order to obtain reliable estimates of parameters like surface areas and lengths, isotropic orientation of the structure of interest is required. Depending on the particular problem, isotropy can be achieved for example, by means of the vertical sectioning technique [14] or the isector method [15].

---

## Material and equipment

### List of equipment

The materials and equipment necessary for the procedure described are given in Table 17.1.

### *Solutions*

(use a fume hood, safety goggles and safety gloves during preparation, handle with great care because most of the ingredients are toxic, irritating, and/or allergenic – *see* manufacturer's information):

### *Primary fixative for conventional TEM and SEM (1.5% formaldehyde and 1.5% glutaraldehyde in 0.1 M cacodylate buffer)*

To make a volume of 5 l of primary fixative (e.g. for fixation and storage of a single dog lung) we need 2500 ml of 0.2 M cacodylate buffer, 300 ml of 25% aqueous formaldehyde, 300 ml of 25% aqueous glutaraldehyde, and 1900 ml bidistilled water. After addition of all the ingredients thoroughly stir the solution, adjust the pH to 7.35, and finally determine the total osmolality of the fixative (800–900 mOsmol/kg).

To make a stock solution of 0.2 M cacodylate buffer, which can be stored for months in a refrigerator, dissolve 107 g of sodium-dimethylarsenic salt in bidistilled water to give a final volume of 2500 ml. Adjust pH with 1N HCl to 7.35. Add NaCl to adjust osmolality to 600 mOsmol/kg using a freezing-point depression osmometer (we will need about 5.8 g NaCl per 1000 ml). Equal parts of the stock solution and bidistilled water are mixed to prepare about 100 ml of 0.1 M cacodylate rinsing buffer (control osmolality of 300 mOsmol/kg). (The total osmotic pressure of glutaraldehyde fixatives has early been recognized to be of less importance for

*Table 17.1. List of materials and equipment*

| Materials | | Type of study |
|---|---|---|
| **Chemicals for** | | |
| primary fixation | 25% glutardialdehyde, EM-grade* | general |
| | paraformaldehyde, extra pure | general |
| | dimethylarsinic acid sodium salt trihydrate, for synthesis-grade | c-TEM |
| | HEPES | immuno-TEM |
| sampling | agar-agar | general |
| secondary fixation | osmium tetroxide, crystalline | c-TEM, SEM |
| processing | uranyl acetate dihydrate, for analysis-grade | c-(immuno-)TEM |
| | thiocarbohydrazide | SEM |
| embedding | ethanol or acetone (absolute) | c-TEM, SEM |
| | glycol methacrylate | LM |
| | Araldite, Epon | c-TEM |
| | methanol (absolute) | immuno-TEM |
| | Lowicryl (HM 20, K4M) | immuno-TEM |
| **Equipment for** | | |
| primary fixation for general purposes | reservoir with outlet and tubing, e.g. buret (rat: 100–200 ml; dog: 1000 ml) | |
| | processing tray | |
| | laboratory stand | |
| | appropriate tracheal catheter | |
| | dissecting scissors | |
| | disposable dissecting scalpel with blades | |
| | several clamps, forceps, small cotton ribbons | |
| | histology storage container (rat: 100–200 ml; dog: 5000 ml) | |
| additionally for vascular perfusion | pulmonary artery or right ventricle catheter | |
| | roller pump | |
| | device to control airway pressure | |
| sampling | self-made spiral-like basket [21] | |
| | glass beaker (rat: 500 ml; dog: 5000 ml) | |
| | dissecting board | |
| | autopsy knife or blades | |
| | needles | |
| | transparent sheets with test grid | |
| secondary fixation | snap cap vials, pasteur pipettes | |
| processing | critical point dryer | SEM |
| embedding | laboratory oven | c-TEM |
| | freeze-substitution unit | immuno-TEM |

* *Glutaraldehyde is commercially available from a number of companies as an EM grade solution of 25% aqueous glutardialdehyde. However, quality has been shown to be quite different [16].*

proper fixation than the osmotic pressure of the fixative vehicle [17]. Griffiths ([5] p. 58) pointed out that although the highly complex process of fixation is not fully understood "at least in the first seconds and minutes of fixation the aldehyde fixative is free to enter cells, whereas most charged buffer ions are not." Therefore, "buffer ions, and not fixative molecules, will be primarily responsible for the effective osmotic pressure of the buffered fixative solutions," and "the effects of the charged buffer ions in use must be primarily extracellular.")

To make 25% aqueous formaldehyde, which should be freshly prepared (commercially available solutions contain methanol as a stabilizer, the effect of which on ultrastructure is unclear ([5] p. 63)), weigh out 75 g paraformaldehyde in a glass jar (be careful during handling not to inhale the powder). Be careful while filling in bidistilled water to give about 250 ml. Heat up to 65 °C using a magnetic stirrer. As soon as 65 °C have been achieved, remove jar from heating plate and add 1N NaOH until the solution becomes almost clear. Cool to room temperature (solution becomes clearer), and fill in bidistilled water to get a total volume of 300 ml.

### Primary fixative for immunocytochemistry (4% formaldehyde and 0.1% glutaraldehyde in 0.2 M HEPES buffer)

To make a volume of 5 l, dissolve 260.28 g HEPES in 4480 ml bidistilled water. Add 20 ml of 25% glutaraldehyde, and 500 ml of 40% formaldehyde. Stir the solution thoroughly. Adjust pH to 7.35, and determine the total osmolality (800–900 mOsmol/kg).

To make a 40% formaldehyde solution, proceed as described above, but use 160 g paraformaldehyde and add bidistilled water to make a final volume of 400 ml. Add the solution to the buffer after it cools to room temperature (RT).

### Cryoprotectant for infiltration of specimens to be frozen in liquid nitrogen (2.3 M sucrose in phosphate buffered saline, PBS)

To make 100 ml cryoprotectant solution, dissolve 78.93 g of sucrose in PBS and adjust volume to 100 ml.

To make 1 l of PBS dissolve 2.25 g of $Na_2HPO_4 \cdot H_2O$, 0.257 g of $NaHPO_4 \cdot H_2O$, and 8.767 g NaCl in 1000 ml bidistilled water. (PBS is also commercially available.)

### Postosmication for SEM/TEM with 1% osmium tetroxide (OsO₄) in 0.1 M cacodylate buffer

Mix equal parts of a 2% aqueous $OsO_4$ solution, and of the stock solution of 0.2 M sodium-cacodylate buffer which has been adjusted to pH 7.35, and 300mOsmol/kg (*see* above).

To make 50 ml of a 2% aqueous $OsO_4$ solution (which can be stored for a few months in a refrigerator), crack a sealed ampoule containing 1 g of $OsO_4$, and put it into a dark sealable bottle. (Sealed ampoules containing 1g crystalline $OsO_4$ are commercially available. $OsO_4$ is extremely volatile, and should only be handled under a fume hood. Use double sealable dark bottle for storage in a separate refrigerator.) Fill in 50 ml of bidistilled water, and use an ultrasound bath to dissolve the $OsO_4$ crystals.

### Postfixation for TEM with half-saturated aqueous uranyl acetate solution

To make a stock solution of 200 ml of saturated (uranyl acetate has a solubility of 77 g/l at 20 °C) uranyl acetate (which can be stored in a dark bottle for months in a refrigerator) weigh out 16.68 g of uranyl acetate, and add 200 ml of bidistilled water. Stir the solution thoroughly, and do not use it before the next day. There will still be some sedimented salt. The final half-saturated solution is prepared upon usage by mixing equal volumes of the stock solution with bidistilled water.

### Postfixation for SEM according to modified OTOTO procedure [18] with 1% aqueous osmium tetroxide and 1% aqueous thiocarbohydrazide (TCH)

To make a 1% aqueous $OsO_4$ solution, mix equal volumes of a 2% aqueous solution (*see* above) and bidistilled water.

To make a 1% aqueous solution of TCH (prepare at the day of usage), add bidistilled water to 1 g of TCH to yield 100 ml of solution. Stir thoroughly. Be extremely careful, because TCH is highly toxic and explosive when heated.

# Methods

## Modes of fixation

*Fixation by airway instillation*

1) Fill in the fixative into the reservoir (buret). Adjust the fixative's upper level at 20–25 cm above the deflated lung. Be sure that the glass olive or catheter inserted into the trachea (or bronchus) is tightly fastened (if you have to remove some of the connective tissue around the trachea be careful not to make an incision). Clamp the pulmonary artery and veins.

2) Let the fixative flow into the lung. Continuously refill the reservoir with fresh fixative (avoid air bubbles). Proceed until the flow stops automatically at a hydrostatic pressure of 20–25 cm fluid column. Fixation might have been successful if all parts of the lung are well expanded and the pleural surface is smooth. (Final evaluation whether the lung has been homogeneously well preserved is only possible at the microscope.) Problems may arise if lobes are twisted so that the fixative cannot pass the ligated bronchus. Gently unwrap the twisting, so as not to disconnect instillation tube and trachea, and finish fixation.

3) Clamp the trachea in addition to the vessels, and immerse the lung into fresh fixative in a sealable container wide enough that the lung is not compressed. Fill the container completely with fixative, and close it tightly so that only minimal gas space is present. Alternatively, fasten some weight at the trachea to ensure that the lung will be submerged.

4) Store the lung in the fixative for 2 h up to 1 day at 4–8 °C. (If working together with an EM partner who is not local, the lung may be transferred into a tightly sealable container filled with pre-cooled fixative, and put into an insulated box together with a cool element (do not use metal coated elements, the lung may freeze). Now the lung is ready for mailing or transportation.)

5) Follow the sampling procedure given below.

Figure 17.1 gives an example of ultrastructural appearance achieved by this method.

435

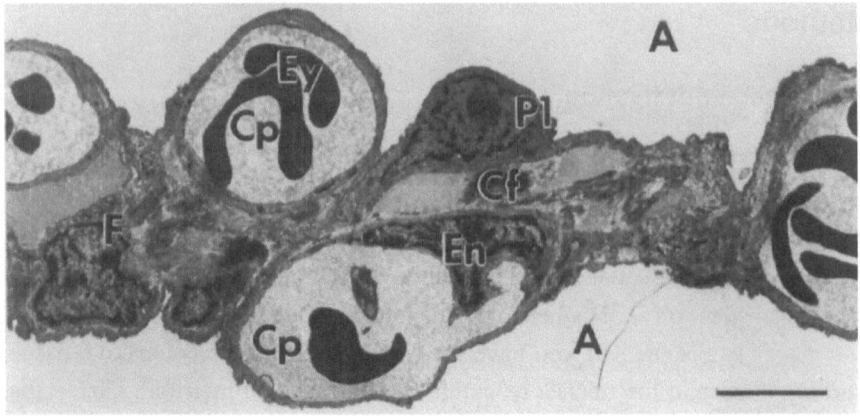

***Figure 17.1. TEM micrograph of canine lung fixed in situ by airway instillation at 25 cm H₂0
within 2 min after cardiac arrest***
*Primary fixative for c-TEM/SEM, sequentially post-fixed with osmium tetroxide and aqueous uranyl
acetate, and embedded in Araldite. Alveolar septum with central collagen fiber strand (Cf), and capillaries (Cp) bulging into the gas containing alveolar space (A). Type 1 pneumocyte (P1) is not covered
with alveolar surfactant, because it is largely removed during instillation fixation. There are no signs of
interstitial or cellular edema. Capillary lumen with erythrocytes (Ey) and flocculent proteinaceous serum material. En=capillary endothelium; F=fibrocyte. Scale bar=4 µm.*

## Fixation by vascular perfusion

1) Connect the trachea to a respirator or other device (*see* [3] Fig. 1.10)
   so that the airway pressure can be adjusted over a range of
   5–30 cm H₂0.

2) Fill in the fixative into the reservoir (buret). Adjust the fixative's
   upper level at 15 cm above the hilum. Be sure that the catheter inserted into the pulmonary artery is tightly fastened.

3) Perform 2–3 inflation/deflation cycles, and finally deflate the lung
   to a constant airway pressure of 10–12 cm H₂0.

4) Start fixation. Fill in fresh fixative into the reservoir by means of a
   roller pump to ascertain constant fixation pressure. Be careful to
   avoid any air bubbles in the perfusion system that might cause an air
   embolus when entering the vessels. Stop flow of fixative after
   2–10 min. Effluate should be clear within 1–2 min. Fixation was

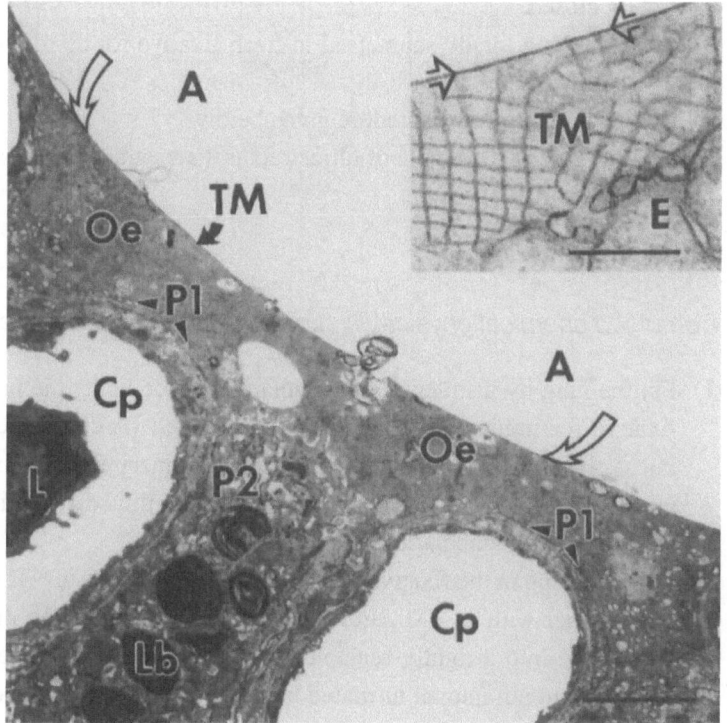

**Figure 17.2. TEM micrograph of rat lung fixed ex situ within 10 min after cardiac arrest by vascular perfusion at a pressure of 15 cm H$_2$0 with airway pressure kept at 12 cm H$_2$0**

Primary fixative for c-TEM/SEM, sequentially post-fixed with osmium tetroxide and aqueous uranyl acetate, and embedded in Araldite. Alveolar epithelium with type 2 pneumocyte (P2) containing surfactant storing lamellar bodies (Lb), and largely fragmented type 1 pneumocytes (P1). Accumulation of protein-rich alveolar edema (Oe) results in separation of air-blood-barrier and alveolar surfactant lining layer (open arrows). Capillary lumen (Cp) is devoid of erythrocytes and flocculent serum material, which are largely removed during vascular perfusion, while lymphocytes (L) may regularly be seen. TM = tubular myelin. Scale bar = 2 µm.

Inset: At higher magnification, a region free of alveolar edema shows alveolar lining layer (open arrows) with closely associated tubular myelin (TM) in direct contact to the alveolar epithelium (E). Scale bar = 0.1 µm.

probably successful, if the lung is no longer soft, but stiff and compact in all the regions. (Final evaluation whether the lung has been homogeneously well preserved is only possible at the microscope.)

5) Tightly ligate trachea, pulmonary artery and veins.

6) To avoid distortion of the lung, use a wide container, which can be tightly closed.

7) Store the lung totally submersed in fresh fixative for up to 1 day at 4–8 °C.

8) Follow the sampling procedure given below.

Figure 17.2 gives an example of ultrastructural appearance achieved by this method.


## Combined chemical/physical fixation for immunocytochemistry

1) Fix the lung by instillation or vascular perfusion using the primary fixative for immunocytochemistry (*see* above). (A combined chemical/physical fixation using conventional primary fixative may be useful, if we are interested in the study of edema fluid distribution rather than in immunocytochemistry.)

2) Store the lung in the fixative for 2 h up to 1 day at 4–8 °C. (If working together with an EM partner who is not local, the lung may be transferred into a tightly sealable container filled with pre-cooled fixative, and put into an insulated box together with a cool element (do not use metal coated elements, the lung may freeze). Now the lung is ready for mailing or transportation.)

3) Cut small (<1 mm$^3$) samples obtained by the sampling procedure given below.

4) Infiltrate samples with cryoprotectant (2.3 M sucrose in PBS) for 1 h.

5) Freeze samples in liquid nitrogen.

6) Store samples in liquid nitrogen until freeze substitution or cryo-sectioning can be performed.


## Fixation by immersion into a chemical fixative

1) The best and most simple way to perform this method is simply not to use it. (In contrast to research purposes, biopsy or autopsy material may be the only specimens available for pathologic diagnosis. For

comprehensive description of methods related to handling of pathology specimens, the reader is referred to the review of Dvorak [19].)

## Sampling of tissue blocks (Fig. 17.3)

Determination of the organ volume, which precedes sampling and is needed for the calculation of absolute stereological parameters, can either be performed by fluid displacement (step 1) or alternatively by application of the Cavalieri principle (step 3).

1) Determination of rat lung volume by means of fluid displacement [21]:

    Put a 500 ml jar filled with 250–350 ml of an isotonic salt solution (e.g., PBS, *see* above) or with fixative with the specific weight $G$ onto a laboratory balance. Immerse a small spiral-like basket (this can easily be made from a piece of stainless steel wire [21]) fixed to a laboratory stand, which will be used for submersion of the lung. Adjust the balance to zero. Remove the lung from fixative, and gently blot it dry with filter paper. Remove all adhering tissue from the lung that are to be excluded from analysis. Submerge the lung with the basket so that neither basket nor lung touch any side of the jar. Read the weight gain $W$ from the balance's display. Calculate the lung volume $V$ to be $V = W/G$, having in mind to subtract the volume of clamps, ligatures etc. determined likewise. Transfer the lung into the fixative again.

2) Generation of organ slices:

    To facilitate sectioning of large organs, the whole lung may be covered with 2% aqueous agar-agar (rat lungs should be completely embedded). Cut the lung from apical to caudal into parallel slices of 2 cm in thickness to get about 10 slices (for rat lungs a thickness of 3 mm will be appropriate; a tissue slicer with equidistant spacings will be very helpful. A device for small lungs is shown by Michel and Cruz-Orive ([14] Fig. 2), one designed for larger lungs is shown by Gundersen and Jensen ([22] Fig. 24)). The position of the first cut should be chosen at random between 0 and 2 cm. Only random posi-

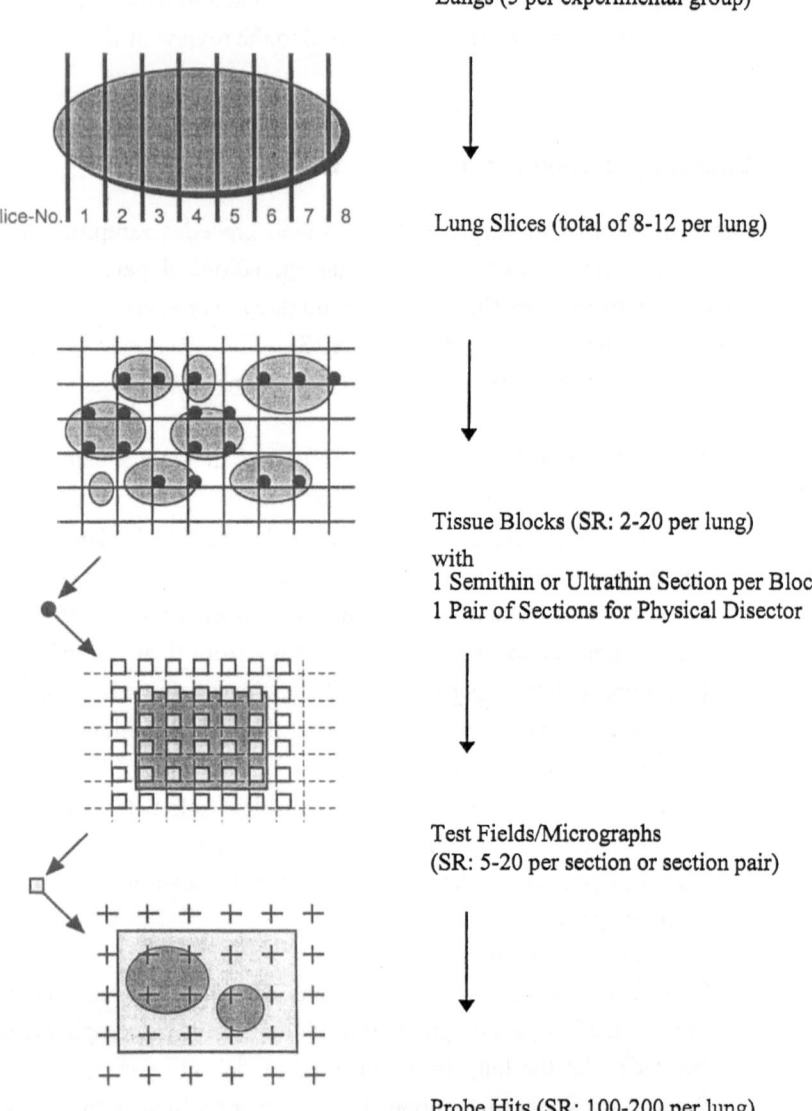

Lungs (5 per experimental group)

Lung Slices (total of 8-12 per lung)

Tissue Blocks (SR: 2-20 per lung)
with
1 Semithin or Ultrathin Section per Block,
1 Pair of Sections for Physical Disector

Test Fields/Micrographs
(SR: 5-20 per section or section pair)

Probe Hits (SR: 100-200 per lung)

**Figure 17.3. Schematic sampling scheme for stereological analysis of lung structures**
*At each level suggested numbers of items are given (modified according to [20]). SR, systematic random sampling.*

tion of the first cut guarantees an equal chance for all regions of the organ to be represented in the slice plane.

3) Determination of canine lung volume by means of the Cavalieri principle:

Lay down the lung slices, which were generated in step 2, apical face up in a processing tray. Superimpose a transparent point grid (e.g. [22], Fig. 19) at random orientation on each slice. A reasonable distance $d$ between any two points will be 1.8 cm (for smaller lungs $d$ should be reduced). Count all the points $P$ falling on the apical section profile of each slice (omit the first slice because it has no apical section profile; do not count points that project on the pleural surface). Since each point $P$ represents a unit area $a(P) = d^2$, we can determine the area $A$ of the apical section profile of each slice. The volume of the lung $V$ may then be estimated by the sum of all section areas $A$ times the slice thickness $t$, i.e. $estV = t \times \sum A = t \times d^2 \times \sum P$. In our case $estV = 2$ cm $\times 1.8$ cm$^2 \times \sum P$. To obtain a reasonable precision, $\sum P$ should be in a range of 100–200 points [22]. (The Cavalieri principle can also be applied using calibrated photographs of the individual slices. This offers the advantages of repeated measurements, and of the possibility to determine the fraction of large non-parenchymal structures. This additional step may be necessary, particularly in the study of large lungs.)

4) For sampling of tissue blocks superimpose a transparent grid with circular, 4 cm spaced holes over all slices, generated in step 2, at random orientation. Use, for example, every second hole for TEM samples, and the others alternating for SEM and LM samples. Insert a needle into the tissue through every hole that projects onto the apical section profile of a lung slice. The position of the needle defines one precise corner (this may be any of the four corners, but must be the same for all tissue blocks of an organ) of the tissue block to be excised.

For TEM, excise a column of 2 cm length (i.e. extending throughout the lung slice). The final tissue blocks should be trimmed from the upper end of the column to get a cube with about 1–3 mm side length (subsequent cubes might be collected if various processing and/or embedding protocols will be used). After processing, samples should be embedded according to the isector method to guarantee IUR-sections (*see* below).

For LM and SEM, excise tissue blocks of a size of $1 \times 1 \times 2$ cm$^3$. Divide the block into two cubes of 1 cm$^3$, and use the upper cube for further sampling for LM stereology purposes. Define x-, y-, and z-plane of the cube e.g., the upper face as "1", the front face as "2" and the right face as "3". Randomly select one of the three numbers, e.g. "2". Cut a 1–2 mm slice from face "2". Go on systematically, i.e. the slice to be cut from the next tissue block will derive from face "3", from the third block from face "1", and so on. By this method we get LM sections in all three dimensions, and although these are not perfect isotropic sections, it takes into account the anisotropy of non-parenchymal components. For all practical reasons this will be okay in a largely homogeneous organ like the lung.

## Processing and embedding of tissue blocks

### For conventional LM

For embedment, the use of a glycol methacrylate (GMA, e.g. Technovit 7100, Heraeus Kulzer, Wehrheim, Germany) instead of paraffin is recommended. Paraffin embedment generally results in extensive tissue shrinkage [23, 24].

1) Rinse tissues blocks with the same buffer used during fixation (about three to six changes during 30–60 min).
2) Successively dehydrate the specimens with 70% (2 h, RT), 96% (2 h, RT), and 100% ethanol (1 h, RT).
3) Transfer the specimens into a 1:1 mixture of 100% ethanol and infiltration medium (GMA + hardener I) for 2 h (RT).
4) Infiltrate specimens with infiltration medium (GMA + hardener I) overnight (RT).
5) Embed specimens in embedding medium (GMA + hardener I + II) using flat embedding molds. (We use embedding molds and corresponding block holders offered by Polysciences Ltd., which we find easier for handling of the polymerized blocks. Therefore, however,

our embedding procedures is slightly different than the one proposed by the manufacturer of Technovit 7100.)

6) Prepare embedding molds by polymerizing a thin layer of embedding medium for 1 h at about 40 °C.

7) Transfer specimens onto polymerized layer, and fill mold with fresh embedding medium.

8) Polymerization is performed for 1–2 h at about 40 °C and subsequently at RT overnight, before microtome holder is fixed.

## For conventional TEM (following [25])

1) Rinsing of tissue blocks in 0.1 M cacodylate buffer (six changes during 30 min, 4–8 °C).

2) Postosmication for 2 h at 4–8 °C with 1 % $OsO_4$ in 0.1 M cacodylate buffer.

3) Rinsing of tissue blocks in 0.1 M cacodylate buffer (four changes during 20 min, 4–8 °C).

4) Two rinses in bidistilled water (5 min each, 4–8 °C).

5) Postfixation overnight (12–18 h) at 4–8 °C with half-saturated aqueous uranyl acetate.

6) Rinsing in bidistilled water (six changes during 30 min, 4–8 °C).

7) Dehydration through an ascending series of alcohols (50 %, 70 % [this is a good point at which to stop the procedure if embedding cannot be immediately accomplished afterwards. Resume the procedure the next day], 90 %, 3×100 %; 10 min each) followed by propylene oxide (two changes, 15 min each). (Propylene oxide may be omitted if an ascending series of acetone is used for dehydration.)

8) Infiltration with a 1:1-mixture of propylene oxide and Araldite or Epon.

9) Infiltration with pure Araldite or Epon overnight.

10) Transfer into embedding capsules or flat embedding molds, and fill with fresh resin. (Preferably use prepared resin of the same charge, which can be frozen until usage.)

11) Polymerize at 60 °C for 3 days.

For generation of IUR-sections modify steps 10 and 11 according to the isector method [15]. After infiltration, embed the specimens in rubber molds with spherical cavities. (Detailed description of how to make the molds is given in the original paper [15].) After polymerization for 2 days at 60 °C, the resulting resin spheres containing the specimens are to be rolled on the laboratory table. Then, the spheres that contain a specimen are embedded in flat embedding molds in precisely the orientation they had when they stopped rolling. This guarantees isotropy of the final sections. Polymerization is continued for 2 days at 60 °C.

Figures 17.1 and 17.2 give examples of ultrastructural appearance achieved by this method.

### For TEM based immunocytochemistry (modified after [26])

1) Transfer cryo-fixed, frozen specimens (under liquid nitrogen) into a freeze-substitution unit (although freeze-substitution may be accomplished in a −80°C refrigerator or in dry ice mixed with acetone (−79°C) in tightly closed vials (*see* Steinbrecht and Müller, 1987 in [27]), the use of a commercially available unit (e.g. from Leica or Balzers) offers more versatility, easier handling, and better reproducibility), which has already been adjusted to −90 °C. Wait for about 10 min so that the specimens can adopt temperature of substitution unit.
2) Transfer the specimens into precooled substitution medium. Carry out freeze-substitution in 0.5% uranyl acetate in methanol at −90 °C for at least 36 h (adjust the time so as to start the washing step in the morning).
3) Raise the temperature to −45 °C at a rate of 5 °C/h.
4) Wash several times with pure methanol.
5) Infiltrate the samples with Lowicryl HM20-methanol 1:1 for 2 h, 2:1 for 2 h, pure Lowicryl for 2 h and pure Lowicryl overnight.
6) Polymerize the samples under UV-light for 2 days at −45 °C.

Figure 17.4 gives an example of ultrastructural appearance achieved by this method.

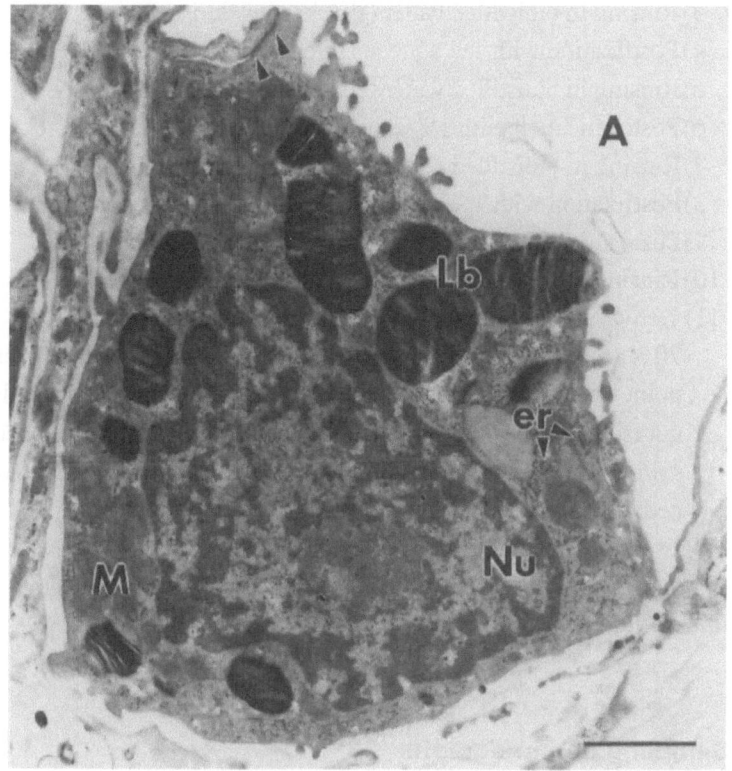

**Figure 17.4. TEM micrograph of porcine lung fixed in situ by airway instillation at 25 cm H₂0 within 2 min after cardiac arrest**
Primary fixative for immuno-TEM, cryoprotected with 2.3 M sucrose in PBS, freeze-substituted with 0.5% uranyl acetate in methanol, and embedded in Lowicryl HM20. Type 2 pneumocyte with surfactant storing lamellar bodies (Lb), mitochondria (M), and nucleus (Nu) showing minimal alterations due to tissue processing and embedding. Lumen of the cisternae of the endoplasmic reticulum (er) filled with moderately dense material. A = alveolar space; arrowheads = cell junctions with neighboring type 1 pneumocytes. Scale bar = 1 µm.

## For SEM modified according to an OTOTO method [18]

1) Rinsing of tissue blocks in 0.1 M cacodylate buffer (six changes during 60 min, 4–8 °C).
2) Postosmication with 1 % OsO₄ in 0.1 M cacodylate buffer for 1–2 h at 4–8 °C.

3) Rinsing in bidistilled water (six changes during 30 min, RT).

4) Postfixation with 1 % aqueous thiocarbohydrazide for 30 min at RT.

5) Rinsing in bidistilled water (six changes during 30 min, RT).

6) Postosmication with 1 % aqueous $OsO_4$ for 1–2 h at 4–8 °C.

7) Rinsing in bidistilled water (six changes during 30 min, RT).

8) Postfixation with 1 % aqueous thiocarbohydrazide for 30 min at RT.

9) Postosmication with 1 % aqueous $OsO_4$ for 1–2 h at 4–8 °C.

10) Rinsing in bidistilled water (six changes during 30 min, RT).

11) Dehydration through an ascending series of alcohols (30 %, 50 %, 70 % (this is a good point at which to stop the procedure if critical point drying cannot be immediately accomplished afterwards. Do not store the specimens for weeks, because extraction will occur, resulting in fine artefactual deposits all over the surfaces to be examined), 90 %, $3 \times 100$ %; 10 min each).

12) Critical point drying.

Figure 17.5 gives an example of ultrastructural appearance achieved by this method.

## Sampling of micrographs

For the stereological investigation of LM and TEM samples usually only one section per block should be used (an exception may be the use of the physical disector method, *see* e.g. [10]). From this section, however, all micrographs selected according to systematic random sampling have to be used for analysis. (Do not simply use the first five or 10 micrographs for stereological analysis, since this collection will yield a biased sample.)

At the LM level, systematic random sampled fields of view can be obtained using the x- and y-axis of the microscope stage micrometers. Starting at a random position outside the section, e.g., at the upper left side, move the microscope stage at fixed intervals along both axes until you have examined the whole section.

For TEM, the squares of the supporting grid or the microscope stage can be used to move at fixed intervals over the whole section. Again, the first field, which should be selected at random, determines the position

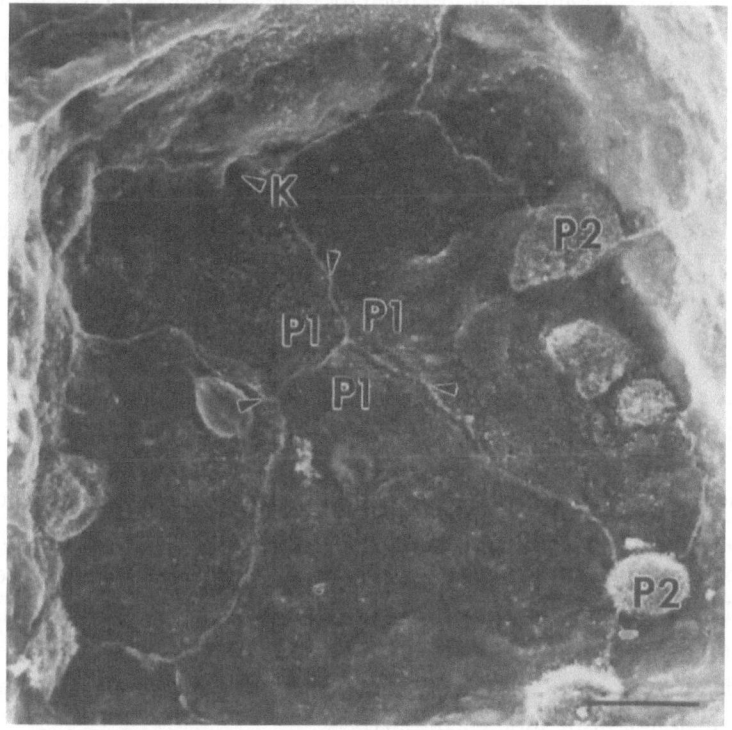

*Figure 17.5. SEM micrograph of human lung fixed by airway instillation at 25 cm H₂0 after clinical organ preservation by pulmonary arterial flush perfusion with modified Euro-Collins solution, and subsequent cold ischemic storage for 5 h*

*Primary fixative for c-TEM/SEM, post-fixed with osmium tetroxide and thiocarbohydrazide (OTOTO method), dehydrated with ethanol, and critical point dried. The look into an alveolus provides a direct view of the alveolar epithelial surface, since alveolar surfactant has been removed by instillation fixation. Cell junctions (arrowheads) between flat and extended type 1 pneumocytes (P1) are clearly delineated. Type 2 pneumocytes (P2) bulge into the alveolar space, and show a dense coverage of microvilli. Pore of Kohn (K) connects neighboring alveoli. Scale bar= 16 µm. (Micrograph by courtesy of D. Riemann, Göttingen).*

of all other fields. These fields of view together represent the appropriate sample to be used for stereological investigation. By means of superimposed test systems, analysis can be performed either on-line using a camera connected to a computer system or off-line using the electron micrographs recorded from the corresponding fields. In any case, however, use a calibration specimen for careful determination of the magnification used. (If analyzing photographic reproductions of micrographs, use a micrograph of the calibration specimen to precisely determine the final magnification during each darkroom session.) Detailed descriptions of the application of stereological methods to the lung are beyond the scope of this chapter. The reader is referred to recent reviews of stereological methods (general: [9–13]; with special emphasis on the lung: [28–30]).

## Discussion

Depending on the information to be obtained from the specimen, the choice of the appropriate method to be used for ultrastructural analysis requires consideration of a number of points related to the various steps of the whole procedure:

i) selection of the mode of fixation, i.e. chemical, physical, or a sequential procedure,

ii) selection of the mode of application, i.e. fixation by immersion, vascular perfusion or instillation via the airways,

iii) selection of the fixing agent, e.g. glutaraldehyde, formaldehyde, acrolein, osmium tetroxide, uranyl acetate, mixtures or sequences thereof (including the appropriate buffer vehicle), or special fixatives for cytochemical or tracer studies,

iv) selection of the sampling procedure (is the interest in precisely located structures or knowledge about the whole organ),

v) selection of the tissue processing procedure for conventional TEM or immunocytochemistry (including decisions about postosmication, postfixation with uranyl acetate, type of embedding resin), and

vi) selection of the appropriate stereological procedures to allow quantification of a parameter of interest.

### Selecting the mode of fixation

Physical fixation of very small pieces of tissue by means of cryo-techniques is the method of choice in time-resolved studies of dynamic cellular events as, for example, ion or other mobile component shifts [31–33], in microanalytical studies of ion distribution [34, 35], in immunocytochemical studies of sensitive antigens [5], or in the study of the aqueous hypophase of the surfactant lining layer [36]. However, cryo-fixation can only be performed on biopsy samples, preferably obtained *in situ* by means of a cryo-snapper or cryo-needle [37, 38], or on cultured cells or suspensions of, for example, surfactant fractions (for review, *see* [27, 39]). At present, there are no cryo-techniques that would allow physical fixation of a whole organ. Therefore, sampling cannot be performed in a way to obtain a representative collection of specimens required for quantitative structural analysis (*see* below) (this is also true for chemical fixation by immersion into a fixative, which is additionally hampered by the fact that the speed of chemical fixation is much slower than of cryo-fixation. Unless high pressure freezing is applied [38], a gradient of ultrastructural preservation is induced with decreasing quality from the outer layers to the centre of a tissue block. Therefore, preservation of the ultrastructure will be all but homogeneous in specimens fixed by immersion [40]). The only way to overcome this problem is to do cryo-fixation on specimens appropriately sampled from a chemically fixed organ. This procedure may be useful in the structural analysis of edema or in immunocytochemistry, since dehydration can be performed at low temperature and/or post-osmication can be avoided.

## Selecting the mode of application

As already noted, immersion fixation is far from being appropriate for scientific purposes. While quick and homogeneous fixation of the whole lung is generally achieved by both vascular perfusion and airway instillation (for review, *see* e.g. [41–43]). Since we have to take into account that the ultrastructure of the compartment (where the fixative enters the organ) might be altered due to fixation, we have to chose whether to be sure of minimal alterations at the gas conducting side or at the blood conducting side of the lung. Instillation via the airways is quite easily performed, and is the method of choice whenever the airways are open and we are not interested in the preservation of any structures present at the gas phase (e.g. surfactant material, alveolar macrophages, alveolar edema). Otherwise, we should do perfusion fixation via the blood vessels (*see* e.g. [28, 42, 43]).

## Selecting the fixing agent

There are a number of different fixing agents available, which can be combined in numberless mixtures, each of which has its own merits and shortcomings. The reader is referred to textbooks of general electron microscopy [1–7].

## Selecting the mode of tissue processing

For conventional TEM, secondary fixatives containing heavy metal atoms as, for example, osmium or uranium, are frequently used as "stains", because they introduce the contrast necessary for microscopic analysis. However, these "stains" clearly act as fixatives since they prevent extraction, particularly of lipids, during the subsequent steps of dehydration and embedding. Postfixation with uranyl acetate has been shown to be a prerequisite for the preservation of pulmonary surfactant for ultrastructural studies [25, 44–47]. Likewise, sequential postfixation with osmium tetroxide and uranyl acetate fixatives has to be performed if the ultrastructural study aims at the examination of alveolar edema [42, 48, 49]. For immunocytochemistry, however, these fixatives have to be omitted because they frequently react with, and thus alter the antigens of interest ([5] p. 77). Over recent years, several techniques for the localization of antigens at the ultrastructural level have been established that can be combined with stereological methods (for detailed review, see [5, 50]). In most cases the use of low-temperature techniques is necessary to maintain the antigenicity of the sample. Besides the well-established Tokuyasu thawed frozen section technique (for detailed description and discussion, see [5]), a new generation of embedding resins in combination with the methods of progressive lowering of temperature (PLT) or of freeze-substitution has proven to be useful (protocols are given in [51]). The choice of the appropriate technique depends on the tissue and the antigen of interest. If, for example, one is interested in the localization of the hydrophobic surfactant protein B in lamellar bodies of type 2 pneumocytes, primary chemical fixation followed by freeze-substitution, embedment in Lowicryl HM 20, and post-embedding antigen labeling is the method of choice [26]. This method results in excellent preservation of the lamellar bodies, which are severely extracted using the Tokuyasu technique [26].

## Stereological analysis

Over the last 10–15 years there have been some major improvements in stereological techniques. By using design-based methods it is now possible to estimate volume, surface, length and number of structures in an unbiased way. In contrast to previous methods, assumptions about the shape, size or orientation of objects are no longer necessary. Therefore, use of design-based methods is recommended [13].

Stereological data are only valid if the samples are representative of the whole organ. Thus, one of the essentials in stereology is to perform systematic random sampling (as described in detail above). Another important point is to obtain absolute rather than relative data, which requires that we know the absolute volume of the respective reference space. Therefore, the volume of the fixed organ has to be determined. This can either be done by fluid displacement or by the application of the Cavalieri method [14]. Although both methods yield almost identical results and are very precise, the Cavalieri method offers some advantages for subsequent stereological investigation [14].

Another important point to notice is that for the determination of certain parameters, isotropy of the structure of interest is required. Length estimation, for example, requires isotropic test planes, i.e. sections through the structures of interest must be randomly orientated in 3-D space. Since one cannot be sure of the given isotropy of a particular structure (never make any assumptions in stereology! [13]), the sampling and embedding procedure has to yield so-called IUR-(isotropic uniform random) sections [12]. An easy method to achieve IUR-sections for LM is the orientator (reviewed e.g. in [11, 12]). For small TEM samples, the isector [15] is the method of choice. Since estimation of surface areas, for example, only requires isotropic test lines, it is sufficient to use the vertical sectioning technique [14]. Although IUR-sections can be used for anything, the advantage of vertical sections is that knowledge of the tissue's orientation can be maintained, which may be of interest, for example, in the study of bronchiolar epithelium or vascular endothelium.

## Interpretation

All the diverse steps mentioned above precede the final analysis at the electron microscope. Although the ultrastructural information will clearly be visible, given that the appropriate methods have been selected, the inexperienced observer may fail to perceive some of the details. The challenge of interpreting an electron micrograph is easily underestimated. An excellent review of some common aspects is given by Elias [52]. The colleagues from the EM unit should be happy to contribute their experience to solving any problems.

## Acknowledgements

We are greatly indebted to J. Richter (University of Göttingen, Germany), head of our division, for helpful discussions and for his generous and continuous support of our work. We are very grateful to J. Nyengaard and H.J.G. Gundersen (University of Aarhus, Denmark) for their valuable advice and critical reading of the manuscript in all aspects of stereology. Many thanks are owed to the laboratory technicians A. Gerken, H. Hühn, and Ch. Rühling for their skillful work, and to all our colleagues for many stimulating discussions, in particular to F. Brasch and A. Schmiedl, and D. Riemann for contribution of Figure 17.5. We thank Th. Wahlers (Hanover Medical School, Germany) for his support and excellent cooperation in the study of human donor lungs. We acknowledge with thanks the financial support of the Deutsche Forschungsgemeinschaft (SFB 330, B12; Bo 172/16-1; Ri 790/1-1).

## References

1   Flegler SL, Heckman JW and Klomparens KL (1993) *Scanning and Transmission Electron Microscopy. An Introduction*, Oxford University Press Oxford

2   Glauert AM (1974) *Practical Methods in Electron Microscopy*, North-Holland Publishing Company Amsterdam

3   Hayat MA (1989) *Principles and Techniques of Electron Microscopy. Biological Applications*, MacMillan Press Hampshire

4   Robards AW and Wilson AJ (1994) *Procedures in Electron Microscopy*, Wiley

& Sons New York

5  Griffiths G (1993) *Fine Structure Immuno-cytochemistry*, Springer-Verlag Berlin

6  Crang RFE and Klomparens KL (1988) *Artefacts in Biological Electron Microscopy*, Plenum Press New York

7  Hayat MA (1993) *Stains and Cytochemical Methods*, Plenum Press New York

8  Kellenberger E, Johansen R, Maeder M, Bohrmann B, Stauffer E and Villiger W (1992) *J. Microsc.* **168**: 181

9  Gundersen HJG, Bagger P, Bendtsen TF, Evans SM, Korbo L, Marcussen N, Moller A, Nielsen K, Nyengaard JR, Pakkenberg B, Sorensen FB, Vesterby A and West MJ (1988) *APMIS* **96**: 857

10  Gundersen HJG, Bendtsen TF, Korbo L, Marcussen N, Moller A, Nielsen K, Nyengaard JR, Pakkenberg B, Sorensen FB, Vesterby A and West MJ (1988) *APMIS* **96**: 379

11  Cruz-Orive LM and Weibel ER (1990) *Am. J. Physiol.* **258**: L148

12  Mayhew TM (1991) *Exp. Physiol.* **76**: 639

13  Mayhew TM and Gundersen HJG (1996) *J. Anat.* **188**: 1

14  Michel RP and Cruz-Orive LM (1988) *J. Microsc.* **150**: 117

15  Nyengaard JR and Gundersen HJG (1992) *J. Microsc.* **165**: 427

16  Prentø P (1995) *Histochem. J.* **27**: 906

17  Arborgh A, Bell P, Brunk U and Collins VP (1976) *J. Ultrastruct. Res.* **56**: 339

18  Malick LE, Wilson RB and Stetson D (1975) *Stain Technol.* **50**: 265

19  Dvorak AM (1987) *J. Electron Microsc. Tech.* **6**: 255

20  Lucocq J (1993) *TICB* **3**: 354

21  Scherle W (1970) *Mikroskopie* **26**: 57

22  Gundersen HJG and Jensen EB (1987) *J. Microsc.* **147**: 229

23  Ladekarl M (1994) *J. Microsc.* **174**: 93

24  Ladekarl M and Svanholm H (1996) *Acta Stereol.* **15**: 165

25  Fehrenbach H, Richter J and Schnabel PA (1991) *J. Microsc.* **162**: 91

26  Voorhout W, Van Genderen I, Van Meer G and Geuze H (1991) *Scanning Microscopy Suppl.* **5**: S17

27  Steinbrecht RA and Zierold K (1987) *Cryotechniques in Biological Electron Microscopy*, Springer-Verlag Berlin

28  Gehr P and Crapo JD (1988) Morphometric Analysis of the Gas Exchange Region of the Lung. In: *Toxicology of the Lung*, Gardner DE, Crapo JD and Massaro EJ (eds), p. 1, Raven Press New York

29  Davies P (1991) *Pharmac. Ther.* **50**: 321

30  Bolender RP, Hyde DM and Dehoff RT (1993) *Am. J. Physiol.* **265**: L521

31  Zierold K (1991) *J. Microsc.* **161**: 357

32  Ryan KP and Knoll G (1994) *Scanning Microscopy* **8**: 259

33  Zierold K (1992) *Scanning Microscopy* **6**: 1137

34  Eckenhoff RG and Somlyo AP (1988) *Am. J. Physiol.* **254**: C614

35  Eckenhoff RG (1989) J. Clin. Invest. **84**: 1295

36  Bastacky J, Lee CYC, Goerke J, Koushafar H, Yager D, Kenaga L, Speed TP, Chen Y and Clements JA (1995) *J. Appl. Physiol.* **79**: 1615

37  Zierold K (1993) *J. Microsc.* **171**: 267

38  Hohenberg H, Tobler M and Müller M (1996) *J. Microsc.* **183**: 133

39  Nicolas G (1991) *J. Electron Microsc. Tech.* **18**: 395

40  Reith A, Kraemer M and Vassy J (1984) *Scanning Electron Microscopy* **2**: 645

41  Weibel ER (1984) *Resp. Physiol. (Techniques in the Life Sciences)* **P401**: 1

42  Bachofen H, Ammann A, Wangensteen D and Weibel ER (1982) *J. Appl. Physiol.* **53**: 528

43  Gil J (1990) *Models of Lung Disease – Microscopy and Structural Methods*, Marcel Dekker Inc. New York

44  Balis JU, Paterson JF, Haller EM, Shelley SA and Montgomery MR (1988) *Am. J.*

*Pathol.* **132**: 330

45 Balis JU, Paterson JF, Lundh JM, Haller EM, Shelley SA and Montgomery MR (1991) *Am. J. Pathol.* **138**: 847

46 Ochs M, Fehrenbach H and Richter J (1994) *J. Histochem. Cytochem.* **42**: 805

47 Uhlig S, Brasch F, Wollin L, Fehrenbach H, Richter J and Wendel A (1995) *Am. J. Pathol.* **146**: 1235

48 Bachofen H, Schürch S and Weibel ER (1993) *Am. Rev. Respir. Dis.* **147**: 997

49 Bachofen H, Schürch S, Michel RP and Weibel ER (1993) *Am. Rev. Respir. Dis.* **147**: 989

50 Lucocq J (1994) *J. Anat.* **184**: 1

51 Roos N and Griffiths G (1994) Use of Ultrathin Cryo- and Plastic Sections for Immunoelectron Microscopy. In: *Cell Biology. A Laboratory Handbook – Vol. 2*, Celis JE (ed.), p. 168, Academic Press San Diego

52 Elias H (1972) *J. Microsc.* **95**: 59

# Autoradiography in the lung

*R.G. Goldie and*
*P.J. Rigby*

This chapter is an attempt to assemble a set of guidelines that can be followed by investigators interested in using autoradiography as a research tool in lung biology. Different research teams have developed autoradiographic techniques suitable for pulmonary research that vary in detail, but which are substantively similar. The general aim of this document is to provide a summary of the knowledge that we have accumulated regarding the application of autoradiographic methods appropriate to investigations of a range of binding site-ligand interactions in the respiratory tract. While it is true to say that the methods that we have described are not the only ones that work well, it is also the case that these techniques have proven to be reliable in our hands over many years and are thus likely to be of use to the novice and the expert alike.

Autoradiography, particularly as used in experimental biology, refers to a set of techniques which enable the visualisation of sources of radiation associated with sites of radionuclide binding within a tissue specimen. The sources of radiation are detected by photographic emulsion applied in close apposition to the tissue specimen (Fig. 18.1), such that emitted radiation induces a latent image within the film which closely maps the distribution and density of radioactivity in the underlying specimen. Photographic film (e.g X-ray film), or liquid emulsion can be applied and dried onto a flexible matrix such as a glass coverslip which is then apposed to the tissue specimen. Alternatively, the specimen can be dipped into a liquefied photographic emulsion to minimise the distance between the radiation source and the film. The latent image formed is then developed using standard photographic developing methods, resulting in the production of silver grains within the photographic emulsion, which in the simplest case, can be viewed and analysed via light microscopy. To obtain optimum results, the choice of photographic emulsion used in light microscopic autoradiography, whether it be one of several films or one of several nuclear track emulsions, must

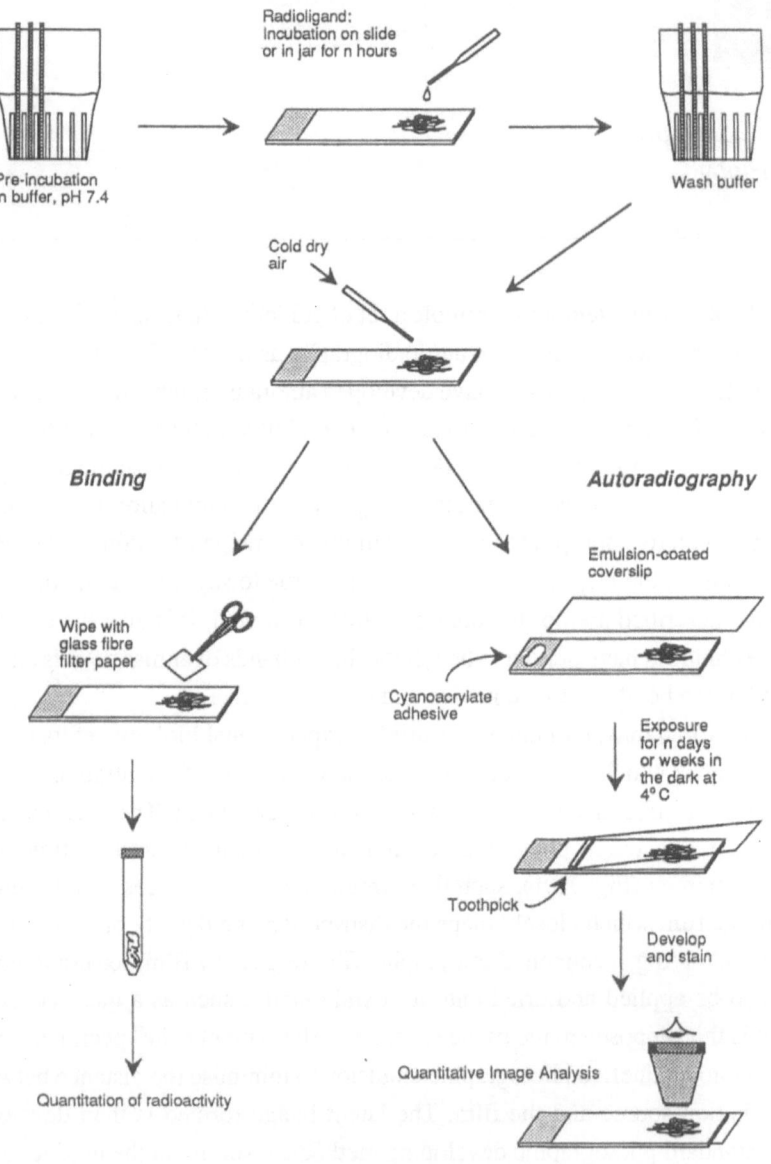

**Figure 18.1. Diagrammatic representation of the procedure for incubating and processing slide-mounted tissue sections for the retrieval of radioligand binding data and the production of autoradiograms**

depend upon several factors including the resolution required and the energy and activity of the emitted radiation.

Autoradiography is a relatively simple technique which can provide extremely powerful information relating to the distribution and localisation of sources of tissue radioactivity. These sources might be sites at which radioligands are bound either strongly or weakly to intracellular or extracellular proteins including receptors for various drugs and bioactive mediators, sites of radioligand incorporation into macromolecules including proteins and nucleic acids or other loci at which there is attachment of a radiolabelled compound. However, it should be remembered that the autoradiogram only provides a visible record of the distribution of autoradiographic silver grains. This record can be assumed to accurately represent the distribution of the binding sites of interest only if it can be shown that the radioligand remains in association with the relevant binding site. In many cases, particularly those involving drug-receptor interactions where binding of a radioligand to a specific site (receptor) is often readily reversible, precautions must be taken to ensure the ligand remains associated with its specific binding site during the process of development of the latent autoradiographic image. Solutions to this important problem will be described in the methods section of this text.

Importantly, quantitative autoradiographic data can also be derived from such investigations. Thus, light microscopic autoradiography has been vital to our current understanding of the distribution, localisation and density of receptors for various endogenously produced ligands including neurotransmitters and hormones. For example, until the early 1980s, relatively little was known concerning the distribution and density of β-adrenoceptors in the lung. By the mid to late 1980s, β-adrenoceptor subtype densities and localisation had been thoroughly assessed in the respiratory tract in the human [1, 2], as well as in animal species [3–6]. These data have played a major role in enhancing our understanding of the actions of β-adrenoceptor agonists in the lung, particularly in relation to their therapeutic effects in diseases such as asthma. A range of other cell surface and intracellular receptor types for various mediators and drugs have subsequently been detected, localised and quantified in the lung using light microscopic autoradiography, adding immeasurably to our knowledge of these systems.

In this chapter, we will summarise the essential tools of trade with respect to conducting light microscopic autoradiographic investigations in tissues of the respiratory tract including trachea, bronchi and lung parenchyma. In addition, the essential methods, experimental procedures, including tissue preparation and sectioning and some of the major methodological pitfalls likely to be encountered with this technique will also be described. We have particularly focussed upon autoradiographic detection of binding sites for drug receptor ligands where often the association between receptor and ligand is readily reversible. However, the processes involved in successfully producing an autoradiographic record of the binding of irreversible receptor-ligand associations or of radiolabelled substrates incorporated into intracellular proteins, nucleic acids etc., are essentially similar.

## Materials and equipment

A list of the essential materials and equipment required for successful light microscopic autoradiography experiments using lung tissue is included in Table 18.1. We have incorporated notes which include suggestions and modifications which we have found valuable and/or time saving without compromising the quality of the final autoradiogram.

## Methods

In autoradiography, it is necessary to establish that the emulsion has recorded radioactive particles reaching it from all parts of the specimen with equal efficiency [7] and that silver grains are specifically derived from the radioactive probe being used. Good experimental design, careful attention to methodological technique and the use of appropriate controls will aid in this process and help to minimise problems.

*Table 18.1. Materials essential for light microscopic autoradiography in lung tissue*

| Materials | Notes |
| --- | --- |
| 1) *Microscope slides* | Must be clean and frosted at one end. Slides may need to be coated or "subbed as described below". |
| 2) *Tissue freezing and cutting* | |
| Vacuum flask | Must be designed to hold liquid nitrogen. |
| Isopentane | Also known as 2-methylbutane. |
| copper vessel | To hold isopentane. Lowered into liquid nitrogen and held in place at the neck of the vacuum flask with a collar. Cylinder opening must be large enough to accept tissue pieces and foil pans. |
| Cryostat microtome | Tissue-Tek II, Miles Laboratories, Naperville, IL USA |
| OCT compound 4583 embedding medium | Tissue-Tek, Miles Inc, Elkhart, IN, USA |
| Macrodex | 6% Dextran 70 in 0.9% (normal) saline (used as a plasma expander in i.v. drips). This is not expensive. |
| 3) *Tissue radiolabelling* | |
| Radioligand and buffers | Individual binding protocols will determine the buffers and other materials used. |
| Labelling containers | Coplin or Hellendahl jars are useful for incubation of slide-mounted tissue with ligand. |
| PAP pen | Where a ligand is expensive, use to circumscribe tissue so that a small volume (up to 300 μl of ligand solution) can be applied directly onto the tissue sections. Available from The Binding Site Inc., San Diego, USA |
| Vacuum line | Incubation solutions including ligand and wash fluids can be removed rapidly via vacuum line with drainage to an isolated reservoir. Fluid replacement is via syringe. |
| Drying equipment | Clean compressed air passed through silica gel and bubbled into acetone chilled with dry-ice. |

(continued on next page)

*Table 18.1. (continued)*

| Materials | Notes |
|---|---|
| 4) *Coverslip preparation* | |
| Coverslips | $75 \times 25 \times 0.10-0.12$ mm (Size 0). These are thinner than normal coverslips (which are size 1 or size 1.5) and may be a special order from your supplier. |
| Emulsion | Kodak Nuclear Track emulsion NTB2 (iodinated ligands) and NTB3 (tritiated ligands). We have found these emulsions to be reliable and readily melted and re-used without significant increases in background grain counts. Other emulsions are available from Ilford and Amersham. |
| Water bath | A thermostatically controlled water bath is essential for melting NTB2 and NTB3 emulsions. |
| Glass dipping chamber | Coplin jar (for large numbers of coverslips) or Amersham Hypercoat dipping vessel (RPN39) |
| Drying rack | Clothes pegs spaced along a semi-rigid wire or bar are ideal for suspending and drying newly dipped coverslips. Prepare in batches of about 100 to minimise the frequency of emulsion remelting. |
| Slide boxes | Must be light tight and able to prevent coverslips from touching each other. |
| 5) *Darkroom facilities* | |
| Location | Well separated from areas involved in the use of radioligands. |
| Separate wet & dry areas | Recommended |
| Stable water temperature | 20 °C recommended |
| Light trap | Entry via a light trap enables entry/exit without compromising light safeness. |
| Safelight | As required for emulsion or film being used. For NTB2 and NTB3, an Ilford 904 safelight works well. Light coloured walls in the darkroom often help to improved illumination. |
| Superglue | Any commercially available cyanoacrylate adhesive will suffice. |

*(continued on next page)*

**Table 18.1. (continued)**

| Materials | Notes |
|---|---|
| 6) *Exposure containers* | Disused X-ray cassettes of various sizes are ideally suited for the purpose. Remove the intensifier screen. Amersham Hypercassettes can also be purchased. |
| 7) *Photographic development* | |
| Developer | Depends on emulsion or film used. Kodak Dektol for coverslips and Kodak D19 for Fuji X-ray and Amers ham Hyperfilm. |
| Stop bath | 1–3% acetic acid containing 2.5% Ilford Hypam hardener. |
| Fixative | Ilford Hypam Rapid Fix containing 2.5% Hypam hardener. |
| 8) *Tissue staining* | |
| Stain | Gill's haematoxylin |
| Dehydration and clearing | Graded ethanol solutions and xylene |
| Mounting | DePeX mounting medium (BDH) |
| 9) *Microscopy and photography* | |
| Photomicroscope | Good quality photomicroscope with manual control of exposure. |
| Condenser | Require both bright and dark-field condensers. |
| Film | General purpose fine grain film for colour and black and white images e.g. Kodak Ektachrome Tungsten balan ced 64 ASA (colour); Ilford Pan F (black and white). |
| 10) *Quantitation of grain densities* | |
| Microscope | Good quality light microscope. |
| Video camera | Best to use a CCD camera |
| Microscope objective lens | High quality ×100 oil immersion lens with high numerical aperture. |
| Computer | PC or Macintosh depending upon image analysis software. |
| Image analysis software | Good general purpose software like Optimas |
| Data analysis software | General spreadsheet such as Microsoft Excel |

## Slide preparation

For convenience, most autoradiography is performed on tissue collected on 75 mm×25 mm glass slides which have one "frosted" end. If you intend to use the "coverslipping" method, do not use slides for tissue collection which have a polished or "painted end", since it is difficult to see these in the darkroom when trying to glue the coverslip to the slide. Furthermore, the bond made with cyanoacrylate adhesive ("superglue") between the frosted end of the slide and the coverslip is stronger than that made when non-frosted slides are used. All slides should be clean and should be checked for blemishes or chips on the surface of the slide. This is particularly important if the preparations are intended to be viewed on the microscope under dark-field illumination. We have found surface blemishes to often be a problem on microscope slides where the frosted end was produced by sand blasting. Slides which have been inadvertently stored in a humid environment should also be checked for the presence of fungal growths.

## Slide cleaning and subbing

Depending upon the tissue and the type of experiment to be performed, slides may need to be coated or "subbed" to aid the adherence of tissue sections to the glass slide during subsequent labelling and washing procedures. Chrome alum/gelatin coated slides provide a simple yet effective substrate for most frozen sections.

## Preparation of chrome alum/gelatin solution (adapted from [8])

Dissolve 2.5 g gelatin in 400 ml of distilled water with gentle heating. Allow to cool. Dissolve 0.25 g chrome alum (chromic potassium sulphate: $CrK(SO_4)_2 \cdot 12\,H_2O$) in 100 ml distilled water. Mix the two solutions. Since this solution quickly becomes infected, it should be used the same day, but may be stored overnight at 4 °C and used the next day.

## *Application*

Dip microscope slides approximately 50 mm into acetone ×3 (to remove any oil/grease film), distilled water ×3 (to wash acetone off slides), and subbing solution ×3 changes for approximately 5 s each and then place slides vertically onto an absorbent, clean and dust-free surface to allow excess subbing solution to drain and the slides to dry. Make sure that a thick area of chrome alum/gelatin does not form at the bottom of the slide and that subbing solution does not contact the frosted end of the slide. Dry subbed slides can be stored for several months in a non-humid environment before use. Be particularly careful to prevent bubbles from forming over the area to be covered by tissue, and to prevent extra thick areas of gelatin solution from drying on the slide.

## Preparation of emulsion-coated coverslips

### *Safelight illumination*

Always make sure that the safelight to be used in the darkroom is of the correct type for the emulsion that you are using and that the power of the globe is no higher than 15 W. If in doubt about how safe the safelight is, perform the following simple test: place a sample of the emulsion you intend to use at about the usual working distance from the safelight. Shade half of the emulsion with an opaque substance such as a coin or piece of aluminium foil, taking care to not directly touch the emulsion. Allow this preparation to "expose" for the period of time that your autoradiographs would normally be exposed to the safelight and then develop the emulsion normally. When processed and dried, examine the emulsion and count the silver grains to assess any difference between the exposed region and the shaded region. Any increase in silver grain density over the unshaded region indicates that the safelight is in fact not "safe". Accordingly, you should change the filter type, use a globe of lower power, increase the usual working distance from the safelight, or decrease the time your autoradiographs are exposed to the safelight. As a rough guide, recommended safelights are safe provided a 15 W globe is used at a distance of no less than 1 metre for no longer than 20 min.

Remember also that while "emulsion safe" safelights are essential, adequate levels of illumination are also required to enable procedures to be performed efficiently and safely. Often, light coloured walls and using indirect lighting (where the safelights are pointed towards the ceiling or walls) rather than direct lighting will achieve this is.

## Emulsion coating of coverslips

Coverslips 75 mm × 25 mm × size 0 (0.10–0.12 mm thick) which are clean and free from blemishes and chips should be selected. Under a suitable safelight, liquid emulsion should be melted in a waterbath and diluted, as recommended by the manufacturer. For Kodak Nuclear Track emulsions (NTB2 and NTB3), we use 43 °C and dilute 1:1 with distilled water. After very gentle mixing, aliquot emulsion and store the portion not being used immediately at 4 °C. Small air bubbles floating on the surface of the liquefied emulsion should be removed. Leaving the diluted liquefied emulsion undisturbed in the waterbath for 30–60 min helps and dipping several "test" coverslips into the emulsion also picks up and removes many of the surface bubbles. Only when you can consistently produce an even, blemish-free film of emulsion on test coverslips should you proceed to produce a batch of "working" coverslips. Avoid unnecessary remelting of the emulsion as this can contribute to increases in the background grain count.

Coverslips should only be handled by their edges and gently dipped approximately 50 mm into the liquefied emulsion and then slowly and evenly withdrawn. Suspend these preparations by spring clips attached to the non-emulsion end of the coverslip and allowed to dry slowly in the dark. Wooden clothes pegs make ideal clips as they are cheap and do not stress the fragile glass. Drying usually takes 2 to 3 h after which time completely dry coverslips should be stored on their edge in light-tight slide trays at 4 °C where they remain useable for many weeks. By not using desiccant during storage, you may help to reduce background grain counts.

## Tissue preparation

Autoradiography in the respiratory tract primarily involves airway tissues including trachea, bronchi and peripheral structures such as bronchioles and alveolar wall. The following tissue preparation regimes for major and peripheral airways result in good preservation of tissue which can be successfully sectioned as frozen specimens. We have found no practical benefit from fixing frozen tissue specimens in routine fixatives like paraformaldehyde either before, during or after autoradiogram preparation.

### Tracheal and bronchial tissue

Tracheal and bronchial tissues to be frozen sectioned can be treated similarly, since they are both essentially hollow, cartilaginous tubes. Following dissection, tube segments should be cut into 8–10 mm lengths and placed vertically into small (approximately 10 mm × 10 mm × 10 mm) aluminium foil pans filled with Macrodex solution, taking care to ensure that luminal air bubbles are released. Adjust the size of foil pans to suit the size or number of tissue pieces being frozen in a single block. These pans are then slowly lowered into liquid isopentane which is cooled (quenched) with liquid nitrogen. Initially, do not completely immerse the block since freezing of the top Macrodex surface will likely result in splitting of the block. Store specimens in liquid nitrogen or at −70°C.

### Peripheral lung tissue

Inflation of lung parenchyma with diluted OCT or Macrodex before freezing can aid frozen sectioning. Inflation involves the instillation via an airway of either 20% OCT embedding medium in saline or neat Macrodex. Care must be taken to ensure that this fluid does not contain air bubbles. Inflation should occur under a standard head of pressure, although in most instances, careful passive inflation via a hand-held syringe may be sufficient. Once inflated, pieces of parenchymal tissue (whole lung lobe in the case of a small laboratory animal) are frozen by immersion in isopentane quenched with liquid nitrogen. Store the tissue as described above.

## Cutting frozen sections

It is not our intention here to teach you how to cut frozen sections and the only recipe which we can offer for good sectioning is good technique, good equipment and lots of practice. However, always remember to use a sharp knife and make sure that the tissue and knife are locked firmly in place. We have found that Macrodex and OCT blocked respiratory tissues section well when cut at between −20 °C and −25 °C. Collect the sections by thaw-mounting onto the lower 25 mm of subbed microscope slides and allow them to dry completely. Adequately label all slides with graphite pencil (not solvent based pens) before storing at −70 °C until use. We have found that short storage of the tissue sections at −70 °C helps adhesion of tissue to the slide.

## Radioligand binding procedures

The binding of diffusible, reversibly bound radioligands such as the β-adrenoceptor antagonist [125I]-iodocyanopindolol to respiratory tissues have been described in detail in several publications [1, 2, 5, 9] and will not be described exhaustively here. Briefly, slide-mounted frozen sections of tissue are incubated for specified periods of time in a buffer containing the radioligand of interest (Fig. 18.1). In most cases, binding is performed at room temperature, although for other ligands, incubation at 4 ° or at 37 °C may be more appropriate. Usually, adjacent serial tissue sections will be incubated simultaneously in the presence of substances that would be expected to displace ligand from specific binding sites in order that the level of non-specific binding can be determined. For example, in the case of [125I]-iodocyanopindolol binding to airway β-adrenoceptors, non-specific binding is assessed in the presence of the β-adrenoceptor antagonist propranolol (1 µM) or the β-adrenoceptor agonist (-)-isoprenaline. Other tissue sections may be incubated with radioligand in the presence of β-adrenoceptor subtype-selective antagonists, where an evaluation of the contribution to specific binding from receptor subtypes is required. Additionally, extra slide-mounted total binding sections should always be included for "tester" autoradiograms. Some radioligands including [$^{125}$I]-iodocyanopindolol degrade when exposed to ultraviolet light which may come from overhead fluorescent lights. In such cases, experiments must be conducted under conditions of reduced illumination via an incandescent light source.

Following incubation in radioligand, wash in buffer, rinse in distilled water to remove excess unbound ligand and buffer salts, and thoroughly dry sections under a stream of cold, dry air where compressed air is first passed through silica gel and then bubbled through acetone chilled with dry-ice. It is important to remove moisture to dryness in a chilled atmosphere, as this precaution minimises any tendency for the diffusible ligand to dissociate from its specific binding sites (receptors). When all tissue sections are completely dry, attach emulsion-coated coverslips or dip in liquefied emulsion. Some radioligands associate with specific binding sites in a non-reversible manner. For example, [$^{125}$I]-endothelin-1 binds pseudo-irreversibly to at least two receptor subtypes in airway smooth muscle [10–14]. In this case, drying of labelled tissue sections can be conducted at room temperature.

Additionally, slides that have been incubated in buffers containing radioligand can also be used to estimate total tissue levels of radioactivity. This tissue is wiped from slides using glass fibre filter paper (Whatman GF/A or GF/C) and radioactivity estimated in a gamma radiation counter (e.g [$^{125}$I]) or in a liquid scintillation counter (e.g. [$^{3}$H]) (Fig. 18.1).

## Attachment of emulsion-coated coverslips

Allow stored coverslips to come to room temperature before opening the light-tight container under safelight conditions. Holding the microscope slide by the edges (tissue uppermost) between the thumb and index and middle fingers, place a small stripe of cyanoacrylate adhesive (superglue) across the frosted portion of the slide. Place an emulsion-dipped coverslip over the slide, suspending it above the slide using the fingers which are simultaneously holding the slide. Gently lower the coverslip, making sure that approximately 4 mm of the emulsion-coated end overhangs the non-frosted end of the slide. This end of the coverslip usually has a considerably thicker emulsion coating, and if this thickened region was placed over the microscope slide, the emulsion over the radio-labelled tissue would be elevated slightly above the tissue leading to a significantly inferior autoradiogram. Press the coverslip and slide together using the thumb and index finger of the other hand, squeezing excess superglue out of the preparation. Remove this excess glue. The finished preparation should have the entire frosted area under the coverslip covered with superglue. This is readily visible under safelight because the frosted portion becomes transparent where glue is present. Too little glue will result in preparations coming apart during development and staining, while too much glue causes bonding beyond the frosted region. Place the coverslipped tissue preparations onto a thin foam rubber sheet inside an X-ray cassette, making sure no preparations are overlapping. Close the cassette and seal inside a container with silica gel.

## Emulsion-dipped autoradiograms

In some cases, localisation of autoradiographic grains over tissue can be optimised by dipping slide-mounted radioactive tissue into liquefied emulsion, rather than by attaching emulsion-coated coverslips. However, care should be exercised when examing data collected this way. If the radioligand used is reversibly bound to its specific binding sites, dipping slide-mounted specimens into warm, liquefied photographic emulsion might promote the dissociation of ligand from its receptor. This would be predicted for ligands such as $[^{125}I]$-iodocyanopindolol. Interestingly, however, we found that this was not a problem with this ligand when used in human peripheral lung tissue [15]. Success with this ligand under these conditions might relate to its high lipid solubility which aids its retention in the cell membrane. However, for other potentially more mobile ligands, the issue of ligand-receptor dissociation during the dipping process might rule out the use of this technique.

The dipping technique is essentially the same as that used in the preparation of emulsion-coated coverslips. It is vital that all air bubbles be removed from the emulsion before specimen dipping begins and excess emulsion is removed by draining preparations in a vertical position, allowing emulsion to collect onto absorbent paper. Emulsion can also be wiped from the back of the slide using tissue paper. Dipped autoradiograms should be left to dry vertically for several hours, then exposed at 4°C in light-tight slide boxes containing silica gel.

## Film autoradiograms

Various types of film available in sheets can be used in autoradiography. Where high energy radionuclides have been used (e.g. [$^{125}$I]-iodinated ligands), standard X-ray film such as Fuji Nif Rx, provides a convenient detection system. However, if lower energy radionuclides like $^{3}$H are used, a more sensitive film may be necessary such as Amersham Hyperfilm-$^{3}$H. Greater sensitivity is, in part, conferred to this product by not having a protective anti-scratch layer over the emulsion, which would otherwise retard the passage of low energy β particles into the emulsion. However, the absence of this layer makes it very easy to scratch and careful handling is essential since pressure artefacts are easily induced and fingerprints are commonly also imaged. Hyperfilm can be used in complete sheets layered over slides in X-ray cassettes.

## Exposure of autoradiograms

Incubation conditions should be optimised to reduce fading of the latent image which is more likely to be a problem under conditions of prolonged exposure, increased temperature or humidity, or in the presence of oxidising agents [7]. Good results are achieved after short periods of incubation of autoradiograms at 4 °C in the presence of silica gel to produce and maintain a dry atmosphere. Optimum exposure time should be determined by preparing "tester" autoradiograms, which are incubated in separate X-ray cassettes (slide boxes for dipped autoradiograms) and which are developed and assessed before the primary experimental slides are processed. When assessing testers, pay attention to both the background level and the maximum grain density over tissue, such that the optimum signal-to-noise ratio is achieved. This is particularly pertinent where quantitation of autoradiographic data is required and where grain densities must be kept within the limits of analysis.

When using high specific activity radiolabelled compounds like [$^{125}$I]-iodinated ligands, and where binding levels may be expected to be relatively high, autoradiograms might need to be incubated at 4 °C for only 1–4 days. In contrast, autoradiograms involving the binding of tritiated, low energy ligands usually have to be incubated for periods of several months. In such cases, it is particularly important to ensure that the preparations are moisture-free and that they remain so for the duration of the exposure.

## Development and staining of autoradiograms

### Preparation for development and tissue staining

Allow X-ray cassettes and slide boxes to reach room temperature before opening under appropriate safelight conditions. For coverslipped preparations, take each autoradiogram and very gently bend the flexible coverslip away from the slide. Gently slide a 30 mm length of a toothpick (approximately 1 mm × 1 mm in cross section) between the coverslip and slide above the slide-mounted tissue, taking care not to scratch the emulsion which overlies the tissue region (Fig. 18.1). Release the coverslip and the toothpick should stay firmly in place, leaving the coverslip elevated at one end. This wedge must be placed such that it is not easily dislodged during further manipulation and processing of the autoradiogram. Insert the glued end of the autoradiogram into a clip held in a staining rack.

## Processing solutions

All solutions, including wash water, should be at 20°C. Higher temperatures can result in softening of the emulsion with possible total loss of emulsion from the coverslip. We have not found lower temperatures to be necessary.

1) *Developer*. Kodak Dektol developer, diluted 1:1 with water. This should be freshly diluted before each development session. Stock, undiluted developer should be stored tightly capped in a dark bottle to minimise oxidation, which is indicated by the developer turning brown. Fresh developer should be a light straw colour.

2) *Stop Bath*. 1–3% acetic acid in water containing 2.5% Ilford Hypam Hardener. This solution can be reused several times. It should be discarded when it fails to remove the soapy feel of the developer and/or turns cloudy.

3) *Fixer*. Ilford Hypam Rapid Fixer diluted 1:4 with water containing 2.5% Ilford Hypam Hardener. This solution can be reused several times. The fixer is becoming exhausted when the clearing time for the emulsion becomes more than approximately 60 s.

4) *Water*. Clean tap water at the correct temperature is adequate for washing autoradiograms. In our experience, there is no advantage in using distilled or deionised water. If using running water, make sure the temperature does not change during the washing cycle. This is a common problem when the external building temperature varies significantly from the internal room temperature.

## Photographic development

Develop the emulsion by immersion of the tissue end of the slide/coverslip assembly (or dipped autoradiogram) in developer at 20°C for 3 min with agitation for 5 s every 30 s. Drain excess developer (include draining time in total development time) and continuously agitate in stop bath solution for 20–30 s. Transfer assemblies to fixative for 120–150 s with agitation for 5 s every 30 s. Do not overfix, particularly when using rapid fixers, as this can lead to bleaching and loss of some of the silver grains. Wash assemblies in several changes of water, or in running tap water for a minimum of 20–30 min. Insufficient washing can lead to loss of silver grains, particularly if the emulsion is subsequently placed in an acidic staining solution.

## Tissue staining and mounting

### *Materials*

1) *Gill's haematoxylin.* Gill's haematoxylin (minus acetic acid) is a good general nuclear and cytoplasmic stain for lung tissues as it has a non-critical staining time and does not precipitate onto the autoradiogram. Precipitation is a potential problem when viewing autoradiograms under darkfield illumination, where small crystals and silver grains can look very similar. Furthermore, haematoxylin-stained tissue has a muted neutral appearance under dark-field illumination, whereas some other stains (e.g. toluidine blue) make tissue appear brightly coloured.
   Preparation: To make 1 litre – add in the following order:

   | | |
   |---|---|
   | Distilled water | 750 ml |
   | Ethylene Glycol (Ethanediol) | 250 ml |
   | Haematoxylin | 4.0 g |
   | Sodium Iodate $NaIO_3$ | 0.4 g |
   | Aluminium Sulphate $Al_2(SO_4)_3 \cdot 18\ H_2O$ | 35.2 g |

2) *Tap water wash.* If the pH of tap water to be used after staining is not sufficiently alkaline to "blue" the haematoxylin, add a few drops of ammonium hydroxide to 500 ml of water and leave the washed preparations in this for 30–60 s [8].
3) *Dehydrating solutions.* Usually solutions of 50%, 70%, 95% and 2×absolute ethanol are sufficient.
4) *Transition solvent.* Absolute ethanol in xylene (1:1).
5) *Clearing agent.* 2×changes in xylene.
6) *DePeX mounting medium.*

## Procedure

Freshly developed autoradiograms which have not been dried (for coverslipped preparations, with the toothpick still in place), should be placed individually in Gill's haematoxylin for 30–60 s (vary this time depending upon requirements). For coverslipped autoradiograms, a staining rack which can be used to stain tissue but not emulsion is recommended. Rinse excess stain from the preparations in tap water, place in alkaline tap water for 30–60 s then dehydrate autoradiograms with graded solutions of ethanol (10–15 s per solution is usually sufficient). It is important to allow a little more time in absolute ethanol to ensure complete tissue dehydration. For coverslipped autoradiograms, beware of water trapped at the top of the autoradiogram where the coverslip is glued to the slide. Rinse in absolute ethanol/xylene and then finish clearing in 2×changes of xylene.

At this stage it is advisable to examine autoradiograms for the presence of small immiscible droplets of water on the preparations which may not be removed from high on the slide near the glued junction of the slide and coverslip. If water is visible, replace the xylene and take the autoradiogram in the reverse direction back to absolute ethanol, thoroughly dehydrate, then clear again. Failure to do this will result in small round water droplets in your autoradiogram, which will show up very clearly, particularly under darkfield illumination. Once cleared successfully, drain excess xylene onto a paper towel and place a small amount of DePeX (approximately 0.3 ml) directly onto the tissue area, taking care not to introduce any air bubbles. Slowly withdraw the toothpick, allowing the coverslip to contact the DePeX. For dipped autoradiograms, a standard coverslip is attached. Place the preparations with their coverslip side down onto absorbent paper and allow to dry for a minimum of 36 h.

After preparations have dried, gently remove these assemblies from the paper backing, and using a scalpel or other blade, remove any dried DePeX from the coverslip surface. Using approximately 1 M NaOH solution on a cotton bud, wipe the outer surface of the coverslip to soften and remove the emulsion and then wash the preparation with tap water. For coverslipped autoradiograms, score the portion of the coverslip overhanging the end of the slide with a diamond pencil and snap this portion off.

## Chemography controls

Controls for both positive and negative chemography, which are treated and developed identically to test preparations, should be included in autoradiography experiments. A suitable positive chemography control is to prepare an autoradiogram where the tissue has had no exposure to radiation. The detection of non-background silver grains in the autoradiogram is an indication of some event producing latent images unrelated to radiation from the radioligands being tested. A suitable negative chemography control would be a test preparation which is briefly illuminated with light prior to exposure in the X-ray cassette. After development, any pale regions in the uniformly dense black layer of silver grains indicates the presence of some substance in the autoradiogram which is causing the loss of the latent image.

# Discussion

Where an autoradiographic image of the binding of a potentially diffusible ligand (e.g. $[^{125}I]$-iodocyanopindolol) to its receptor(s) in lung or airway tissue is required [9], the ligand must be allowed to bind to tissue sites after the relevant specimen has been frozen sectioned and thaw-mounted onto glass slides. Thereafter, precautions must be taken to ensure maintenance of the association between ligand and receptor. If tissue pieces were exposed to such a radioligand and the specimen then processed using standard fixation, paraffin embedding and histological staining techniques, the preservation of tissue architecture would be greatly improved, but the probability of ligand-receptor dissociation would also be greatly increased. This could result in inappropriately low levels of tissue radioactivity and/or relocation of ligand to non-receptor sites. Thus, autoradiography involving frozen sections compromises tissue architecture in exchange for accurate mapping of reversible radioligand binding to receptors. However, often the radioligand of interest is bound tightly to its receptor (e.g. $[^{125}I]$-endothelin-1 [12, 16]), or is incorporated into a protein, nucleic acid or some other macromolecule (e.g. free $[^{125}I]$-Iodine [17, 18]), or deposited at an extracellular site in an insoluble form (e.g. $[^{125}I]$-fibrin [19]), in which case, precautions against ligand-binding site dissociation can be ignored. In such instances, tissue specimens including cultured cell preparations or whole mounts in which the radiolabel is already incorporated, can be processed using standard histological methods if desired, followed by autoradiography involving emulsion-coated coverslips, emulsion dipping [19], or the use of X-ray film.

## Controls

In all autoradiography experiments, it is essential that appropriate controls be included with every experiment. When analysing autoradiographs, you must be able to establish that silver grains on autoradiographs are due to radioactivity in the specimen and are not the result of some other process. For example, chemical vapours can induce the production of autoradiographic grains (positive chemography) or the loss of autoradiographic grains (negative chemography). Silver grains can also be induced in autoradiograms by the application of undue pressure or scratching of the emulsion surface.

## Choosing the appropriate autoradiographic method

### Emulsion-dipped preparations

The methods employed in light microscopic autoradiography will largely be determined by the requirements of the investigation and the nature of the ligand-binding site interaction. For example, in many cases, autoradiography will be employed to determine the distribution and localisation of binding sites without the need for quantitation of these data i.e. the production of a photographic image/record of the population of binding sites is the primary reason for using an autoradiographic technique [20]. In this case, various options are open to the investigator. If localisation of the binding image (autoradiographic grains) to the tissue sites of radiation (binding sites) is to be optimised, the distance between the photographic emulsion and the radioactive tissue must be minimised. This is best achieved by dipping the slide-mounted tissue specimen (e.g. frozen section) containing the bound ligand into liquefied emulsion, allowing the preparation to dry with subsequent storage in a cooled light-tight environment while the autoradiogram exposes. Autoradiographic grains develop in the emulsion very close to the plane of focus for the underlying tissue and can be viewed under either bright- or dark-field illumination [15, 19].

However, this approach has the potential to deliver erroneous results, since two major assumptions are made when interpreting the data. The first assumption is that the emulsion layer remains evenly distributed across the tissue specimen after application. For solid tissue sections, this assumption is usually correct, but in the case of sections that are not uniformly dense like lung alveolar tissue, the possibility of uneven distribution of emulsion arises. For example, emulsion might pool in alveolar spaces and be only very thinly coated across alveolar wall tissue which contains the ligand of interest. Should this occur, fewer autoradiographic grains would be observed over alveolar wall tissue than would otherwise have been produced, perhaps leading to erroneous conclusions.

Secondly, if the ligand binds reversibly and thus can readily dissociate from its binding site, such dissociation may be promoted during the emulsion dipping procedure. This is possible in the case of solidified emulsions that must be liquified by melting at approximately 43 °C and which must be maintained at this temperature during the dipping process. Ligand-receptor dissociation of this kind can lead to poor localisation of autoradiographic grains over tissue and/or in the worst case, to completely erroneous conclusions concerning the sites of ligand binding.

The third assumption is that the closeness of the contact between emulsion and tissue in dipped assemblies will not give rise to either negative or positive chemography. The extent to which these issues might give rise to errors must be assessed in parallel pilot experiments using a different approach to apposing tissue and emulsion, e.g. using emulsion-coated coverslips. Negative and positive chemography control autoradiograms must also be included in experiments using both types of assemblies.

The tissue within autoradiograms must be stained to reveal appropriate histological features. Radiolabelled tissue to be dipped in photographic emulsion can be stained before dipping, or after dipping, storage and photographic development, by allowing the stain to diffuse through the emulsion to the underlying tissue. It has been our usual practice to stain tissue that contains a reversibly bound ligand after dipping and development, to minimise the exposure of tissue to another aqueous phase and thus increase the risk of diffusion of the ligand from its binding sites during the staining process. However, in the case of tightly or irreversibly bound ligands (e.g. ligands hybridised *in situ*, covalently bound DNA aducts, etc.) tissue sections can be stained before dipping and development of emulsion. The major concern that must be controlled for in this case is that of stain-induced positive or negative chemography, problems that are avoided in post-stained autoradiograms.

## Emulsion-coated coverslip preparations

The use of emulsion-coated coverslips attached to slide-mounted tissue specimens provides high quality autoradiograms for most applications in lung tissue. However, the localisation of autoradiographic grains over tissue is poorer than with dipped autoradiograms and with appropriate pressure between the coverslip and slide, this decrement in the "tightness" of binding localisation can be minimised. Importantly, several advantages are afforded by using this approach over the emulsion dipping technique, including the fact that quantitative data can also be retrieved using well established computer-assisted image analysis techniques as described in detail by Henry et al. [6, 16]. Briefly, fields in a histologically stained tissue plane of focus can be identified and their areas measured. Autoradiographic grains developed in the emulsion lie in a plain significantly above the tissue plane of focus and can thus be imaged in focus under brightfield illumination and counted in isolation using a grain counting algorithm [21]. Estimates of autoradiographic grain densities (grains/1000 $\mu m^2$) can then be calculated. Features in the underlying stained tissue would interfere with the grain counting process if they were imaged with grains in the same plane. It is the closeness of the planes of focus for tissue and grains in dipped autoradiograms that usually precludes the quantitation of autoradiographic data in this way.

Photographic development of the emulsion and tissue staining occur as separate processes in "coverslipped" autoradiograms, further reducing the potential for the production of chemographic artifacts. In this case, the emulsion associated with the coverslip can be temporarily levered away from the tissue and exposed to photographic developer, hardener and fixative but not to either the tissue stains or the washing solutions to which the tissue section is independently exposed at a later time.

## Film imaging

Autoradiographs can also be obtained using sheets of film that are sensitive to the radiations emitted by radioligands. Autoradiographs are produced similarly to that described for coverslip autoradiograms, in that sheets of film can be placed over radiolabelled, slide-mounted tissue sections and compressed as a sandwich between flat plates in a light-tight box or X-ray cassette. Film imaging is ideal for the production of autoradiographs in large tissue sections where only low magnification images are required without an accompanying detailed image of the cellular sources of radiation e.g. where the image resolves binding site populations in main and lower order bronchial walls. Importantly, quantitative data can also be derived from such images using densitometry procedures.

## Microscopy

For most applications, autoradiograms can be viewed under either bright-field or dark-field illumination on a light microscope. Probably the major benefit from brightfield viewing is that the underlying stained tissue can be seen at the same time as the developed silver grains, although these grains usually have to be present in reasonable numbers before they become obvious. Low grain densities are usually difficult to see except at higher magnifications. With dark-field illumination, silver grains are visible even at low magnification. This is partly because, under dark-field illumination, individual silver grains appear larger than they are in reality. Dark-field illumination is also often preferred when a "panoramic" low magnification view of the binding is required. However, exact localisation of grains with respect to tissue components is usually more difficult under dark-field illumination.

## Photography

The primary consideration of microscope photography is "does the final print look like the original autoradiogram?" This is especially important when images from different autoradiograms must be compared with each other and for example, is critical for the determination of relative levels of receptor binding in lung tissues which have been exposed to different binding displacement agonists or antagonists. In these situations, the relative brightness of the images is often the most important visual cue. Since photographic light meters are usually calibrated to provide settings for "normal" subjects, the use of automatic exposures will invariably result in inadequate results, especially if using darkfield illumination. One possible solution to this dilemma is to measure the exposure required for the "master" image (to which all of the other images are compared – this might be the "total" treatment) and to manually expose other autoradiograms (which might be the agonist/antagonist or non-specific treatments) for identical times.

Occasionally, to give optimum results, minor corrections may be required to the "master" exposure recommended by the automatic exposure system. Bracketing (which is a process of taking deliberately underexposed, "correctly" exposed, and overexposed photographs of the same autoradiogram under the same lighting conditions) is a good way to determine the best exposure for your conditions. As a guide, if using negative film for photography, try three exposures where the first is the recommended or "correct" exposure, the second receives half the recommended exposure (underexposed by one $f$ stop) and the third receives double the exposure (overexposed by one $f$ stop). If using positive or slide film, smaller increments will likely be required.

The choice of which photographic film to use is often the result of personal preference. The films mentioned here are by no means exclusive and are only mentioned because we have had considerable success with these products. A general purpose, fine grained black and white negative film like Ilford Pan F (50 ASA) is a good starting point to obtain black and white prints, while Kodak Ektachrome (tungsten light balanced) (64 ASA) is good for colour slides. A note of caution – unless you intend to develop and process your own photographs, select a good processing laboratory that understands "scientific" photography (or is prepared to reprint your material if it is not adequate). This is because most printing machines do not "know" what a correct print should look like and thus microscope images invariably are printed incorrectly.

One element of photography that is often either overlooked or completed incorrectly is the determination of final print magnification. The best way to determine magnification correctly is to photograph a micrometer slide using the same microscope objective as used to photograph the autoradiogram and to then print this image along with the images from the autoradiograms. Measure the divisions on the print with a ruler and calculate the final magnification. Display the magnification as a bar on the photograph rather than quote a magnification in the legend. This gives more information to the reader and is not distorted if the publisher changes the print size for publication.

## Image analysis

Quantitative data (grain densities) can be determined from autoradiographic images under some circumstances. In our laboratory, we use a computer-assisted image analysis system in conjunction with the grain counting algorithm of Reep and Creegan [21]. This system utilises a video camera attached to a light microscope and can discriminate between individual grains and non-grain image artefacts within prescribed fields of interest (e.g. airway smooth muscle, epithelium). However, this discrimination is limited to a maximum grain density, beyond which significant inaccuracies occur. Such quantitation can only be done in emulsion-coated coverslip autoradiograms, in which the grains are resolved in a plane of focus above the underlying tissue. Many commercially marketed image analysis packages are available and, with the assistance of a computer programmer, the Reep and Creegan algorithm [21] could be simply implemented to work on many digital image file formats.

Another way in which quantitative data can be obtained is to measure optical densities in film images. Low magnification images of high grain densities in film are particularly suited to such analysis. Suitable radiation standards like Amersham Microscales should be included in these analyses.

## References

1   Spina D, Rigby PJ, Paterson JW and Goldie RG (1989) *Br. J. Pharmacol.* **97**: 701

2   Spina D, Rigby PJ, Paterson JW and Goldie RG (1989) *Am. Rev. Respir. Dis.* **140**: 1410

3   Barnes PJ, Basbaum, CB, Nadel JA and Roberts JM (1982) *Nature* **299**: 444

4   Carswell H and Nahorski SR (1983) *Br. J. Pharmacol.* **79**: 965

5   Goldie RG, Papadimitriou JM, Paterson JW, Rigby PJ and Spina D (1986) *Br. J. Pharmacol.* **88**: 621

6   Henry PJ, Rigby PJ and Goldie RG (1990) *Br. J. Pharmacol.* **99**: 136

7   Rogers AW (1979) *Techniques of*

*Autoradiography*. 3rd Ed. Elsevier/North Holland Biomedical Press Amsterdam

8　Kiernan, J.A. (1990) *Histological and Histochemical Methods. Theory and Practice*. 2nd Ed. Pergamon Press Oxford UK

9　Henry PJ, Rigby PJ, Mackenzie JS and Goldie RG (1991) *Br. J. Pharmacol.* **104**: 914

10　Henry PJ. (1993) *Br. J. Pharmacol.* **110**: 435

11　Carr MJ, Goldie RG and Henry PJ (1996) *Br. J. Pharmacol.* **117**: 1222

12　Goldie RG, Grayson PS, Knott P G, Self GJ and Henry PJ (1994) *Br. J. Pharmacol.* **112**: 749

13　Goldie RG, D'Aprile AC, Cvetkovski R., Rigby PJ and Henry PJ (1996) *Br. J. Pharmacol.* **117**: 736

14　Goldie RG, D'Aprile AC, Self GJ, Rigby PJ and Henry PJ (1996) *Br. J. Pharmacol.* **117**: 729

15　Knott PG, D'Aprile AC, Henry PJ, Hay DWP and Goldie RG (1995) *Br. J. Pharmacol.* **114**: 1

16　Henry PJ, Rigby PJ, Self, GJ, Preuss JMH and Goldie RG (1990) *Br. J. Pharmacol.* **100**: 786

17　Self, GJ, Rigby PJ, Passarelli M and Goldie RG (1990) *Eur. J. Pharmacol.* **176**: 169

18　Rigby PJ, Self GJ and Goldie RG (1992) *Eur. J. Pharmacol.* 228 (Environ. Tox. Pharmacol.), **1**: 141

19　Pedersen KE, Rigby PJ, Self GJ and Goldie RG (1991) *Br. J. Pharmacol.* **104**: 128

20　Rigby PJ, Passarelli MC, Self GJ, Preuss JMH and Goldie RG (1988) *Biochem. Pharmacol.* **37**: 1421

21　Reep RL and Creegan WJ (1988) *Comp. Biomed. Res.* **21**: 244

# Further methods

# 19 Application of aerosols

*W. Koch*

Inhalation is a very efficient pathway to bring airborne material into the human body. For aerosols it is almost the only way to interact with the biological system. Aerosols are liquid or solid particles suspended in air. They are applied for local lung therapy as well as for systemic therapy. Furthermore, they serve as a diagnostic tool for the study of lung morphometry, lung physiology and clearance mechanism. Frequently, experimental animals such as rodents and dogs are used to investigate pulmonary effects of inhaled aerosols, particularly in view of particle related toxic effects. Particles as they are inhaled will be transported through the respiratory system and will be deposited in various regions in the lung depending on the particle size, the breathing pattern and the lung morphology, i.e. species. The applied dose is determined by the (mass) concentration and the size distribution of the inhaled aerosol and the regional deposition efficiency which is a function of particle size. The respiratory system can be divided into three compartments: the extrathoracic region (nose, mouth cavity, pharynx, larynx), the tracheo-bronchial airways and the alveolar airspace. In order to maximize the expected effect of the aerosol and to minimize side-effects it is often required to deliver the particles only to one specific region of the lung. For example, substances designed to get into the systemic circulation should be preferentially deposited in the alveolar space whereas bronchio dilatators act locally in the bronchial region and, thus, should be deposited preferentially in this region. As can be seen from Figure 19.1 showing the regional deposition efficiency as a function of particle size the deposition of aerosols in a certain target region requires quite different sizes for different species [1, 2]. In rodents, for example, particles with diameters smaller than 1 μm will be deposited preferentially in the alveolar region. In humans the corresponding deposition maximum is for particles with diameters at 3–4 μm.

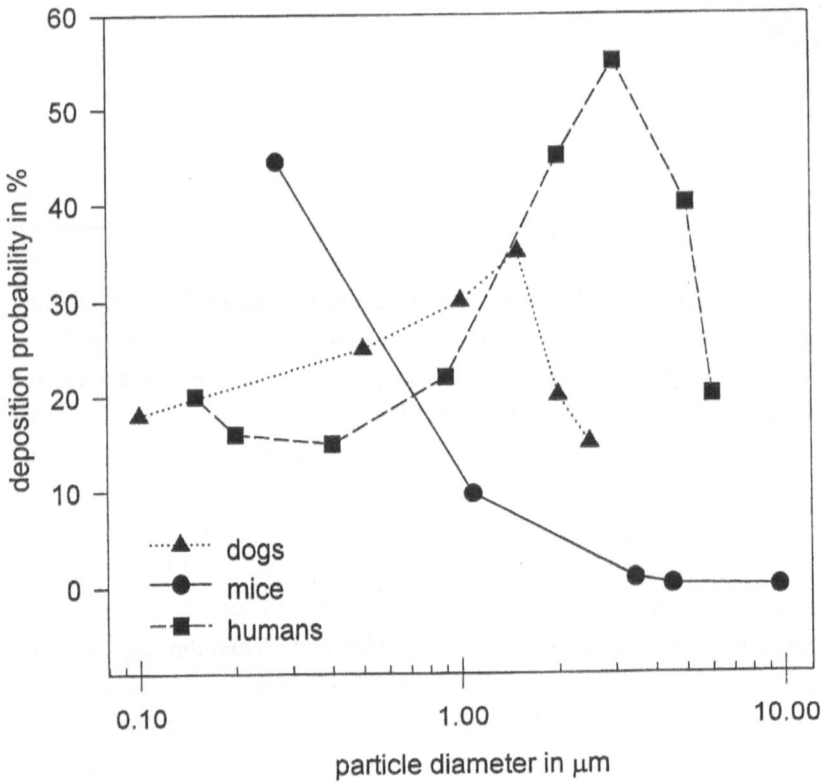

**Figure 19.1. The probability of particle deposition in different lung compartments**
*The total deposition is obtained from a superposition of the three regional deposition curves.*

In the following paragraphs we describe techniques of how to generate aerosols of known particle size, how to measure concentration and size and how to introduce the aerosols into the lung. Before starting with technical details some important definitions and a description of basic properties of aerosols will be presented. Understanding these quantities is of great importance for experimental design in lung research using aerosols as well as for a proper dose estimation.

# Methods

## Physical characterization of aerosols

Aerosols are liquid and/or solid particles suspended in air. A basic dose determining aerosol property is the mass concentration, $C_M$, measured in units of microgram of aerosol material (active substance) per liter of air. In case of spherical particles (nebulized droplet aerosols) the particle size is simply the geometric diameter, $d_g$. Irregularly shaped particles (most powders) are characterized by the so called aerodynamic diameter, $d_{ae}$. This is equal to the geometric diameter of a sphere of unit density ($\rho_0$) i.e. a water sphere, with the same settling velocity in air as the particle under consideration. For spheres composed of material with density $\rho_p$ the aerodynamic diameter and the geometric diameter are related through [3]:

$$d_{ae} = \sqrt{\frac{\rho_p}{\rho_0}} \, d_g$$

For particles larger than a few tenths of a micron the aerodynamic diameter determines the transport and deposition properties of particles in the respiratory tract. In this so-called aerodynamic size regime the deposition probability increases as the particle size and the volumetric flow rate increase. For very small sizes the Brownian (diffusional) motion of the particles becomes the dominating mechanism responsible for particle deposition in the lung. In this size regime nonspherical particles are described by their diffusion equivalent diameter. The deposition probability increases with decreasing particle size.

Estimation of the aerosol uptake in the lung requires information about the size distribution. The mathematical description of the size distribution can be either in terms of particle number concentration as function of particle size, $c_N(d_p)$, or in terms of mass concentration, $c_M(d_p)$. The coexistence of these two different concepts often leads to misunderstanding and confusion. An important parameter of the distribution is the median diameter (50-percentile), i.e. count median diameter, CMD, for the number distribution, respectively mass median diameter, MMD, for the mass distribution. Fifty percent of the total number respectively mass concentration belongs to particles with diameters smaller than the CMD, respectively MMD. Except for strictly monodisperse distributions, the count median diameter is always smaller than the mass median diameter. The difference depends on the width of the distribution characterized by the geometric standard deviation, $\sigma_g$ defined as:

$$\sigma_g = \sqrt{\frac{84 - \text{percentile}}{16 - \text{percentile}}}$$

The geometric standard deviation is a dimensionless number. Its value denotes that 68 % of the aerosol number/mass concentration is in the size range between between $GMD * \sigma_g > d_p > GMD/\sigma_g$, where GMD is the geometric mean diameter of the distribution, either count or mass. An aerosol is called monodisperse for $\sigma_g < 1.15$, quasimonodisperse for $1.15 < \sigma_g < 1.5$ and polydisperse for $\sigma_g > 1.5$. The size distribution of many laboratory aerosols can be approximated mathematically quite well by a lognormal function (Fig. 19.2). In this special case, the count median diameter and the mass median diameter are related through:

$$MMD = CMD \exp\left[3\ln^2 \sigma_g\right]$$

Assume a collision nebulizer generates a droplet distribution with a geometric standard deviation $\sigma_g \approx 2$ and a mass median diameter around 8 µm. From the above equation the count median diameter is calculated to be 2 µm. Thus, characterizing the aerosol distribution by the CMD instead of the MMD lets it look much better in view of aerosol therapy targeted to the alveolar region of the human lung because the CMD well meets the maximum of the alveolar deposition and the MMD does not (see Fig. 19.1). However, the choice of the suitable parameter characterizing the average particle size is directly coupled to the dose-determining quantity. If the deposited mass is the relevant dose quantity (which is commonly the case in aerosol therapy) then the mass median diameter should be used. If the biological effect is related to the number of particles such as in fiber carcinogenicity, the count median diameter is a better parameter to characterize the average size of the aerosol particles.

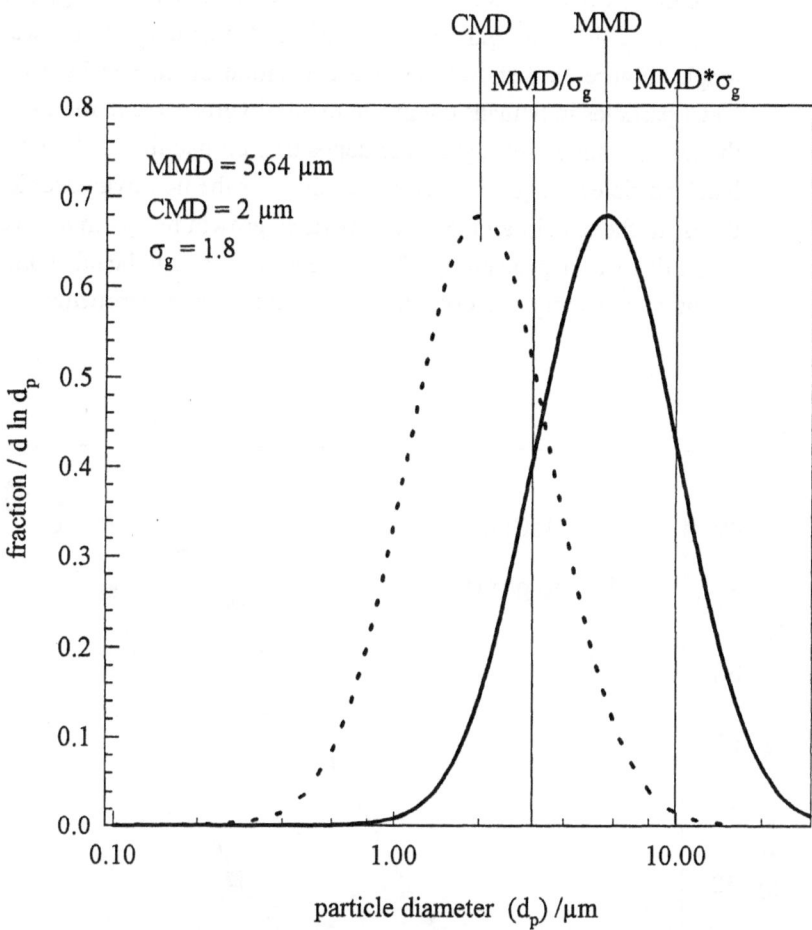

*Figure 19.2. The two different representation of a lognormal aerosol distribution: Number distribution density, mass distribution density*
*The two curves coincide only when $\sigma_g = 1$.*

Many pharmacological aerosols contain or consist of hygroscopic substances, usually a mixture of inorganic and organic salts. Salts dissolved in water cause a reduction of the vapor pressure. This is why dry salt particles will liquify and start growing at relative humidities below 100%. Therefore, dry pharmaceutical aerosols generated by MDIs (metered dose inhalers) or DPIs (dry powder inhaler), for example, can grow substantially upon inhalation because they enter a region of high relative humidity. This has a significant effect on the deposition pattern. As an example, Figure 19.3 shows the total deposition of inhaled hygroscopic NaCl particles in humans compared to non-hygroscopic particles [4]. In the aerodynamic size regime the deposition probability of the growing NaCl particles is significantly higher than for the non-hygroscopic particles. In the small particle regime particle growth results in a lowering of the deposition probability. These effects have also to be taken into account when testing hygroscopic aerosols in animal experiments.

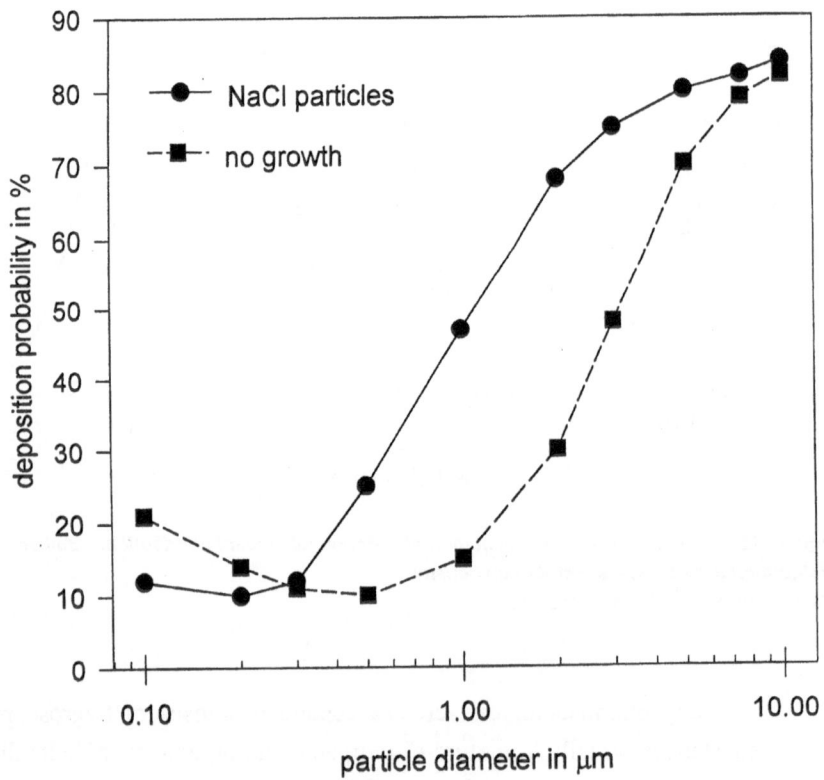

**Figure 19.3. Total deposition curve for growing (NaCl) and non-growing particles**
Lung capcity 1000 ml, inspiration time 2.5 s.

Another physical process that has to be taken into account, particularly when dealing with aerosols at high number concentrations, is coagulation. Coagulation means the collision between two particles resulting in a larger particle. This process leads to a decrease in the number concentration of the aerosol population and to a shift of the CMD towards larger sizes. The mass concentration is not affected by the coagulation process. The overall effect of coagulation depends on the number concentration and the observation time, for example, the residence time in the generator and the exposure chamber. It is particularly pronounced under conditions of high number concentrations. As a rule of thumb the time, $t_{1/2}$, after which the number concentration, $C_N$, has decreased to half its initial value, $C_{N, 0}$, is given by [3]

$$t_{1/2} = \frac{2 \cdot 10^9}{C_{N,0}} \ [s],$$

where the number concentration is measured in units of particles per cubic centimeter. This formula is useful to estimate, for a given situation, whether coagulation is important or not. For example if the aerosol number concentration, $C_{N, 0}$, entering an inhalation chamber is $10^7 \ cm^{-3}$ the coagulation half-time would be 200 s. For a monodisperse aerosol composed of unit density spheres the number concentration of $10^7 \ cm^{-3}$ corresponds to a mass concentration of 5 mg/m$^3$. Thus the number concentration is significantly reduced when the aerosol flows through an inhalation chamber at an exchange rate less then 10-fold per hour, which corresponds to an average residence time larger than 360 s. In aerosol generators the local aerosol number concentration can be extremely high so that the emerging aerosol is coagulation controlled although the residence time in the instrument is short.

## Methods of aerosol generation

For the generation of aerosols there exist two principally different groups of mechanisms: comminution and growth, i.e., "making big things small", respectively, "making small things big".

An example of the first group is the dispersion process. Particle generation starts from the bulk material, which is either a liquid or a powder. Mechanical energy is introduced into the system and is transformed into surface energy by either disintegrating a liquid or by dispersing the powder. Nebulization of liquids can be achieved either by interaction with a pressurized gas, usually air, or by focusing ultrasonic energy onto the surface of the liquid. Compressed air nebulizers, also called collision nebulizers, are widely in use. The working princinple of all of the existing devices is essentially the same (Fig. 19.4). The liquid with the active solvent is sucked from a reservoir into high speed air emerging from a nozzle. The liquid jet is disintegrated by the action of pressure and shear forces. Usually, the energy input is not very efficient so that a droplet spectrum with a large fraction of noninhalable coarse particles are generated. These particles are removed from the air stream by impinging them against a baffle. It is the combination of the disintegration and the removal process that determines the initial droplet spectrum of the nebulizer. The large droplets flow back into the reservoir. Usually more than 90 % of the droplets have to be removed so that, on the average, the liquid is recirculated and disintegrated more than 10 times before leaving the device as an inspirable aerosol. The repeated dispersion process can cause stability problems for substances sensitive to external mechanical stress such as surfactants. During the nebulization process a substantial

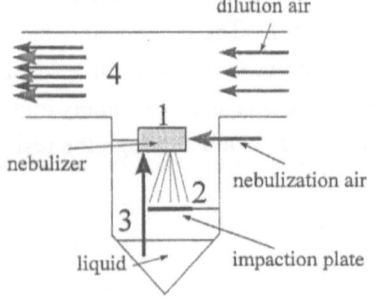

1   generation of droplets

2   removal of large droplets

3   partial evaporation, saturation

4   dilution, further evaporation

**Figure 19.4. The operating principle of a compressed air nebulizer**
This type of nebulizer can be either incorporated into a forced ventilation system, or also be used as a nebulizer for spontaneous breathing. The humidity of the dilution air determines the degree of evaporation of the droplets.

part of the liquid water will be evaporated because the nebulization air is usually dry and the droplets provide a large surface area for the evaporation of water. The solvent concentration will therefore increase continuously as the nebulization time proceeds and the inhaled dose will increase with time. The increase in solvent concentration can eventually lead to an increase in the viscosity of the liquid or crystallization of the solvent and, therefore, may clog the liquid nozzle. Table 19.1 shows the MMD and the geometric standard deviation of various commercially available nebulizers operated under their intended conditions. The droplet spectrum can also be influenced to some extent by changing the operating conditions of the nebulizers. An example is shown in Figure 19.5. The mass median diameter of the droplets generated by the nebulization system "Inhalette" (Drägerwerk AG, Lübeck, Germany) can be adjusted between 7 and 2.5 μm depending on the air flow rate through the device [5]. After nebulization, the aerosol flow is introduced into the breathing air, which can either be preconditioned to 37 °C and nearly 100% relative humidity in case of forced ventilation, or can just be room air when the nebulizers are used at home and the patient sucks through the device.

**Table 19.1. Characteristics of the initial droplet spectrum generated by various commercially available compressed air nebulizers**

| Nebulizer, producer | Parameters of the initial size distribution | |
|---|---|---|
| | MMD (μm) | $\sigma_g$ |
| Micro-Cirrus, Intersurgical | 1.0 | 1.7 |
| Respigard, Marquest M.P. | 2.0 | 2.0 |
| Cirrus, Intersurgical | 2.5 | 2.0 |
| IS-2, Pari | 2.8 | 2.3 |
| Turret, Turbo | 3.0 | 2.0 |
| Sidestream, Medic Aid | 3.0 | 2.0 |
| Inhalierboy, Pari | 4.7 | 2.0 |
| Master, Pari | 4.7 | 2.0 |
| Respi-Jet, Kendall | 5.0 | 2.0 |
| Davos, Wenger | 6.0 | 2.0 |
| Pulmoneb, DeVilbiss | 9.3 | 1.7 |

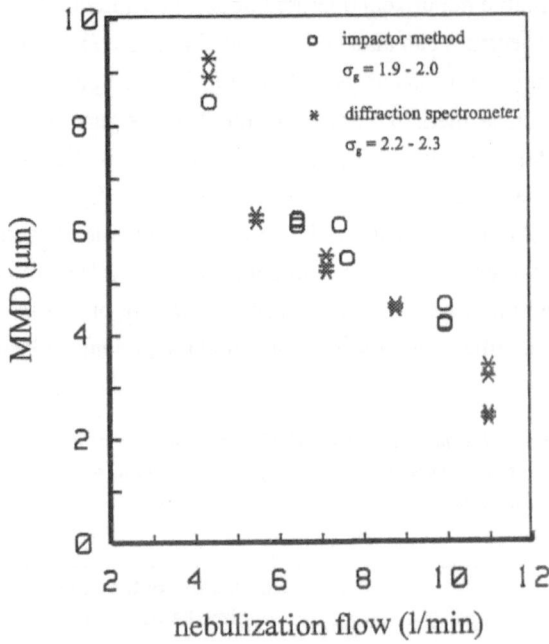

**Figure 19.5. The MMD of droplets generated by a compressed air nebulizer under different conditions**

When being mixed with the dilution air the droplets will partly evaporate depending on the relative humidity. This may lead to an increase in the MMD since smaller droplets evaporate more rapidly than larger ones.

A second method to generate droplets is by ultrasonic nebulization. Nebulization air is not required for these devices. The liquid is aerosolized by focusing an ultrasonic sound wave generated by a piezoelectric oscillator on the surface of a liquid. Droplets are emitted from the surface waves which are induced by the ultrasound. The droplets are then carried away by the carrier air flow. The geometric mean diameter of the droplets is predictable from the surface tension, $\sigma_l$, and the density, $\rho_l$, of the liquid and the frequency of oscillation, $v$, according to [6]:

$$d_{dr} = 0.34 \sqrt[3]{\frac{8\pi\sigma_l}{\rho_l v^2}}$$

Typical ultrasonic nebulizers operate in the frequency regime between 100 kHz and 1 MHz. Droplet spectra with MMDs as small as 2 µm can be generated. The big advantage of ultrasonic nebulizers is that no air is required for the nebulization process. This enables the generation of highly concentrated aerosols in small air streams as it is often required in experiments with intubated animals. A large amount of energy is continuously fed into the liquid which may cause a breakdown of organic molecules for example surfactants.

In view of pulmonary research with laboratory animals, especially with small rodents, the primary droplet spectrum generated by the devices described above may be too coarse. High particle deposition rates in the alveolar airspaces of small rodents can only be achieved using submicron particles. A significant reduction of the particle size can be achieved in case of nebulization of (aqueous) solutions of nonvolatile substances by complete evaporation of the solvent. The final aerosol consists of dry solute particles. The size reduction is determined by the solute concentration, $c_l$, the densitiy of the solvent, $\rho_0$, (which is assumed to be the same as the density of the solution), and the density of the dry solute, $\rho_r$. The geometric diameter, $d_p$, of the residual particles is calculated from the droplet diameter, $d_{dr}$, using:

$$d_p = \sqrt[3]{\frac{\rho_0 c_l}{\rho_r}} d_{dr}$$

where $c_l$ is the non-dimensional mass fraction of the solute in the solution. For unit densities, spraying a 0.1 % solution of a nonvolatile substance with subsequent drying leads to a size reduction by a factor of 10 for all droplets. A droplet spectrum with MMD of 5 µm would then be transformed into an aerosol spectrum with a MMD of .5 µm. The geometric standard deviation, $\sigma_g$, remains unchanged. The maximum dry aerosol concentration that can be generated by this method is limited by the saturation concentration of the evaporated solvent in the carrier gas. The saturation concentration of water vapor at room temperature is 25 g/m³. In the above example a maximum concentration of the corresponding dry aerosol of 25 mg/m³ would therefore be possible. The spraying evaporation method can be extremely variable when the volume flow and the mass flow of the nozzle can be adjusted independently from each other. An experimental set-up suitable for this technique of aerosol generation is shown in Figure 19.6. The droplets are dispersed by a pneumatic nozzle with an air flow rate of 4 l/min in this example. The liquid feed rate is adjusted via the speed of the syringe pump or by any other low flow rate pump, for example, a peristaltic pump. The spray is

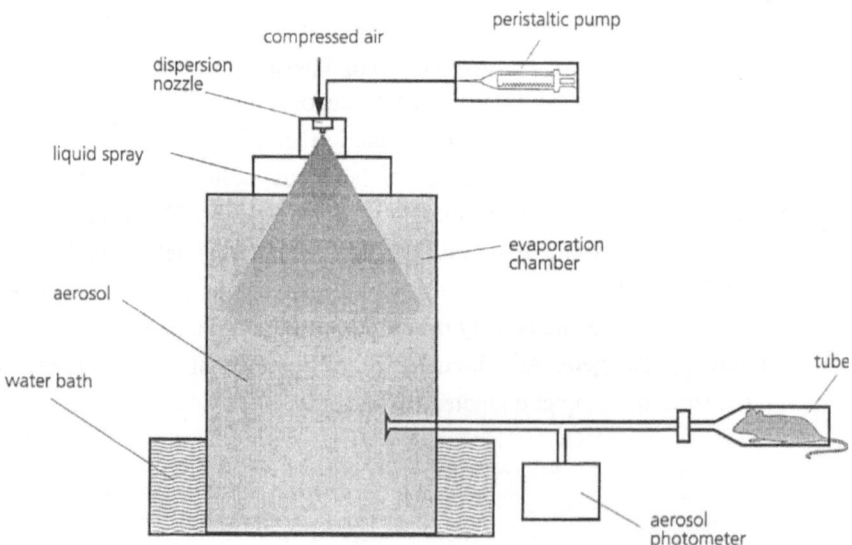

*Figure 19.6. A possible experimental set-up for aerosol generation from the liquid phase and a route of aerosol administration to a small rodent*

blown into an evaporation chamber where the droplets evaporate. The dry aerosol leaves this chamber via a tube and can be administered directly to an experimental animal. A computerized unit housing nebulization and dilution air supply as well as a liquid pump is the Bronchy H developed at Fh-ITA.

In case the aerosol material to be suspended is not soluble in water or any other non-toxic solvent the generation has to be performed by dry dispersion methods. There are various generators available to perform this task. A widely used system is the rotating brush generator (Palas GmbH, Karlsruhe, Germany) where a piston filled with the dust to be dispersed is pressed against a rotating brush. The brush scrapes off material which is then dispersed by a pressurized air nozzle. With some modifications, this principle can also be used to generate fibrous aerosols. The rotating brush generator requires a certain minimum amount of material (1–2 g), and is therefore not useful if the test substances are available only in very small quantities. Small amounts of material can be redispersed continuously by an apparatus shown in Figure 19.7. The bulk material is transported from a reservoir to an aspiration tube via the holes drilled into a rotating disk. The individual dust portions are levitated and finally dispersed by a pressurized air dispersion nozzle [7]. The feed rate can be as low as 5 mg/h and the minimum amount of material required for proper operation is 50–100 mg. This instrument was developed at the Fraunhofer-Institute (Fh-ITA) and was successfully used in numerous toxicity tests with expensive pharmaceutical screening substances.

The second basic physical principle for the generation of aerosols is gas-to-particle conversion. Particles are formed from the gas phase by condensation of a supersaturated vapor. With this principle rather narrow aerosol distributions with MMDs significantly below 1 μm can be produced. The vapor of the aerosol material is generated by heating a liquid or solid substance. The saturated carrier gas is then mixed with condensation nuclei generated for example by a collision nebulizer. This mixture is cooled and the vapor condenses onto the nuclei. If the supersaturation profile is homogeneous over the condensor cross-section, size distributions with a geometric standard deviation as small as 1.1 can be generated. Particles of low volatile liquids and even solid particles can be generated using the evaporation condensation method. Commercial

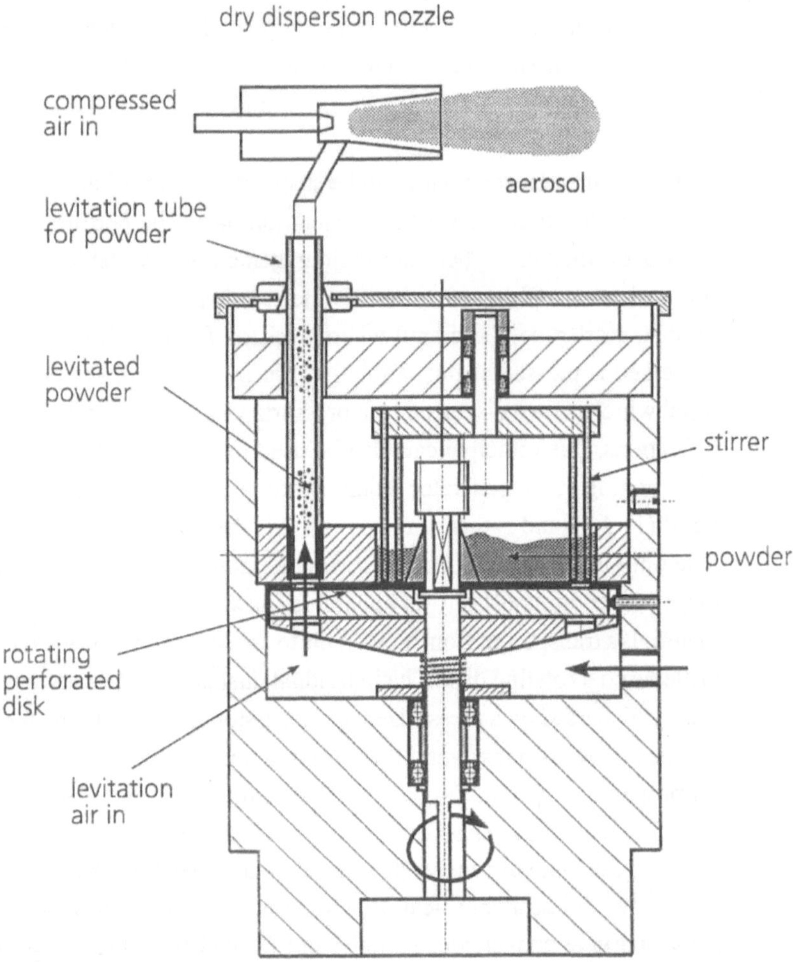

Figure 19.7. Small scale powder feeding and dispersion system (Fh-ITA)

versions of the condensation aerosol generator are available from Palas GmbH, Karlsruhe and TSI, Deutschland GmbH, Aachen.

Solid particles from non-volatile bulk material such as soot can be produced from electrically conducting solids by the spark technique. Spark discharges are generated in an inert gas flow by a high voltage between two electrodes made of the aerosol substance. The high energy density of the sparks vaporizes some of the electrode material, which re-condenses shortly afterwards to form small primary particles. The primary particles are electrically charged and may undergo coagulation to form chain-like agglomerates. The degree of agglomeration depends on the rate of primary particle generation, on the volumetric flow rate of the inert gas and on the subsequent mixing with a dilution gas. The spark generator (Palas GmbH, Karlsruhe) is frequently used to produce soot particles in the diameter range between 0.05 and 0.2 μm, but particles composed of other conductive materials can be generated as well.

## Methods of aerosol measurement

The detailed properties (size distribution, concentration) of the aerosols produced by the generation systems described above depend on the oper-ating conditions of the generators. Therefore the measurement of the ac-tual concentration and the particle size distribution is of great importance in aerosol inhalation. In this chapter we will describe only a few out of a huge variety of experimental methods for aerosol characterization.

The mass concentration of low or non-volatile aerosol particles is usually measured by the filter method. The aerosol is sucked at a known flow rate through a glass fiber or a membrane filter. The weight of the filter is determined before and after sampling and the concentration is calculated from the deposited mass and the total volume passed through the filter. For optical inspection of the particles by optical or electron mi-croscopy the samples have to be taken on surface membrane filters such as nucelopore filters [3]. Using a critical orifice it is particularly easy to set a constant volume flow rate through the filter (see Fig. 19.8). The ori-fice is simply connected to a vacuum line. When the absolute pressure behind the orifice is 40% or less of the pressure before the orifice the ori-fice is operated in the critical regime and the volume flow rate is con-stant, independent of pressure fluctuations in the vacuum line. Glass ca-pillaries are frequently used as critical orifices. The critical flow rate depends on their diameter and their length. Useful data are given in Table 19.2. The filter size has to be chosen such that the pressure drop

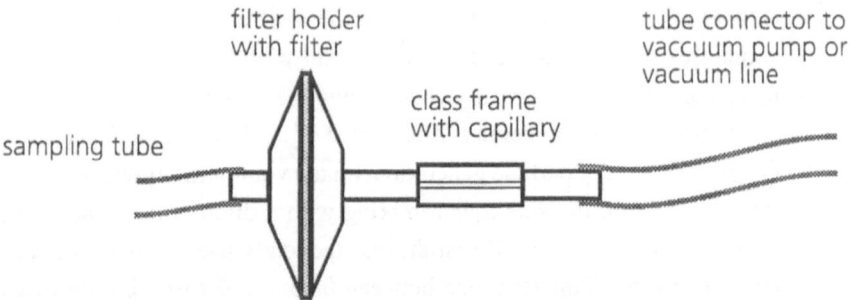

**Figure 19.8. Measurement of aerosol concentration using a critical orifice**
*The sample volume is calculated from the sampling time and the flow rate through the orifice specified by its length and its diameter.*

**Table 19.2. Critical flow rates of glass capillaries**

| Flow rate [l/min] | Diameter [mm] | Length [mm] |
|:---:|:---:|:---:|
| 0.5 | 0.3 | 13.0 |
| 1.0 | 0.4 | 14.5 |
| 2.0 | 0.55 | 18.5 |
| 4.0 | 0.8 | 30.0 |

across the filter, $\Delta p_{filter}$, for the intended flow rate is small compared to the pressure drop across the critical orifice, $\Delta p_{orifice}$ (which is 50 kPa), i.e. $\Delta p_{filter} < 1$ kPa.

When the sampling time is equal to the total exposure time the filter method gives the time average of the mass concentration. However, it is often desirable to have information about the temporal concentration pattern, particularly for intermittent or short-term exposure. For this purpose, on-line monitors based on light scattering can be used. These instruments are called aerosol photometers. They either take a sample from the aerosol stream (SAD, Fh-ITA, sample flow rate adjustable between 0.2 and 1.5 l/min) as it is shown in Figure 19.5, or they are integrated in the aerosol transport line in a way that the entire aerosol passes through the photometer (SAD II, Fh-ITA). The devices have an excellent time resolution with time constants as small as 100 ms. This high time resolution allows, for example, a detailed monitoring of an intermittent aerosol application under forced ventilation. The photometers have to be calibrated using the basic filter method in order to convert the voltage output into a mass concentration reading. The calibration constant depends on the optical properties and the size distribution of the aerosol to be monitored. Therefore, a separate calibration has to be performed for each type of aerosol to be monitored. The photometers can easily be incorporated into a computer controlled exposure system and the signals are used for example to estimate the dose or to control the aerosol generator.

The standard instrument to measure the mass size distribution as a function of the aerodynamic equivalent diameter is the cascade impactor. In the instrument, particles are separated from the air stream by inertial impaction in a stagnation point flow. In this flow type generated by a jet impinging on a surface the flow direction suddenly changes. All particles with aerodynamic diameters smaller than a certain critical size will follow the streamlines and will remain airborne. Particles larger than the critical size are deposited on a removable surface (aluminum foil, glass or thin metallic plate). The cascade impactor consists of a staggered layer of nozzle plates and deposition surfaces. A well defined size fraction of the aerosol sucked through the instrument is deposited on each surface. The size of the removed particles decreases as the aerosol flows through the cascade, i.e. the coarser particles are found on the top stages whereas the finer ones are on the bottom stages. A back-up filter collects all particles below the smallest size removable by impaction in the lowest stage. A very popular type of cascade impactor is the "Berner" low pressure impactor which comes in different versions (Gesellschaft für Innovative Verfahrenstechnik, Breuberg, Germany). The type LPI, 30, 0.06 is particularly suitable for the measurement of inhalation atmospheres. The instrument has nine stages covering the overall size range between 0.06 µm and 16 µm. The flow rate is 30 l/min and is stabilized by a built-in critical orifice which makes the operation extremely easy. Particles are deposited on thin aluminum, plastic, or Teflon foils. In order to avoid that particles bounce upon impaction it is advised to cover the foils with a sticky non-vaporizable surface, for example, with silicon (Silicon Release Spray, Dow Corning). For some applications the sampling flow rate of the Berner impactor is too high. A low flow rate cascade impactor is the "Marple personal cascade impactor" (Gesellschaft für Innovative Verfahrenstechnik, Breuberg, Germany) operating at a flow rate of 2 l/min and covering a size range between 0.25 and 20 μm with seven stages. Particles smaller than 0.25 μm are sampled on a built-in back-up filter. The flow rate through the instrument can be controlled using an external critical orifice as for filter sampling.

Time-resolved mass size distribution measurements can be done with a new instrument called Electrical Low Pressure cascade impactor (Gesellschaft für Innovative Verfahrenstechnik, Breuberg, Germany). In this instrument the particles are electrically charged before being collected on the impaction stages. The temporal pattern of the mass accumulation rate on each stage can be determined from the charge accumulation rate measured by an electrometer. The flow rate through the instrument is 10 l/min. The size range between 0.03 and 20 μm is distributed on, in total, 10 stages. A less expensive instrument for time- and size-resolved aerosol measurements is the newly developed "Respicon" (Fh-ITA, Hund GmbH, Wetzlar, Germany) [8]. The instrument samples the aerosol at a flow rate of 3.1 l/min. Using a combination of inertial classification via a two-stage virtual impactor and aerosol photometry, three size fractions (<4 μm, 4–10 μm, and >10 μm) are deposited on filters and are monitored on-line.

There exists a variety of particle counting devices suitable for number distribution measurements. Among them the Aerodynamic Particle Sizer (TSI-Deutschland GmbH, Aachen) will be mentioned here. The aerosol is sucked into the instrument at a flow rate of 5 l/min and passed through a nozzle where the particles are accelerated. The particles lag behind the gas depending on their aerodynamic diameter. The velocity of each particle at the nozzle exit is measured and the counts are evaluated by a multichannel analyzer. The instrument's software then transforms the velocity spectrum into the number distribution as a function of the aerodynamic particle diameter. The instrument allows for a very detailed size resolution in the range between .5 and 15 μm. To avoid coincidences of counting events and data processing the aerosol number concentration is limited to a maxmimum value of about $10^3$ particles/cm$^3$ for a coincidence error smaller than 5%. Higher aerosol concentrations have to be properly diluted prior to the measurement with the particle counter (Fig. 19.9). A very simple way of aerosol dilution is the injection method where the aerosol is mixed with particle free air in an injection nozzle. Using a cascade of injection nozzles dilution ratios up to $10^4$ can be easily achieved. However, the system has to be designed very carefully in order to avoid extensive particle losses. A commercialized and well

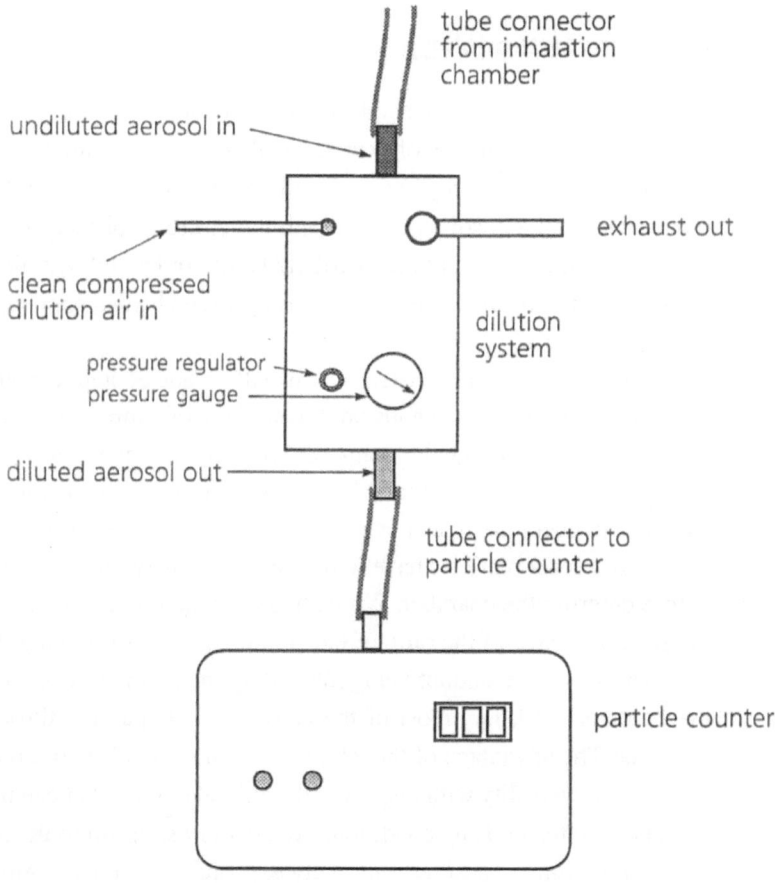

**Figure 19.9. Measurement of the aerosol number distribution using a particle counter and a dilution system**

characterized version of the injection type dilution system is available from Palas GmbH, Karlsruhe. Each dilution unit has a fixed dilution factor of 10. Higher dilution factors can be achieved by building a cascade of several single stage dilutors.

A detailed description of the various generation, measurement and dilution techniques can be found in the VDI guideline #3491. This guidelines contain also many practical hints about operation and possible difficulties.

## Exposure methodology

There are many possibilities to bring the aerosol into the lung of the test species. In view of the use of experimental animals these are [10]: whole body exposure, head-only and nose only exposure systems. In this type of exposure the aerosol passes through the entire respiratory tract with the effect that the particles are distributed more or less all over the respiratory system. The upper airways can be bypassed by using an implanted tracheal cannula.

Whole body exposure systems are usually made of stainless steel and glass. The overall size depends on the numbers of animals to be housed. The air flow rate through the chambers is either vertical or horizontal. Air exchange rates between 10 and 20 per hour are tolerable as long as the chamber temperature does not exceed the comfort level of the test species. The aerosol particles have to be homogeneously mixed with the air before entering the chamber. Whole body inhalation chambers are very inefficient in view of the ratio of the amount of aerosol flowing through the chamber to the amount being inhaled by the animals. The ratio is of the order of 1:60, i.e., most of the aerosol is just passing through the chamber. The advantage of the whole body chambers is their simplicity and their universality with respect to the animal species that can be used. Furthermore the housing conditions are not very stressful to the animals so that long time exposures with daily exposure durations of more than 10 h can be done using whole body chambers.

The aerosol is used in a more efficient way when it is administered to the animals via the nose/head-only only exposure route. A widely used design consists of a concentric cylinder where the freshly generated aerosol flows vertically downwards. Aerosol exits are provided at different levels in a ring arrangement. The aerosol is blown directly into the breathing region of the rodent sitting in a tube attached to the cylinder. The exhaled air is sucked away from the animal and flows into the outer cylinder (Fig. 19.10). The flow rate through the system depends on the number of animals attached to the tube. As a rule of thumb an air flow rate of 1 l/min has to be provided per animal. For rats the breathing flow rate is 0.2 l/min. This means that the ratio of supplied to inhaled aerosol for the nose only devices is 5:1 compared to 60:1 for whole body chambers. Versatile nose-only chambers of the type drawn in Fig. 19.8 are available from C.R. Equipment, Tanney, Switzerland. Head only expo-

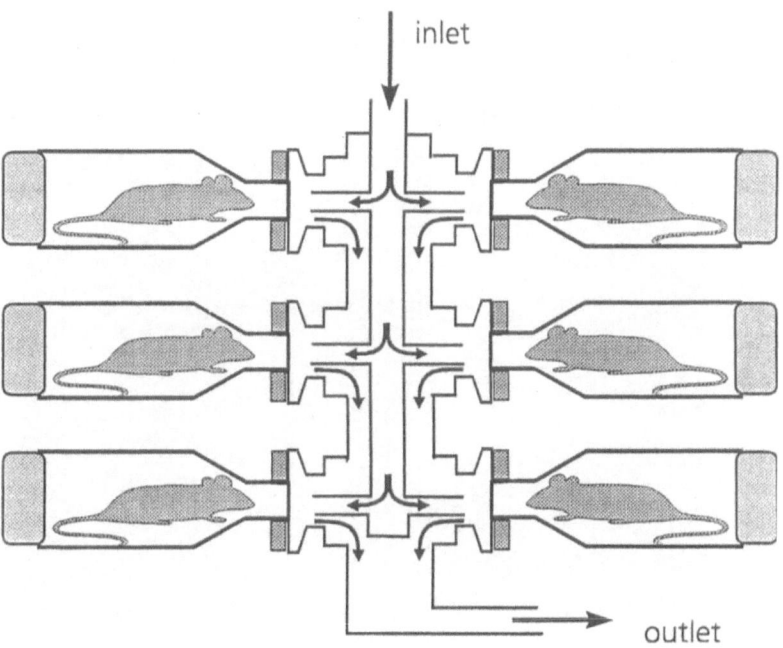

*Figure 19.10. Schematic drawing of a concentric tube nose-only inhalation chamber*

sure systems are also available for dogs (Fig. 19.11). One unit can handle four dogs. It consists of the aerosol generation system and a distribution chamber. The four dogs are connected to the chamber vial frills, so that their entire head is exposed. The dogs are fixed by a leather harness attached to an adjustable supporting frame. The total air flow through the chamber is 50 l/min. Use of nose/head-only system is restricted to shorter exposure durations: 4 h per day for the rodents in the tubes and maximum 1 h for the dogs (Fig. 19.10).

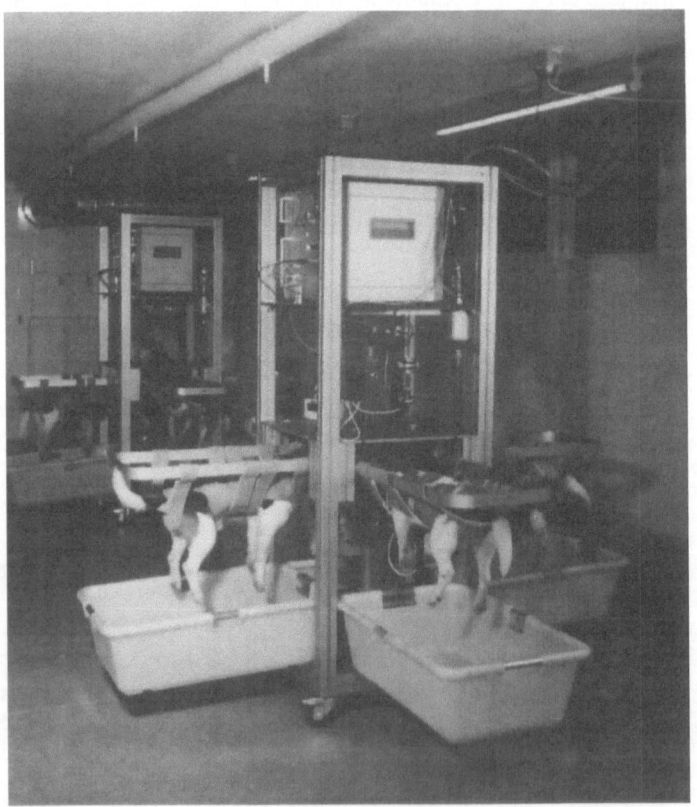

*Figure 19.11. Photograph of a head-only inhalation system for beagle dogs*

# References

1 Schlesinger RB (1985) *Toxicol. Environm. Health* **15**: 197

2 Raabe OG, Al-Bayati MA, Teague SV and Rasolt M (1988) *Ann. Occup. Hyg.* **32**: 53

3 Hinds WC (1982) *Aerosol Technology*, John Wiley & Sons New York

4 Ferron GA, Kreyling WG and Haider B (1988) *J. Aerosol Sci.* **19**: 611

5 Koch W, Pohlmann G and Uta J (1994) *J. Aerosol Sci.* **25**: S315

6 Drews WD (1979) *Elektronik* **10**: 83

7 Windt H, Oenning G and Ott W (1995) *Patentschrift DE195 00 726A1*

8 Koch W, Dunkhorst W and Lödding H (1997) *Gefahrstoffe-Reinhaltung der Luft*, **57**: 177

9 Verein Deutscher Ingenieure (1996) *Particulate Matter Measurement*, Beuth Verlag Berlin

10 Phalen RF, Kleinmann MT, Mautz WJ and Drew RT (1994) Inhalation Exposure Methodology. In: *Respiratory Toxicology and Risk Assessment*, Jenkins PG, Kayser D, Muhle H., Rosner G and Smith EM (eds), p. 59, Wissenschaftliche Verlagsgesellschaft mbH Stuttgart

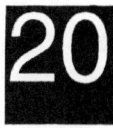

# Cryopreservation of human pulmonary tissues

*E. Müller-Schweinitzer*

Pharmacological studies normally require freshly obtained tissues. These are usually taken from various animal species, although results obtained from human tissues are naturally the most predictable for human pharmacology. However, the main problems with use of human tissues are the irregularity of its supply and the quantity of material that can be utilized at one time, as the tissues change their *in vitro* characteristics progressively and deteriorate rapidly after removal from the body [1, 2]. Furthermore, while the usefulness of human tissues may be limited by factors such as age of the patient, concomitant disease, anaesthesia and medication, certain pharmacological questions can be only addressed when rare tissues, e.g., bronchi from asthmatic patients are available. Cryopreservation allows storage of living cells for virtually indefinite time and has become an important tool for the storage of human vascular tissues in pharmacological research [3, 4]. Recently, evidence has been presented that human airway smooth muscle preparations may also be stored by this technique with a wide variety of functional activities being well preserved [5–8].

## Mechanisms of freezing injury

Freezing of living mammalian cells without cryoprotective additives generally induces severe cell damage and only few if any cells survive [9–11]. During cooling to subzero temperatures water tends to flow out of the cell to freeze externally and the cells shrink during this process (Fig. 20.1). If cooled too fast, cells are injured by the formation of intracellular ice crystals; if cooled too slowly, the cells will be injured by the "solution-effect", i.e., by changes in the composition of extra- and intracellular solutions since the concentration of extracellular salts in the residual unfrozen medium increases as ice is formed [9].

# Ice formation during freezing of cells at different cooling rates

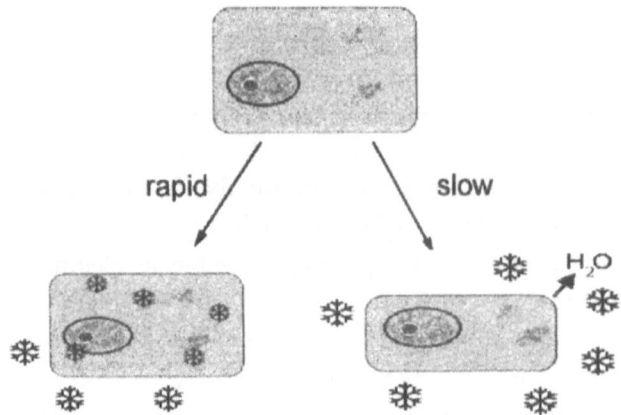

**Figure 20.1. Ice formation during freezing of cells at different cooling rates**
*Ice nucleation is initiated around −5 °C outside the cell. If cooling is performed rapidly, small ice crystals form within the cell. During thawing these small ice crystals will fuse to form larger crystals and damage the cell membrane. If cooling is performed slowly, ice crystals are formed outside the cell and the environment of the cell becomes hyperosmotic. Consequently, the cell loses water and shrinks. During thawing these cells will be rehydrated.*

## Cryoprotective agents and cryomedia

To reduce the freezing injury during cryopreservation tissues must be suspended in a cryomedium consisting of a vehicle solution containing the cryoprotecting agents. Optimal protection against cryoinjury will be obtained by the combined action of a permeating and a nonpermeating cryoprotectant. The most commonly used permeating cryoprotectants are dimethyl sulfoxide (DMSO) and glycerol. It is assumed that these agents protect the cell from cryoinjury by entering the cell, thereby replacing some water [10]. Nonpermeating cryoprotectants such as sucrose, trehalose and hydroxyethyl starch, are suggested to stabilize the cell volume by retaining more liquid water at low temperatures, thereby reducing the external electrolyte concentration [9]. Both types of cryoprotectants act directly at the level of the cell membrane, yet their protective action may be synergistic

[12]. Most commonly used vehicles for the cryomedia are Dulbecco's modified Eagle's medium [13–15], fetal calf serum [7, 8, 12, 16] and Krebs-Henseleit solution [5, 6, 17, 18]

## Freezing procedure and storage temperature

The optimal cooling rate differs from cell to cell and is dependent on both the water permeability of the cell membrane and the surface area to volume ratio of the cell. The presence of many different cell types within a tissue or organ implies, therefore, that no single freezing/thawing procedure can satisfy them all [10]. Moreover, in many peripheral arteries cells are quite densely packed together which may also reduce cell survival. Veins and pulmonary vessels are considerably less compact and show often better post-thaw recovery than peripheral arteries. To minimize the effects of cryoinjury, tissues must equilibrate for 10–30 min with the cryomedium before being slowly frozen. Prolonged pre-freezing exposure to a DMSO-containing medium may attenuate the post-thaw functional activity [17, 18]. For mammalian cells the optimal cooling rate may range from 0.3 to 10 °C per minute, but once a sample is cooled to about −70°C, it can be transferred directly into liquid nitrogen (−196°C) and stored there for virtually infinite time until use [9, 10]. Although storage at higher temperatures (−70 to −85 °C) of both vascular [19] and airway tissues [14] has been shown to allow short-term storage for 3–4 weeks, this temperature range does not provide truly long-term survival of mammalian cells [15, 20].

## Thawing procedure

During thawing ice is converted into free water, cells are exposed to an extra-cellular hypotonic solution and the dehydrated cells must rehydrate in order to remain in osmotic equilibrium. Serum or other high molecular weight polymers in the medium are suggested to reduce the damaging effect of this dilution shock [9]. Indeed, experimental evidence suggests that for many cell types, e.g., for endothelial cells in dog coronary arteries, it seems to be important to have at least 20% serum in the cryomedium [21]. However, considerable species and/or organ differences appear to exist. Thus, in human mesenteric and coronary arteries endothelium-dependent responses to bradykinin and substance P are not modified by serum supplementation of the cryomedium [22]. The same applies for human bronchi, the post-thaw functional recovery of which is unchanged by the addition of serum to the cryomedium [5].

With isolated cells in general a rapid rate of warming, which limits the growth of ice crystals in the frozen samples, is applied. Thawing of isolated tissues at a high warming rate, however, may lead to mechanical stress inducing fractures which occur at temperatures between –100 °C and –150 °C [23]. This can be prevented by a slow rewarming procedure, i.e., by allowing the sample to reach slowly a temperature of about –70 °C prior to thawing in a 40 °C waterbath [23–25].

## Temperature courses during freezing and thawing

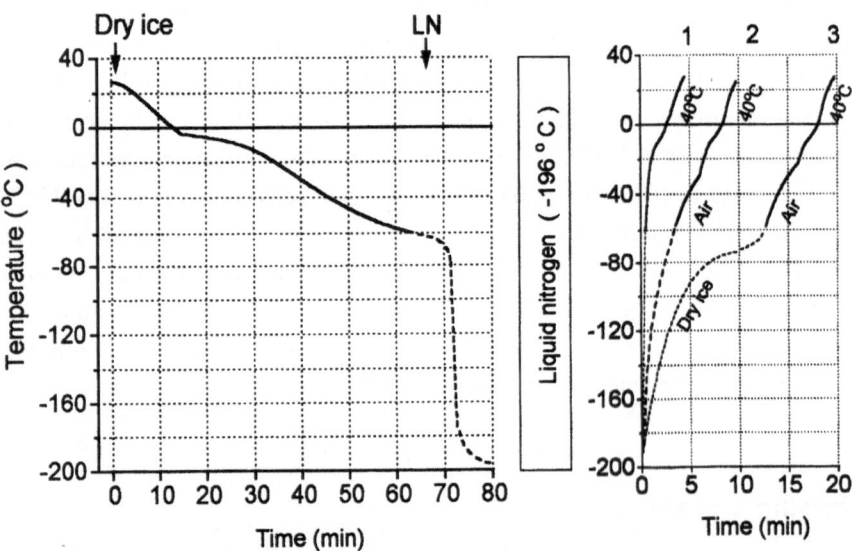

Figure 20.2. *Temperature changes recorded during freezing and thawing within small segments of human internal mammary artery suspended in 2 ml plastic cryotubes containing Krebs-Henseleit solution with 1.8 M DMSO and 0.1 M sucrose*

Left: The samples were placed in a polystyrol box and slowly frozen to –70 °C (dry ice) before being transferred into liquid nitrogen (LN). Right: Different thawing procedures: 1) the samples were thawed rapidly by placing the cryotubes during 4 min into a 40 °C waterbath, or 2) samples were first exposed for 6 min to room temperature before being thawed within 4 min in a 40 °C waterbath, or 3) samples were placed during 10 min on dry ice and then exposed for 6 min to room temperature before being thawed within 4 min in a 40 °C waterbath. The dotted lines indicate extrapolated time-courses.

Temperature courses during freezing and different thawing procedures are illustrated in Figure 20.2. After thawing of isolated mammalian cells often a stepwise dilution protocol is used, in order to avoid osmotic shock which may kill cells when returned to isotonic solution [10]. In isolated venous tissues such as canine saphenous and rat portal veins, which had been frozen in fetal calf serum containing 1.8 M DMSO, this procedure did not improve the post-thaw contractile function (E. Müller-Schweinitzer, unpublished observations). However, recent experiments on arterial tissues have shown that adding and removing cryoprotectants in a manner that avoids severe osmotic consequences, may improve the post-thaw function of both smooth muscle and endothelial cells in rabbit carotid arteries [25].

# Methods, material and equipment

Material and equipment for cryopreservation of isolated tissues are summarized in Table 20.1.

## Cryopreservation

### Freezing procedure

1) Specimens of human lung, (obtained from surgery or multiple organ donors), are immersed in buffered physiologic salt solution, e.g., Krebs-Henseleit solution (composition mM: NaCl 118, KCl 4.7, $MgSO_4$ 1.2, $CaCl_2$ 1.2, $KH_2PO_4$ 1.2, $NaHCO_3$ 25, glucose 11, pH 7.4), to be transported to the laboratory as soon as possible (within 24 h) after retrieval.

2) Small bronchi and/or pulmonary blood vessels (inner diameter $\approx 1-4$ mm) are excised and cleaned of surrounding tissue.

3) Tissues are cut into segments or rings suitable for an *in vitro* experiment and placed in 2 ml Liquid Nitrogen Storage Ampoules (Nunc Products) containing about 1.5 ml cryomedium.

4) After an equilibration time of 10–30 min at room temperature the samples are frozen slowly to –70 °C at a mean cooling rate of

**Table 20.1.** *Material and equipment for cryopreservation*

| Tissues, media and equipment | Facts | Comments |
|---|---|---|
| Human tissues | Lung samples containing bronchi and pulmonary arteries (2–4 mm Ø) obtained from surgery for cancer or from multiple organ donors | Material should be processed as soon as possible (<24 h) after retrieval |
| Cryomedium | Krebs-Henseleit solution (with 1.2 mM $CaCl_2$ pH 7.4) containing 1.8 M DMSO + 0.1 M sucrose | Higher concentrations of $CaCl_2$ will precipitate |
| Cryotubes | 2 ml plastic cryotubes with screw-top closure (internal threads). | To minimize explosion potential during thawing. |
| | Single-use volumes of 1–1.5 ml cryomedium may be prepared and stored at −20 °C to be readily available if required | This volume is sufficient to store material for up to six rings for *in vitro* studies |
| Polystyrol box (outer size about 5×7×15 cm) | Wall thickness about 1–2 cm required for slow freezing of the samples to −70 °C in a freezer or in dry ice | Cryotubes must be densely packed, empty space filled with paper tissue |
| −70 °C Freezer | For slow freezing of samples in a polystyrol box | If a programmable freezing apparatus is not available |
| Cryocanister | Container filled with liquid nitrogen to store the samples at −196 °C | The level of liquid nitrogen must be continuously monitored and refilled regularly |
| Liquid nitrogen | | One cryocanister for 600 samples requires about 750 l liquid nitrogen per year |
| Dry ice (−70 °C) | For transportation and slow re-warmingof the samples before use | |

1 °C/min. The ideal cell cooling rate can be provided by a programmable-rate freezing apparatus. If this is not available, slow freezing can be achieved by packing the ampoules into a polystyrol box (5×7×15 cm) which then is placed in a freezer maintained at −70 °C.

# Freezing procedure

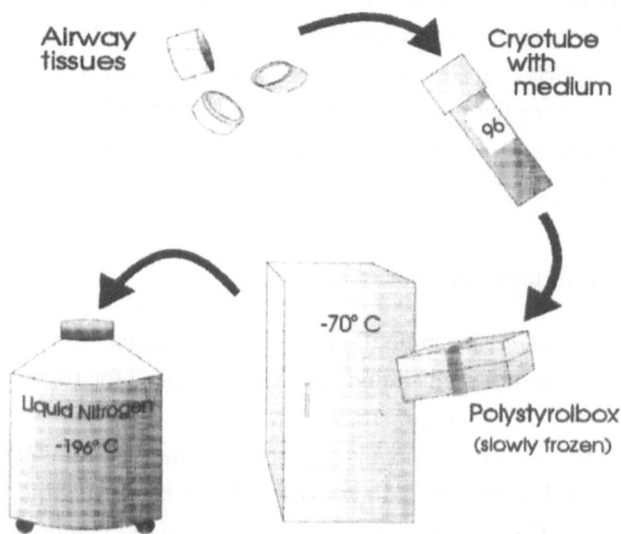

Airway tissues

Cryotube with medium

-70° C

Liquid Nitrogen -196° C

Polystyrolbox (slowly frozen)

*Figure 20.3. Illustration of the freezing procedure for isolated tissues to be used for* in vitro *experiments*

5) About 1.5–15 h later the ampoules are transferred into liquid nitrogen (–196 °C) where they can be stored until used for *in vitro* experiments.

## *Temperature and sample handling during storage*

The level of liquid nitrogen in the cryocanister must be continuously monitored and refilled if required. Make a note on a calendar whenever liquid nitrogen was added to the unit. Each time when a frozen sample is exposed to a warmer environment, even briefly, it experiences a change in temperature (Fig. 20.2) which may have detrimental effects on the viability of the frozen sample. Box stacking systems necessitate exposure of boxes at the top to warmer temperatures when retrieving samples from lower boxes. If possible, use a cryocanister with aluminum canes to store the samples. The cryotubes are pressed onto the cane which is then placed into an aluminum or cardboard cryosleeve to eliminate the potential for the tubes to fall from the cane. This system maximizes the available space and needs considerably less liquid nitrogen than a box stacking system. When retrieving a frozen sample the cane should be lifted only to a level that exposes the requested sample without removing the remaining ampoules from the cryosleeve. Work as quickly as possible!

## Thawing procedure

1) The selected sample (2 ml cryotube containing the frozen tissue) is removed from the liquid nitrogen and placed for 10 min on dry ice to warm up slowly to $-70\,°C$.
2) Thereafter the sample is exposed for 6 min to room temperature.
3) Rapid thawing is achieved within 4 min by placing the ampoule into a 40 °C waterbath. Some gentle agitation of the tube during this period may accelerate the thawing process.
4) The whole content of the cryotube is then added to about 20 ml Krebs-Henseleit solution at room temperature before the tissue samples are transferred into fresh Krebs-Henseleit solution to be prepared for the *in vitro* experiment.

## Inventory control

Numerous information may be important for the future and should be kept on appropriate records. Each vial must be labeled, e.g., by consecutive numbering, to allow identification of type and origin of the content, preservation methodology used, and location of the stored material in the cryocanister. Ideally three records are kept:

1) One record (*"donor record"*) lists informations about each patient or organ donor such as age, sex, disease, drug therapy and time between retrieval and cryopreservation of the tissues.

# Thawing procedure

1. 10 min at -70° C on dry ice

2. 6 min at room temperature

3. 4 min in a 40° C water bath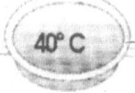

4. Washout in Krebs-Henseleit solution at room temperature

*Figure 20.4. Illustration of the thawing procedure for the frozen samples to be used for* in vitro *experiments*

2) A second record (*"sample record"*) should contain the identification numbers of the samples, patient's identification number, source, type and amount of the tissue, date of cryopreservation, applied freezing procedure and date of use.

3) A third record (*"location record"*) shows the location of each frozen sample in the cryocanister allowing rapid retrieval of a cryopreserved tissue with minimal risk of warming other samples.

## Post-thaw functional recovery

Following suspension of *human bronchi* in the organ bath the tissues normally develop spontaneous tone. After cryopreservation this spontaneously developed tone amounts to about 50% of that observed in unfrozen bronchi [26]. However, the same is true for unfrozen human bronchi after storage overnight at 4 °C [27]. In some studies, after maximal relaxation of cryopreserved human bronchi by the combined action of papaverine with isoprenaline or bimakalim, the remaining passive resting tension in frozen/thawed bronchi was about 70% higher than in unfrozen controls suggesting that the cryopreservation process attenuated the bronchial elasticity [5]. However, other investigators found no evidence for any cold-induced reduction in the elasticity of human bronchi [7].

Functional responses of cryopreserved human bronchi to a large variety of contractile and relaxant agonists and antagonists have been tested and compared to those of unfrozen control tissues. Though eventually maximal responses to some agonists of cryopreserved bronchi tended to be slightly diminished, these differences rarely reached statistical significance. The same was true for the sensitivity as assessed by the $pD_2$ values (negative logarithm of the molar concentration of an agonist producing 50% of maximal response) of these agents [5–8]. It has been shown, furthermore, that accumulation of [3H]-inositol phosphate during incubation with acetylcholine was similar in both unfrozen and frozen/thawed human bronchi indicating well preserved phosphoinositide turnover in cryopreserved human bronchi [7]. In addition to a well maintained preservation of post-thaw smooth muscle function, the integrity of human bronchial epithelium has been shown to be largely maintained after cryopreservation as well. Evidence for this has been presented by both light microscopy [7] and by demonstration of the ability to produce epithelium-derived inhibitory factor(s) (EpDIF) of cryopreserved human bronchi [6]. However, in spite of a good preservation of post-thaw contractile and relaxant responses to various agonists, the contraction following application of antigen to bronchi from sensitized donors was not preserved when tested after cryopreservation, indicating that cryopreserved airway tissues would be unsuitable for studies in which the effect of sensitization status is pertinent [8].

As has been documented for various human blood vessels [1, 3, 4, 18, 19, 22], well preserved functional activity has also been shown for cryopreserved *human pulmonary arteries* [16]. These comparative studies were performed with a cryomedium consisting of fetal calf serum containing 1.8 M DMSO without addition of sucrose. Moreover, in that study no attention was paid to the pre-freezing equilibration time. Despite some reduction, by about 25%, of the contractile responses to various agonists of the cryopreserved pulmonary arteries, there was a significant correlation of the apparent $pD_2$ values. The same was true for different relaxant agonists tested on arterial rings which had been precontracted by a submaximal concentration of the stable thromboxane analogue U46619. Although in these comparative experiments the preservation of endothelial function was not specifically investigated, a relaxant response to low concentrations of histamine in some of the frozen/thawed arteries suggested that the endothelial function may also be preserved after cryostorage of human pulmonary arteries [16].

## Conclusion

Despite the relevance of human isolated tissue for human pharmacology, its use is still very much the exception rather than the rule. The major reason for this is that the supply of fresh human material is both irregular and unpredictable, and once removed from the patient, the tissue has a very short life span. Storage of isolated blood vessels in physiologic salt solution at 4 °C induces rapid and progressive changes of physiologic and functional properties within a few days. The method of cryopreservation and storage at −196 °C offers the prospect of virtually indefinite storage of both human airway and vascular tissues and may be used in pulmonary research and drug development. It may also be used to investigate pathophysiological mechanisms in diseased airway tissues such as bronchi from asthmatics and from patients who died during an asthmatic attack [26]. The method ensures the availability of human vascular and airway smooth muscle preparations with well maintained functional activity of enzymes, contractility and epithelial function.

In summary, despite certain problems such as maintenance of responses to antigen and some reduction in contractile force, affinities of most agonists and antagonists, phosphoinositide turnover and epithelial function have been shown to be well preserved in human bronchi after cryopreservation. Hence, this technique offers clear potential for ensuring the supply of both human airway and vascular material for pharmacological studies.

# Safety recommendations

- Use buffered salt solution or culture medium (never 0.9% NaCl solution) for storage and transportation of tissues before cryopreservation.
- Avoid accidental rewarming during handling of frozen samples, e.g., when transferring ampoules from −70 °C into liquid nitrogen or when retrieving a selected sample for an experiment.
- Use plastic ampoules with internal thread screw-top closures to minimize explosion potential during thawing.
- Be cautious when handling human material which might contain infectious viral agents.
- Be cautious when handling DMSO which is quickly absorbed through the skin and might facilitate transport of potentially harmful substances into the body.
- Wear isolating gloves and a fullface shield whenever working with liquid nitrogen.

# References

1  Nataf P, Hadjiisky P, Lechat P, Mougenot N, Peuchmaurd M, Gouezo R, Gerota J, Cabrol C and Gandjbakhch I (1995) *Cryobiology* **32**: 327

2  Carbognani P, Spaggiari L, Rusca M, Cattelani L, Sollo P, Romani A, Alessandrini F, Dell'Abate P, Valente M and Bobio P (1995) *J. Intern. Med. Res.* **23**: 200

3  Müller-Schweinitzer E (1994) Vascular Tissue Preservation Techniques. In: *The Human Brain Circulation: Functional Changes in Disease,* Bevan JA and Bevan R (eds), p. 319, The Humana Press Inc Clifton

4  Müller-Schweinitzer E (1994) *Cryobiology* **31**: 57

5  Müller-Schweinitzer E, Hasse J and Swoboda L (1993) *J. Asthma* **30**: 451

6  Vacciana A, Ebeigbe AB, Hasse J, Swoboda L and Müller-Schweinitzer E (1994) *Exp. Physiol.* **79**: 409

7  Sarriá B, Naline E, Cortijo J, Moreau J, Cerdá JM, Morcillo EJ and Advenier C (1995) *Br. J. Pharmacol.* **116**: 2569

8  Johnson PRA, McKay KO, Armour CL and Black JL (1995) *Pulmon. Pharmacol.* **8**: 43

9  Mazur P (1977) Slow Freezing Injury in Mammalian Cells. In: *The Freezing of Mammalian Embryos,* Elliott K and Whelan J (eds), p. 19, Elsevier Amsterdam

10  Pegg DE (1985) Principles of Tissue Preservation. In: *Progress in Transplantation,* Morris PJ and Tilney NL (eds), p. 69, Churchill Livingstone, Edinburgh-London- Melbourne-New York

11  Pegg DE (1987) Ice Crystals in Tissues and Organs. In: *The Biophysics of Organ Cryopreservation*, Pegg DE and Karow AM Jr. (eds), p. 117, Plenum Publishing Corp.

12  Müller-Schweinitzer E and Ellis P (1992) *Naunyn-Schmiedeberg's Arch. Pharmacol.* **345**: 594

13  Deschamps C, Trastek VF, Ferguson JL, Martin WJ, Colby TV, Pairolero PC and Payne WS (1989) *Ann. Thorac. Surg.* **47**: 208

14  Yokomise H, Inui K, Wada H, Hasegawa S, Ohno N and Hitomi S (1995) *J. Thorac. Cardiovasc. Surg.* **110**: 382

15  Yokomise H, Inui K, Wada H, Ueda M and Hitomi S (1996) *J. Thorac. Cardiovasc. Surg.* **111**: 930

16  Ellis P and Müller-Schweinitzer E (1991) *Br. J. Pharmacol.* **103**: 1377

17  Müller-Schweinitzer E (1994) *Cryobiology* **31**: 330

18  Müller-Schweinitzer E, Stulz P, Striffeler H and Haefeli WE (1997) *J. Vasc. Surg.*, in press

19  Ku DD, Liu Q, Norton P and Caulfield JB (1994) *Cryobiology* **31**: 82

20  Malinin TI, Pegg DE, Perry VP and Brodine CE (1970) *Cryobiology* **7**: 65

21  Ku DD, Willis WL and Caulfield JB (1990) *Cryobiology* **27**: 511

22  Müller-Schweinitzer E, Mihatsch JM, Schilling M and Haefeli WE (1997) *J. Vasc. Surg.* **25**: 743

23  Pegg D, Boylan S and Wusteman M (1995) *Cryobiology* **32**: 553

24  Wassenaar C, Wijsmuller EG, Van Herweden LA, Aghai Z, Van Tricht CLJ and Bos E (1995) *Ann. Thorac. Surg.* **60**: S165

25  Song YC, Pegg DE and Hunt CJ (1995) *Cryobiology* **32**: 405

26  Müller-Schweinitzer E, Schilling M and Haefeli WE (1998) *J. Asthma* **35**: 177

27  Ellis JL, Hubbard WC, Meeker S and Undem BJ (1994) *Am. J. Resp. Crit. Care. Med.* **150**: 717

# Appendix I
# Physiological data of various mammalian species

|  | Mouse A | Mouse NA | Rat A | Rat NA | Guinea Pig A | Guinea Pig NA | Rabbit A | Rabbit NA | Dog A | Dog NA | Man A | Man NA |
|---|---|---|---|---|---|---|---|---|---|---|---|---|
| Body Weight (kg) | 0.03 | 0.03 | 0.2–0.4 | 0.2–0.4 | 0.7–0.9 | 0.2–0.6 | 2.4–4.0 | 1.5–2.5 | 10–18 | 11 | 70 | 70 |
| Lung weight (g) | 0.2 | – | 1.6 | – | 3.2 | – | 9.1 | – | 82 | – | 1065 | – |
| Tidal Volume (ml) | 0.16 | 0.13[2], 0.18[1] | 1.55, 0.22[3] | 1.46[4] | 3.7 | 1.7[5] | 16, 2.8[6] | 4[8], 21[7] | 140 | 200[10], 250[9] | 400 | 620[11] |
| TV pressure swing (cm H$_2$O) | 3.6 | – | 4.3 | – | 3.2 | – | 2.9 | – | 3.8 | – | 4.5 | – |
| Frequency (Hz) | 110 | 250[12], 330[12] | 97, 110[13] | 170[14], 75[13] | 42, 90[9] | 81[5], 56[15] | 39, 160[15] | 105[8], 21[13] | 18 | 22[10] | 15 | 11–26[16] |
| Minute volume (l/min) | 0.021 | 0.048[2,3] | 0.16 | 0.16[4] | 0.13 | 140[5] | 0.62 | 0.44[8] | 3.1 | 4.1[10] | 6.4 | 9[16] |
| Pulmonary compliance (ml/cm H$_2$O) | 0.022[17] | – | 0.26[18], 0.42[19] | 0.39[20] | 0.43[21] | 0.53[9] | 0.64[7] | 0.53[6] | 29[22] | 62[10] | 140[13], 88[23] | 140[11], 110[23] |
| Pulmonary resistance (cm H$_2$O/l/sec) | 480, 630[17] | – | 250[18], 480[19] | 250[20] | 59, 100[21] | 73[5], 46[9] | 25, 37[7] | 130[24], 460[6] | 1.3, 4.3[22] | 12[10] | 0.9, 1.9[25] | 1.5[26], 2.0[25] |
| Cardiac output (ml/min) | 15[27] | – | 97[28] | 123[28] | 170[29] | 150[30] | 300[15], 310[38] | 500[31] | 2200[32] | 2200[32] | 4400[33] | 5800[34] |
| Heart reate (1/min) | 450[27], 545[35] | – | 290[28] | 360[28] | 200[36] | 300[37] | 250[15] | 260[15] | 80[32] | 96[39], 120[32] | 60[40], 100[40] | – |
| Systemic arterial pressure (mm Hg) | 100[35] | – | 86[28] | 107[28] | 81[41] | 87[41] | 96[38] | – | 91[32] | 85[32] | 98[42] | – |
| Pulmonary artery pressure (mm Hg) | – | – | 16[43] | 24[44] | 15[45] | 15[30] | 18[46] | – | 20[47] | 19[39] | 15[42] | – |

*Shown are data for anaesthetised (A) and non-anaesthetised (NA) animals. Since anaesthetics vary considerably in their effect on lung functions, the data for anaesthetised animals are given mainly to illustrate the degree of variation that anaesthesia may induce. In addition, for some species only data for anaesthetised animals are available.*

# References

All data without superscript reference have been taken from Corsfill ML and Widdicombe JG (1961) *J Physiol* **158**: 1

1  Yee WFH and Scarpeli EM (1986) *Pflügers Arch* **406**: 615
2  Depledge MH (1985) *Respir. Physiol.* **60**: 83
3  Schenker EH (1985) *Comp. Biochem. Physiol.* 82A: 293
4  Leong KJ, Dowd GF and MacFarland (1964) *Can. J. Physiol. Pharmacol.* **42**: 189
5  Amdur MO and Mead J (1958) *Am. J. Physiol.* **192**: 364
6  Silbaugh SA and Mauderly JL (1984) *J. Appl. Physiol.* **56**: 1666
7  Davidson JT, Waserman K, Lilington GA and Schmidt RW (1966) *J. Appl. Physiol.* **21**: 1094
8  Gregoretti SM and Pleuvry BJ (1977) *Br. J. Anaesth.* **49**: 323
9  Zin WA, Böddener A, Silva PRM, Pinto TMP and Milic-Emili J (1986) *J. Appl. Physiol.* **61**: 1647
10  Mauderly JL (1974) *J. Gerontol.* **29**: 282
11  Attinger EO, Monroe RG and Segal MS (1956) *J. Clin. Invest.* **35**: 904
12  Travis EL, Down JD, Hall L, Vojnovic B and Holmes SJ (1981) *Brit. J. Radiol.* **54**: 50
13  Agostini E, Thimm FF and Fenn WO (1959) *J. Appl. Physiol.* **14**: 679
14  Haston CK, Newcomb CH, Grant K, Hill RP and van Dyk J (1993) *Int. J. Radiation. Oncology.* **27**: 651
15  Neutze JM, Wyler F and Rudolph AM (1968) *J. Appl. Physiol.* **215**: 486
16  Mead J (1960) *J. Appl. Physiol.* **15**: 325
17  Martin TR, Gerard NP, Galli SJ and Drazen JM (1988) *J. Appl. Physiol.* **64**: 2318
18  Diamond L and O'Donnell M (1977) *J. Appl. Physiol.* **43**: 942
19  Palecek F (1969) *J. Appl. Physiol.* **27**: 149
20  Tepper JS, Wiester MJ, Weber MJ, Weber MF and Ménache MG (1990) *J. Appl. Toxicol.* **10**: 7
21  Watson JW, Jackson AC and Drazen JM (1986) *J. Appl. Physiol.* **61**: 304
22  Hull WE and Long EC (1961) *J. Appl. Physiol.* **16**: 439
23  Gold MI and Helrich M (1965) *Anesthesiology* **26**: 281
24  Schlesinger RB, Zeccardi AV and Monahan J (1980) *J. Appl. Physiol.* 48:1092 (includes nose)
25  Clements JA, Sharp JT, Johnson RP and Elam JO (1959) *J. Clin. Invest.* **38**: 1262
26  DuBois AB, Bothelo SY and Comroe JH (1956) *J. Clin. Invest.* **35**: 327
27  Hartley CJ, Michael LH and Entman ML (1995) *Am. J. Physiol.* 268 : H499
28  Wada DR, Harashima H, Ebling WF, Osaki EW and Stanski DR (1996) *Anesthesiology* **84**: 596
29  Thompson BT, Steigman DM, Spence CL, Janssens SP and Hales CA (1993) *J. Appl. Physiol.* **74**: 916
30  Thompson BT, Hassoun PM, Kradin RL and Hales CA (1989) *J. Appl. Physiol.* **66**: 920
31  Warren DJ and Ledingham JGG (1974) *J. Appl. Physiol.* **36**: 246
32  Manders WT and Vatner SF (1976) *Circ. Res.* **39**: 512
33  Esten B and Li TH (1955) *J. Clin. Invest.* **34**: 500
34  Brantwhaite MA and Bradley RD (1968) *J. Appl. Physiol.* **24**: 434
35  Dalkara T, Irikura K, Huang Z, Panahian N and Moskowitz MA (1995) *J. Cerebral Blood Flow Metabolism* **15**: 631
36  Liu CTL and Zhong-Mao G (1992) *Lab. Animal Sci.* **42**: 275

37  Feuerstein G, Goldstein DS, Ramwell PW, Zerbe RL, Lux WE, Faden AI and Bayorh MA (1985) *J. Pharmacol. Exp. Therap.* **232**: 786

38  Mott JC (1965) *J. Physiol.* **181**: 728

39  Hammon JW, Smith PK, McHale PA, Vanbenthuysen KM and Anderson RW (1981) *J. Appl. Physiol.* **50**: 805

40  Borg G and Noble BJ (1974) In: *Excercise and Sports Sciences Review*, Wilmore J (ed.), **2**: 131, Academic Press London

41  Hart MV, Rowles JR, Hohimer AR, Morton MJ and Hosenpud JD (1984) *Am. J. Vet. Res.* **45**: 2328

42  Grossmann W (1980) *Cardiac catheterization and angiography*, 2nd Ed., Lea & Febinger Philadelphia

43  Raffestin B, Adnot S, Eddahibi S, Macquin-Mavier I, Braquet P and Chabrier PE (1991) *J. Appl. Physiol.* **70**: 567

44  Chang SW, Sakai A and Voelkel NF (1989) *Am. Rev. Respir. Dis.* **140**: 1814

45  Spence CR, Thompson BT, Janssens SP, Steigman DM and Hales HA (1993) *Am. Rev. Respir. Dis.* **148**: 241

46  Bhattacharya S, Glucksberg MR and Bhattacharya J (1989) *Circulation Res.* **64**: 167

47  Barnas GM, Randalls PB, Forrest FC, Hoff BH, Donahue PL, Kong CS and MacKenzie CF (1994) *J. Appl. Physiol.* **76**: 560

## Appendix II
## List of suppliers

The following list shows the full addresses of the suppliers that have been mentioned throughout the book.

**Alabama Research and Development**, Munford, Alabama, 36268, USA

**Axon Instruments Inc**, 1101 Chess Drive, Foster City, CA 94404, USA

**BDH Merck Ltd.**, Hunter Boulevard, Magna Park, Lutterworth, Leicestershire LE17 4XN, UK

**Becton and Dickinson**, Parsippany, NJ 07054, USA

**Branch Technology**, 9500 North Territorial Road, Dexter, MI 48130, USA

**Buxco Electronics**, Westwoods Road, Sharon, Ct. 06069, USA; 635 Second Avenue, Troy, NY 12182 USA

**Calbiochem-Novabiochem**, Boulevard Industrial Park, Padge Road, Beeston, Nottingham NG9 2JR, UK

**Conair Churchill Ltd.**, Riverside Way, Uxbridge, Middlesex UB8 2YF, UK

**C. R. Equipment SA**, 5 Chemin de la Fin, 1295 Tanney, Switzerland

**Cryo Logic Pty Ltd.**, Unit 3, 179 Forster Rd, Mt Waverly, Vic 3149, Australia

**Datex Engström Division**, Instrumentarium Cooperation, PO Box 900, FIN-00031, Datex-Engström in Finland

**Drägerwerk AG**, Moislinger Allee 53/55, 23542 Lübeck, Germany

**EMKA Technologies**, 53 Bd du General Martial Valin, 75015 Paris, France

**Electronetics Cooperation**, 525 Aero Drive, Buffalo, NY 14225, USA

**Ethikon Lmt.**, PO Box 408, Bankhead Avenue, Edingburgh EH11 4HE, UK

**Fraunhofer-Institut für Toxikologie und Aerosolforschung,**
Nikolai-Fuchs-Str. 1, 30625 Hannover, Germany

**Gesellschaft für Innovative Verfahrenstechnik**, Burgstr. 17, 64747 Breuberg,
Germany

**Gibco BRL Life Technologies**, PO Box 35, 3 Fountain Drive, Inchinnan
Business Park, Paisley PA4 9RF

**Gould Incorporated**, 8333 Rockside Road, Valley View, Ohio 44125, USA

**Grass Medical Instruments**, 101 Old Colony Avenue, PO Box 516, Quincy,
MA 02269-0516, USA

**Haake Mess-Technik**, Dieselstr. 6, 76227 Karlsruhe, Germany

**Harvard Apparatus**, Pleasant Street, South Natick, MA 01760, USA

**Helmut Hund GmbH**, Wilhelm-Will-Str. 7, 35580 Wetzlar, Germany

**HI-TECH Ltd.**, Brunel Road, Salisbury SP2 7PU, UK

**Hoyer Bremen Medizintechnik Handelgesellschaft mbH**, Parkalle 44,
28209 Bremen, Germany

**Hugo Sachs Elektronik**, PO Box 138, 79232 March-Hugstetten, Germany

**IG Instrumentengesellschaft A.G.**, Kluserstr. 25, 4054 Basel, Switzerland

**Intracel**, Unit 4, Station Road, Shepreth, Royston, HERTS SG8 6PZ, UK

**Kipp & Zonen**, Mercuriusweg 1, 2624 BV Delft, The Netherlands

**Life Technologies A.G.**, Uferstr. 90, 4019 Basel, Switzerland

**Lorne Worthington Laboratories Lmt.**, PO Box 6, Twyford, Reading,
Berkshire RG10 9NL, UK

**Med-Science Electronics**, 1455 Page Industrial Boulevard, St. Louis,
Missouri 63132, USA

**Meßgerätewerk Zwönitz**, Von Otto Str. 13, 08095 Zwönitz, Germany

**Millipore**, 80 Ashby Road, Bedford, MA 01730, USA

**Molecular Probes**, 4849 Pitchford Avenue, Eugene, OR 97402-9165, USA

**Nikon Europe B.V.**, Schipholweg 321, PO Box 222, 1170 AE Badhoevedorp, The Netherlands

**Palas GmbH**, Greschbacher Str. 3b, 76229 Karlsruhe, Germany

**Photon Technology Instruments Inc.**, Suite 3, The Sanctuary, Oakhill Grove, Surbiton KT6 6DU, UK

**Portex Ltd**, Hythe, Kent CT21 6JL, UK

**Surgipath**, 18 Bunting St., Winnipeg, Manitoba, R2X 2P6, Canada

**Taylor-Wharton Cryogenics**, 4075 Hamilton Boulevard, Theodore, AL 36590-0568, USA

**TSE**, Technical & Scientific Equipment GmbH, Ludwigstr. 10, 61348 Bad Homburg, Germany

**TSI Deutschland GmbH**, Zieglerstr. 2, 52078 Aachen, Germany

**World Precision Instruments**, Liegnitzer Str. 15, 10999 Berlin, Germany; 15, Dudley Road, Hastings, East Sussex TN35 5JP, UK

**Validyne Engineering Corporation**, 8626 Wilbur Avenue, Northridge, California, USA

# Subject index

**U**-46.619 73
ultrasonic nebulization 494
urea 340
urethane 235, 256

**v**agus nerve 232, 239, 240, 241, 248
vascular compliance, *see* compliance, vascular
vascular permeability, *see* permeability 231
vasoactive intestinal peptide (VIP) 78
vasoconstriction 44, 51
vehicle solution 510
venous occlusion, in measurement of microvascular pressure 181
venous pressure 38, 42, 178
ventilation 36
ventilation, mechanical 373, 374
ventilation, negative pressure 48
ventilation, positive pressure 49
venule 101
verapamil 85
vesicular transport 169
vessel mechanics 29
video camera 259, 461
video equipment 94
video image analysis 260, 268
viral culture 337

visceral pleura 165
vital capacity (VC) 17, 20
voltage-activated $K^+$ current 307
volume density ($V_V$), aveolar 376
volume determination, by Cavalieri principle 441, 451
volume determination, by fluid displacement 439, 451

**w**arming rate 512
water channel 164
water 460, 471, 472
wedge position 314
Weibel-Palade body 404
weight gain 43, 171
weight transducer 39
wheezing 343
whole body exposure 504
Wilhelmy balance 364, 365, 367, 379

**x**ylazine 116
xylene 461, 472, 473

**z**ardaverine 21
Ziehl-Neelsen stain 337
zig-zag tracheal strip, guinea pig 76
zone 2 140
zone 3 4, 140, 185

D.A. Isenberg, University College, London, UK /
S.G. Spiro, Middlesex Hospital, London, UK (Eds)

# Autoimmune Aspects of Lung Disease

1997. 288 pages. Hardcover • ISBN 3-7643-5719-3
(Respiratory Pharmacology and Pharmacotherapy)

The lung forms an integral part of the body's immune system and is subject to a range of diseases which are either autoimmune in nature or have clear-cut immunological abnormalities. *Autoimmune Aspects of Lung Disease* provides a concise review of the lung's role in the immune system and a detailed account of both primary and secondary lung diseases which are characterised by immunological perturbation or frank autoimmunity.

The volume presents a detailed, up-to-date account of disorders ranging from infection to neoplasia and is written in both an informative and stimulating style by a prestigious group of authors. The chapters are extensively referenced and provide numerous insights into the aetiopathogenesis and clinical features and treatment of immunologically-linked pulmonary disease.

The book is intended as both an overview for physicians and scientists with an established interest in diseases of the lung, immunologists seeking to learn more about relevant disorders in the lung and general physicians, whether specialists or in training, seeking to enrich their knowledge of the links between the pulmonary and immune systems.

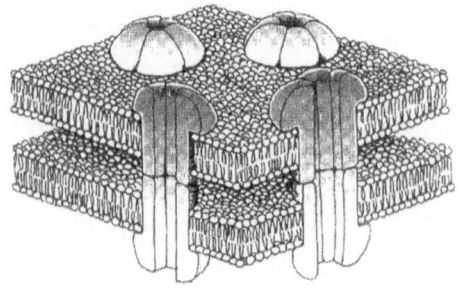

For detailed information please see
http://www.birkhauser.ch
or mail to
sales@birkhauser.ch

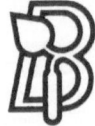

# Birkhäuser Verlag • Basel • Boston • Berlin